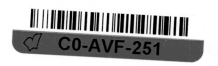

# Cerebral Blood Flow Measurement
## Measurement
—— with ——
## Stable Xenon-Enhanced
## Computed Tomography

# Cerebral Blood Flow Measurement
## — with —
## Stable Xenon-Enhanced Computed Tomography

Editor

### Howard Yonas, M.D.

*Departments of Neurological Surgery
and Radiology
Montefiore University Hospital
Pittsburgh, Pennsylvania*

**Raven Press**   **New York**

**Raven Press, Ltd., 1185 Avenue of the Americas, New York, New York 10036**

Made in the United States of America

**Library of Congress Cataloging-in-Publication Data**

Cerebral blood flow measurement with stable xenon-enhanced computed tomography/editor, Howard Yonas.
     p.  cm.
    Based on papers presented at the First International Conference on Xe/CT CBF in Orlando, Fla., Feb. 8–11, 1990.
    Includes bibliographical references and index.
    ISBN 0-88167-853-8
    1. Cerebrovascular disease—Tomography—Congresses.  2. Blood flow—Measurement—Congresses.  3. Brain—Blood-vessels—Tomography—Congresses.  4. Cerebral circulation—Congresses.  5. Xenon—Diagnostic use—Congresses.  I. Yonas, Howard.  II. International Conference on Xe/CT CBF (1st:  1990:  Orlando, Fla.)
    [DNLM:  1. Cerebrovascular Circulation—physiology—congresses.
2. Cerebrovascular Disorders—physiopathology—congresses.
3. Tomography, X-Ray Computed—methods—congresses.  4. Xenon—diagnostic use—congresses.  WL 302 C4134 1990]
    RC388.5.C373  1992
    616.8'107572—dc20
    DNLM/DLC
    for Library of Congress                                91-28790
                                                   CIP

9  8  7  6  5  4  3  2  1

# Contents

**Part I Theory and Methodology**

## Part III  Neurological Applications

**Part IV   Neurosurgical Applications**

# Contributing Authors

**Seisho Abiko, M.D.**
*Department of Neurosurgery*
*Yamaguchi University School of*
*   Medicine*
*1144 Kogushi Ube*
*Yamaguchi 755, Japan*

**Masaru Aoyagi, M.D.**
*Department of Neurosurgery*
*Tokyo Medical and Dental University*
*1-5-45 Yushima Bunkyo-ku*
*Tokyo 113, Japan*

**Stephen Ashwal, M.D.**
*Department of Pediatrics*
*Loma Linda University School of*
*   Medicine*
*Loma Linda, California 92350*

**Assaad Assaad, M.D.**
*Department of Pediatrics*
*Loma Linda University Medical Center*
*Loma Linda, California 92350*

**Jean C. Baron, M.D.**
*Service Hospitalier Frederic Joliot*
*4, place du General Leclerc*
*Orsay, France*

**Hartmut Becker, M.D., Ph.D.**
*Department of Neuroradiology*
*Hannover School of Medicine*
*Konstanty-Gutschow-Straße 8*
*D-3000 Hannover 61, Germany*

**Thomas Berger, M.D.**
*Department of Neuroradiology*
*Hannover School of Medicine*
*Konstanty-Gutschow-Straße 8*
*D-3000 Hannover 61, Germany*

**Anne M. Bidabé, M.D.**
*Service de Neuroradiologie*
*Place A. Raba-Leon*
*CHR-33076 Bordeaux, France*

**Gerrit J. Bouma, M.D.**
*Department of Neurosurgery*
*Medical College of Virginia*
*Virginia Commonwealth University*
*Box 631*
*MCV Station*
*Richmond, Virginia 23298*

**Ira F. Braun, M.D.**
*Department of Radiology*
*Baptist Hospital of Miami*
*8900 N. Kendall Drive*
*Miami, Florida 33176-2197*

**Heidi Brestowsky, Dipl. Inf.**
*Siemens Medical Systems*
*Henkestr. 127*
*8520 Erlangen, Germany*

**Karl Broich, M.D.**
*Department of Neurology*
*University of Bonn*
*Sigmund Freud Str. 25*
*D-5300 Bonn 1, Germany*

**Wes Brown, M.D.**
*Department of Pediatrics*
*Loma Linda University Medical Center*
*Loma Linda, California 92350*

**Peter Bülau, M.D.**
*Department of Epileptology*
*University of Bonn*
*Sigmund Freud Str. 25*
*D-5300 Bonn 1, Germany*

**Jean M. Caillé, M.D.**
*Service de Neuroradiologie*
*Place A. Raba-Leon*
*CHR-33076 Bordeaux, France*

**Joni M. Clark, M.D.**
Department of Surgery
Montefiore University Hospital
3459 Fifth Avenue
Pittsburgh, Pennsylvania 15213

**Gary R. Conrad, M.D.**
Department of Radiology
University of Kentucky
Albert B. Chandler Medical Center
Lexington, Kentucky 40536

**Eugene E. Cook, B.S.**
Department of Surgery
Montefiore University Hospital
3459 Fifth Avenue
Pittsburgh, Pennsylvania 15213

**Stafford J. Cothran, B.S.**
Department of Radiology
Medical College of Virginia
Virginia Commonwealth University
Box 72
MCV Station
Richmond, Virginia 23298

**Joseph M. Darby, M.D.**
Departments of Anesthesiology/
    Critical Care Medicine and
    Neurological Surgery
University of Pittsburgh School of
    Medicine
Pittsburgh, Pennsylvania 15213

**Bruce L. Dean, M.D.**
Department of Radiology
University of Kentucky
Albert B. Chandler Medical Center
Lexington, Kentucky 40536

**Christian Dettmers, M.D.**
Department of Neurology
University of Bonn
Sigmund Freud Str. 25
D-5300 Bonn 1, Germany

**Douglas S. DeWitt, Ph.D.**
Department of Neurosurgery
Medical College of Virginia
Virginia Commonwealth University
Box 508
MCV Station
Richmond, Virginia 23298

**Hermann Dietz, M.D., Ph.D.**
Department of Neurosurgery
Hannover School of Medicine
Konstanty-Gutschow-Straße 8
D-3000 Hannover 61, Germany

**Burton P. Drayer, M.D.**
Department of Neuroradiology
Barrow Neurological Institute
St. Joseph Hospital and Medical Center
350 W. Thomas Street
Phoenix, Arizona 85013

**Toshihiro Ebisawa, M.D.**
The Second Department of Medicine
Jikei University School of Medicine
3-25-8 Nishishinbashi, Minato-ku
Tokyo 105, Japan

**Christian E. Elger, M.D.**
Department of Epileptology
University of Bonn
Sigmund Freud Str. 25
D-5300 Bonn 1, Germany

**Janet R. Emery, M.D.**
Department of Pediatrics-Neonatology
Loma Linda University Medical Center
Loma Linda, California 92350

**Dieter R. Enzmann, M.D.**
Department of Diagnostic Radiology
Stanford University Medical Center
300 Pasteur Drive
Stanford, California 94305

**Panos P. Fatouros, Ph.D.**
Department of Radiology
Medical College of Virginia
Virginia Commonwealth University
Box 72
MCV Station
Richmond, Virginia 23298

**Marco Fiorelli, M.D.**
*Service Hospitalier Frederic Joliot*
*4, place due General Leclerc*
*Orsay, France*

**Naomi Fukai, M.D.**
*Tokyo Metropolitan Geriatric Medical*
*    Center*
*35-2 Sakae-cho Itabashi-Ku*
*Tokyo 173, Japan*

**Michael Gaab, M.D., Ph.D.**
*Department of Neurosurgery*
*Hannover School of Medicine*
*Konstanty-Gutschow-Straße 8*
*D-3000 Hannover 61, Germany*

**Denis Gense de Beaufort, M.D.**
*Service de Neuroradiologie*
*Place A. Raba-Leon*
*CHR-33076 Bordeaux, France*

**Anne M. Gin, M.D.**
*Service de Neuroradiologie*
*Place A. Raba-Leon*
*CHR-33076 Bordeaux, France*

**Walter F. Good, Ph.D.**
*Department of Diagnostic Radiology*
*    and Radiation Health*
*University of Pittsburgh*
*RC 508 Scaife Hall*
*Pittsburgh, Pennsylvania 15261*

**Yasunobu Gotoh, M.D.**
*Department of Neurosurgery*
*National Cardiovascular Center*
*5-7-1 Fujishiro dai*
*Suita, Osaka 565, Japan*

**Thomas W. Grahm, M.D.**
*Department of Neurosurgery*
*Barrow Neurological Institute*
*St. Joseph Hospital and Medical Center*
*350 W. Thomas Street*
*Phoenix, Arizona 85013*

**Lois M. Gruenauer, Ph.D.**
*Picker International, Inc.*
*595 Miner Road*
*Highland Heights, Ohio 44143*

**David Gur, Sc.D.**
*Department of Diagnostic Radiology*
*    and Radiation Health*
*University of Pittsburgh*
*RC 508 Scaife Hall*
*Pittsburgh, Pennsylvania 15261*

**Munetaka Haida, M.D.**
*Department of Neurology*
*Tokai University School of Medicine*
*Bohseidai, Isehara*
*Kanagawa 259-11, Japan*

**Hitoshi Hamano, M.D.**
*Department of Neurology*
*Tokai University School of Medicine*
*Bohseidai, Isehara*
*Kanagawa 259-11, Japan*

**Alexander Hartmann, M.D.**
*Department of Neurology*
*University of Bonn*
*Sigmund Freud Str. 25*
*D-5300 Bonn 1, Germany*

**Sandra Hartmann**
*Department of Neurology*
*University of Bonn*
*Sigmund Freud Str. 25*
*D-5300 Bonn 1, Germany*

**Bernd Haubitz, M.D.**
*Department of Neuroradiology*
*Hannover School of Medicine*
*Konstanty-Gutschow-Straße 8*
*D-3000 Hannover 61, Germany*

**Masaaki Hayashi, M.D.**
*Department of Neurosurgery*
*Yamaguchi University School of*
*    Medicine*
*1144 Kogushi Ube*
*Yamaguchi 755, Japan*

**Seiji Hayashi, M.D.**
*Department of Neurological Surgery*
*Wakayama Medical College*
*7 Bancho 27*
*Wakayama City 640, Japan*

**Kimiyoshi Hirakawa, M.D.**
*Department of Neurosurgery*
*Tokyo Medical and Dental University*
*1-5-45 Yushima Bunkyo-ku*
*Tokyo 113, Japan*

**John A. Hodak, M.D.**
*Department of Neuroradiology*
*Barrow Neurological Institute*
*St. Joseph Hospital and Medical Center*
*350 W. Thomas Street*
*Phoenix, Arizona 85013*

**Kurt Holl, M.D.**
*Department of Neurosurgery*
*Hannover School of Medicine*
*Konstanty-Gutschow-Straße 8*
*D-3000 Hannover 61, Germany*

**Andreas Hufnagel, M.D.**
*Department of Epileptology*
*University of Bonn*
*Sigmund Freud Str. 25*
*D-5300 Bonn 1, Germany*

**Richard L. Hughes, M.D.**
*Department of Neurology*
*Denver General Hospital*
*777 Banock*
*Denver, Colorado 80204*

**Kathleen Hurwitz, M.D.**
*Department of Pediatrics*
*Loma Linda University School of*
  *Medicine*
*Loma Linda, California 92350*

**Genhachi Hyotani, M.D.**
*Department of Neurological Surgery*
*Wakayama Medical College*
*7 Bancho 27*
*Wakayama City 640, Japan*

**Makoto Ichijo, M.D., Ph.D.**
*Cerebral Blood Flow Laboratory*
*Veterans Affairs Medical Center*
*2002 Holcombe Boulevard*
*Houston, Texas 77211*

**Akira Imai, M.D., Ph.D.**
*Cerebral Blood Flow Laboratory*
*Veterans Affairs Medical Center*
*2002 Holcombe Boulevard*
*Houston, Texas 77211*

**Toru Itakura, M.D.**
*Department of Neurological Surgery*
*Wakayama Medical College*
*7 bancho 27*
*Wakayama City 640, Japan*

**Haruhide Ito, M.D.**
*Department of Neurosurgery*
*Yamaguchi University School of*
  *Medicine*
*1144 Kogushi Ube*
*Yamaguchi 755, Japan*

**Andreas Jacobs, M.D.**
*Department of Neurology*
*University of Bonn*
*Sigmund Freud Str. 25*
*D-5300 Bonn 1, Germany*

**David Johnson, M.D.**
*Department of Radiology*
*University of Pittsburgh School of*
  *Medicine*
*Montefiore University Hospital*
*3459 Fifth Avenue*
*Pittsburgh, Pennsylvania 15213*

**Willi Kalender, Ph.D.**
*Siemens Medical Systems*
*Henkestr. 127*
*8520 Erlangen, Germany*

**Yutaka Kametsu, M.D.**
*Department of Neurology*
*Tokai University School of Medicine*
*Bohseidai, Isehara*
*Kanagawa 259-11, Japan*

**Jun Karasawa, M.D.**
*Department of Neurosurgery*
*Osaka Neurological Institute*
*2-6-23 Shonai-Takara-machi*
*Toyonaka, Osaka 561, Japan*

**Shiro Kashiwagi, M.D.**
Department of Neurosurgery
Yamaguchi University School of
 Medicine
1144 Kogushi Ube
Yamaguchi 755, Japan


**Jun Kawamura, M.D., Ph.D.**
Cerebral Blood Flow Laboratory
Veterans Affairs Medical Center
2002 Holcombe Boulevard
Houston, Texas 77211


**Takeshi Kawase, M.D.**
Department of Neurosurgery
Keio University School of Medicine
35 Shinanomachi, Shinjuku-ku
Tokyo 160, Japan


**Takamasa Kayama, M.D.**
Department of Neurosurgery
Stroke Center
Sendai National Hospital
2-8-8 Miyagino, Miyagino-ku
Sendai, Miyagi 983, Japan


**Richard L. Keenan, M.D.**
Department of Anesthesiology
Medical College of Virginia
Virginia Commonwealth University
Box 695
MCV Station
Richmond, Virginia 23298


**Masato Kimura, M.D.**
Department of Neurosurgery
Fukuoka University
Chikushi Hospital
377-1 Ohaza-Zokumyoin
Chikushino, Fukuoka 818, Japan


**Pulla R. S. Kishore, M.D.**
Department of Radiology
Medical College of Virginia
Virginia Commonwealth University
Box 72
MCV Station
Richmond, Virginia 23298


**Masahiro Kobari, M.D., Ph.D.**
Cerebral Blood Flow Laboratory
Veterans Affairs Medical Center
2002 Holcombe Boulevard
Houston, Texas 77211


**Akira Kobayashi, M.D.**
Department of Neurosurgery
National Cardiovascular Center
5-7-1 Fujishiro dai
Suita, Osaka 565, Japan


**Norihiko Komai, M.D.**
Department of Neurological Surgery
Wakayama Medical College
7 Bancho 27
Wakayama City 640, Japan


**Hideki Koyama, M.D.**
Department of Neurosurgery
School of Medicine, Keio University
35 Shinanomachi, Shinjuku-ku
Tokyo 160, Japan


**Mary Ann Krupper, M.N.S.**
Department of Surgery
Montefiore University Hospital
3459 Fifth Avenue
Pittsburgh, Pennsylvania 15213


**Barton Lane, M.D.**
Department of Diagnostic Radiology
Stanford University Medical Center
Stanford, California 94305


**Richard Latchaw, M.D.**
Department of Radiology
International Resuscitation Research
 Center
3459 Fifth Avenue
Pittsburgh, Pennsylvania 15213


**Charles Lee, M.D.**
Department of Radiology
University of Kentucky
Albert B. Chandler Medical Center
Lexington, Kentucky 40536

**Walter W. Lindstrom, Ph.D.**
*Picker International, Inc.*
*595 Miner Road*
*Highland Heights, Ohio 44143*


**James T. Love, M.D.**
*Departments of Anesthesiology and*
*   Critical Care Medicine*
*University of Pittsburgh School of*
*   Medicine*
*Pittsburgh, Pennsylvania 15213*


**Donald W. Marion, M.D.**
*Department of Neurological Surgery*
*University of Pittsburgh*
*Presbyterian University Hospital*
*230 Lothrop Street*
*Pittsburgh, Pennsylvania 15213*


**Elizabeth C. Marks, M.S.**
*Department of Neurological Surgery*
*University of Pittsburgh School of*
*   Medicine*
*Pittsburgh, Pennsylvania 15261*


**Michael P. Marks, M.D.**
*Department of Diagnostic Radiology*
*Stanford University Medical Center*
*300 Pasteur Drive*
*Stanford, California 94305*


**Anthony Marmarou, Ph.D.**
*Department of Neurosurgery*
*Medical College of Virginia*
*Virginia Commonwealth University*
*Box 508*
*MCV Station*
*Richmond, Virginia 23298*


**John A. Melick, B.S., MLT, P.A.**
*Departments of Anesthesiology and*
*   Critical Care Medicine*
*University of Pittsburgh School of*
*   Medicine*
*Pittsburgh, Pennsylvania 15213*


**John S. Meyer, M.D.**
*Cerebral Blood Flow Laboratory*
*Veterans Affairs Medical Center*
*2002 Holcombe Boulevard*
*Houston, Texas 77211*


**Shahram Mirzai, M.D.**
*Neurosurgical Clinic*
*Nordstadt Hospital*
*Hannover Medical School*
*Haltenhoffstr. 41*
*3000 Hannover 1, Germany*


**Kazuki Miyamoto, M.D.**
*Department of Neurological Surgery*
*Wakayama Medical College*
*7 bancho 27*
*Wakayama City 640, Japan*


**J. Paul Muizelaar, M.D., Ph.D.**
*Department of Neurosurgery*
*Medical College of Virginia*
*Virginia Commonwealth University*
*Box 631*
*MCV Station*
*Richmond, Virginia 23298*


**Kazuo Mulakami, B.E.**
*Anzai Medical Company, Ltd.*
*2-3-4 Higashigotanda*
*Shinagawa, Tokyo 141, Japan*


**Osamu Nakamura, M.D.**
*Department of Neurosurgery*
*Tokyo Metropolitan Komagome*
*   Hospital*
*3-18-22 Honkomagome, Bunkyo-ku*
*Tokyo, Japan*


**Yoshinari Nakamura, M.D.**
*Department of Neurological Surgery*
*Wakayama Medical College*
*7 bancho 27*
*Wakayama City 640, Japan*


**Shigeki Nakano, M.D.**
*Department of Neurosurgery*
*Yamaguchi University School of*
*   Medicine*
*1144 Kogushi Ube*
*Yamaguchi 755, Japan*


**Mohammad-Nabi Nemati, M.D.**
*Department of Neurosurgery*
*Hannover School of Medicine*
*Konstanty-Gutschow-Straße 8*
*D-3000 Hannover 61, Germany*

**Edwin M. Nemoto, Ph.D.**
*Departments of Anesthesiology and*
*  Critical Care Medicine*
*University of Pittsburgh School of*
*  Medicine*
*Pittsburgh, Pennsylvania 15213*


**Hiroshi Niizuma, M.D.**
*Department of Neurosurgery*
*Stroke Center*
*Sendai National Hospital*
*2-8-8 Miyagino, Miyagino-ku*
*Sendai, Miyagi 983, Japan*


**Takashi Nishiguchi, M.D.**
*Department of Neurological Surgery*
*Wakayama Medical College*
*7 bancho 27*
*Wakayama City 640, Japan*


**Walter D. Obrist, Ph.D.**
*Department of Neurological Surgery*
*University of Pittsburgh School of*
*  Medicine*
*9402 Presbyterian University Hospital*
*DeSoto at O'Hara Streets*
*Pittsburgh, Pennsylvania 15213*


**Akira Ogawa, M.D.**
*Division of Neurosurgery*
*Institute of Brain Diseases*
*Tohoku University School of Medicine*
*Sendai, Miyagi 980, Japan*


**Sabina Pappata, M.D.**
*Service Hospitalier Frederic Joliot*
*4, place du General Leclerc*
*Orsay, France*


**Joyce L. Peabody, M.D.**
*Department of Pediatrics*
*Loma Linda University Medical Center*
*Loma Linda, California 92350*


**Susan L. Pentheny, R.N., PA-C**
*Department of Radiology*
*University of Pittsburgh*
*Presbyterian University Hospital*
*DeSoto at O'Hara Streets*
*Pittsburgh, Pennsylvania 15213*

**Ron Perkin, M.D.**
*Department of Pediatrics*
*Loma Linda University School of*
*  Medicine*
*Loma Linda, California 92350*


**Sigrid Poersch**
*Department of Epileptology*
*University of Bonn*
*Sigmund Freud Str. 25*
*D-5300 Bonn 1, Germany*


**Vincent Pointillart, M.D.**
*Service de Neuroradiologie*
*Place A. Raba-Leon*
*CHR-33076 Bordeaux, France*


**Harvey Reich, M.D.**
*Department of Anesthesiology*
*International Resuscitation Research*
*  Center*
*Pittsburgh, Pennsylvania 15213*


**Fernand Ries, M.D.**
*Department of Neurology*
*University of Bonn*
*Sigmund Freud Str. 25*
*D-5300 Bonn 1, Germany*


**Thomas Rommel, M.D.**
*Department of Neurosurgery*
*University of Koln*
*Ostmerheimerstr. 200*
*5 Koln, Germany*


**Ernst Rzesacz, M.D.**
*Department of Neurosurgery*
*Hannover School of Medicine*
*Konstanty-Gutschow-Straße 8*
*D-3000 Hannover 61, Germany*


**Peter Safar, M.D.**
*Department of Anesthesiology*
*University of Pittsburgh School of*
*  Medicine*
*International Resuscitation Research*
*  Center*
*Pittsburgh, Pennsylvania 15213*


**Osamu Sakai, M.D.**
*The Second Department of Medicine*
*Jikei University School of Medicine*
*3-25-8 Nishishinbashi, Minato-ku*
*Tokyo 105, Japan*

**Yoshiharu Sakurai, M.D.**
*Department of Neurosurgery*
*Stroke Center*
*Sendai National Hospital*
*2-8-8 Miyagino, Miyagino-ku*
*Sendai, Miyagi 983, Japan*

**Madjid Samii, M.D.**
*Neurosurgical Clinic*
*Nordstadt Hospital*
*Hannover Medical School*
*Haltenhoffstr. 41*
*3000 Hannover 1, Germany*

**Mark H. Sanders, M.D.**
*Department of Pulmonary Medicine*
*University of Pittsburgh School of*
*Medicine*
*Pittsburgh, Pennsylvania 15261*

**Hiroo Sato, M.D.**
*Department of Neurosurgery*
*Stroke Center*
*Sendai National Hospital*
*2-8-8 Miyagino, Miyagino-ku*
*Sendai, Miyagi 983, Japan*

**Sanford Schneider, M.D.**
*Department of Pediatrics*
*Loma Linda University School of*
*Medicine*
*Loma Linda, California 92350*

**Hiromu Segawa, M.D.**
*Department of Neurosurgery*
*Fuji Brain Institute and Hospital*
*270-12 Sugita*
*Fujinomiya 418, Shizuoka, Japan*

**Hayao Shiga, M.D.**
*Department of Diagnostic Radiology*
*School of Medicine, Keio University*
*35 Shinanomachi, Shinjuku-ku*
*Tokyo 160, Japan*

**Sadatomo Shimojo, M.D.**
*The Second Department of Medicine*
*Jikei University School of Medicine*
*3-25-8 Nishishinbashi, Minato-ku*
*Tokyo 105, Japan*

**Yukito Shinohara, M.D.**
*Department of Neurology*
*Tokai University School of Medicine*
*Bohseidai, Isehara*
*Kanagawa 259-11, Japan*

**Yujiro Shiroyama, M.D.**
*Department of Neurosurgery*
*Yamaguchi University School of*
*Medicine*
*1144 Kogushi Ube*
*Yamaguchi 755, Japan*

**Hisashi Shishido, M.D.**
*Department of Neurosurgery*
*Osaka Neurological Institute*
*2-6-23 Shonai-Takara-machi*
*Toyonaka, Osaka 561, Japan*

**Laszlo Solymosi, M.D.**
*Department of Neuroradiology*
*University of Bonn*
*Sigmund Freud Str. 25*
*D-5300 Bonn 1, Germany*

**Gary K. Steinberg, M.D.**
*Department of Neurosurgery*
*Stanford University Medical Center*
*Stanford, California 94305*

**William Stezoski**
*Department of Anesthesiology*
*International Resuscitation Research*
*Center*
*Pittsburgh, Pennsylvania 15213*

**Warren A. Stringer, M.D.**
*Department of Radiology*
*Medical College of Virginia*
*Virginia Commonwealth University*
*Box 615*
*MCV Station*
*Richmond, Virginia 23298*

**Sadao Suga, M.D.**
*Department of Neurosurgery*
*School of Medicine, Keio University*
*35 Shinanomachi, Shinjuku-ku*
*Tokyo 160, Japan*

**Ryuta Suzuki, M.D.**
*Department of Neurosurgery*
*Tokyo Medical and Dental University*
*1-5-45 Yushima Bunkyo-ku*
*Tokyo 113, Japan*

**Shigeharu Takagi, M.D.**
*Department of Neurology*
*Tokai University School of Medicine*
*Bohseidai, Isehara*
*Kanagawa 259-11, Japan*

**Teiichi Takasago, M.D.**
*Department of Neurosurgery*
*Yamaguchi University School of*
*  Medicine*
*1144 Kogushi Ube*
*Yamaguchi 755, Japan*

**Nobuo Takenaka, M.D.**
*Department of Neurosurgery*
*Ashikaga Red Cross Hospital*
*3-2100 Honjou*
*Ashikaga, Tochigi 326, Japan*

**Akira Tanaka, M.D.**
*Department of Neurosurgery*
*Fukuoka University*
*Chikushi Hospital*
*377-1 Ohaza-Zokumyoin*
*Chikushino, Fukuoka 818, Japan*

**Kimito Tanaka, M.D.**
*Department of Neurosurgery*
*National Cardiovascular Center*
*5-7-1 Fujishiro dai*
*Suita, Osaka 565, Japan*

**Marcos Tatagiba, M.D.**
*Neurosurgical Clinic*
*Nordstadt Hospital*
*Hannover Medical School*
*Haltenhoffstr. 41*
*3000 Hannover 1, Germany*

**Tomoaki Terada, M.D.**
*Department of Neurological Surgery*
*Wakayama Medical College*
*7 bancho 27*
*Wakayama City 640, Japan*

**Yasuo Terayama, M.D., Ph.D.**
*Cerebral Blood Flow Laboratory*
*Veterans Affairs Medical Center*
*2002 Holcombe Boulevard*
*Houston, Texas 77211*

**Joseph Thompson, M.D.**
*Department of Radiation Sciences*
*Loma Linda University Medical Center*
*Loma Linda, California 92350*

**Lawrence Tomasi, M.D.**
*Department of Pediatrics*
*Loma Linda University School of*
*  Medicine*
*Loma Linda, California 92350*

**Ryoichi Toshima, M.D.**
*The Second Department of Medicine*
*Jikei University School of Medicine*
*3-25-8 Nishishinbashi, Minato-ku*
*Tokyo 105, Japan*

**Hajime Touho, M.D.**
*Department of Neurosurgery*
*Osaka Neurological Institute*
*2-6-23 Shonai-Takara-machi*
*Toyonaka, Osaka 561, Japan*

**Shigeo Toya, M.D.**
*Department of Neurosurgery*
*Keio University School of Medicine*
*35 Shinanomachi, Shinjuku-ku*
*Tokyo 160, Japan*

**Keizo Toyohara, M.D.**
*The Second Department of Medicine*
*Jikei University School of Medicine*
*3-25-8 Nishishinbashi, Minato-ku*
*Tokyo 105, Japan*

**Mitsuharu Tsuura, M.D.**
*Department of Neurological Surgery*
*Wakayama Medical College*
*7 Bancho 27*
*Wakayama City 640, Japan*

**Abund O. Wist, Ph.D.**
*Department of Radiology*
*Medical College of Virginia*
*Virginia Commonwealth University*
*Box 72*
*MCV Station*
*Richmond, Virginia 23298*

**Jens P. Witt, M.D.**
*Department of Neurosurgery*
*Hannover School of Medicine*
*Konstanty-Gutschow-Straße 8*
*D-3000 Hannover 61, Germany*

**Sidney K. Wolfson, Jr., M.D.**
*Departments of Surgery and*
 *Neurological Surgery*
*University of Pittsburgh School of*
 *Medicine*
*Montefiore University Hospital*
*3459 Fifth Avenue*
*Pittsburgh, Pennsylvania 15213*

**Masahiro Yamamoto, M.D.**
*Department of Neurology*
*Tokai University School of Medicine*
*Bohseidai, Isehara*
*Kanagawa 259-11, Japan*

**Kousuke Yamashita, M.D.**
*Department of Neurosurgery*
*National Cardiovascular Center*
*5-7-1 Fujishiro dai*
*Suita, Osaka 565, Japan*

**Tetsuo Yamashita, M.D.**
*Department of Neurosurgery*
*Yamaguchi University School of*
 *Medicine*
*1144 Kogushi Ube*
*Yamaguchi 755, Japan*

**Takahito Yazaki, M.D.**
*Department of Neurosurgery*
*Keio University School of Medicine*
*35 Shinanomachi, Shinjuku-ku*
*Tokyo 160, Japan*

**Hideyoshi Yokote, M.D.**
*Department of Neurological Surgery*
*Wakayama Medical College*
*7 Bancho 27*
*Wakayama City 640, Japan*

**Howard Yonas, M.D.**
*Departments of Neurological Surgery*
 *and Radiology*
*University of Pittsburgh School of*
 *Medicine*
*Montefiore University Hospital*
*3459 Fifth Avenue*
*Pittsburgh, Pennsylvania 15213*

**Yasuhiro Yonekawa, M.D.**
*Department of Neurosurgery*
*National Cardiovascular Center*
*5-7-1 Fujishiro dai*
*Suita, Osaka 565, Japan*

**Shinya Yoshinaga, M.D.**
*Department of Neurosurgery*
*Fukuoka University*
*Chikushi Hospital*
*377-1 Ohaza-Zokumyoin*
*Chikushino, Fukuoka 818, Japan*

**Stephan Zierz, M.D.**
*Department of Neurology*
*University of Bonn*
*Sigmund Freud Str. 25*
*D-5300 Bonn 1, Germany*

# Preface

Many techniques in 1991 can provide information about cerebral blood flow (CBF), but due to their different limitations, none have achieved wide acceptance and use. Although Winkler first reported in 1966 that xenon was radiodense enough to be imaged by x-ray transmission (*Nuc Med* 1966;96:1035–1040), not until 1978 did Drayer (*Stroke* 1978;9:123–130) and Kelcz (*Radiology* 1978;127:385–392) describe approaches to measuring cerebral blood flow with stable xenon-enhanced computed tomographic (Xe-CT) imaging. With the improvements in CT technology since then, Xe/CT CBF has evolved significantly. The signal-to-noise ratio has been reduced, better x-ray tubes have enabled more rapid imaging, sophisticated computers now provide more elegant CBF analyses and display, and closed-circuit delivery systems have been developed to recycle and, therefore, save xenon. These advances were possible because of the thoughtful consideration, debate, and research reflected in this book and in the conference that preceded it.

The goal of the First International Conference on Xe/CT CBF (Orlando, Florida, February 8–11, 1990) was to bring together basic scientists, clinicians, proponents, and critics of this relatively new blood flow method for a critical assessment of its current status. Participants included many of the pioneers in CBF measurement with radioactive xenon, who contributed a valuable perspective. The meeting was structured so that a large number of diverse papers could be presented and discussed within the context of the entire body of work currently being conducted around the world.

Response to the meeting was gratifying. More than 70 papers were presented, of which more than 50 were selected for this book. The chapters are presented in sections that parallel the general topics of the meeting. Each section is followed by a discussion section which attempts to capture a portion of the critical debate that accompanied the presentations. The intention of this book is to convey not only the content of the material formally presented at the meeting, but also some of the enthusiasm of the participants about their involvement in the development of an important clinical technology.

*Howard Yonas, M.D.*

# Acknowledgments

I would like to thank all of the individuals and companies that assisted in organizing the meeting and preparing this book. I wish to thank Helene Marion for editorial assistance, Elizabeth Marks and Lauren Mohan for organizational and technical assistance, and Diana Fishman and Bernie Beavers. I would also like to thank the companies that provided the support needed to bring together the meeting. Finally, I would especially like to thank Royce Fishman of Union Carbide, who despite endless criticism of Xe/CT CBF, believed that this method has a positive role to play in clinical medicine.

Cerebral Blood Flow Measurement with Stable
Xenon-Enhanced Computed Tomography,
edited by Howard Yonas. Raven Press, Ltd.,
New York © 1992.

# A Historical Perspective

## Walter D. Obrist

*Department of Neurological Surgery, University of Pittsburgh School of Medicine,
9402 Presbyterian University Hospital, DeSoto at O'Hara Streets,
Pittsburgh, Pennsylvania 15213*

The following was adapted from Dr. Obrist's opening presentation at the International Conference on Stable Xenon/CT CBF, February 8, 1990, in Orlando, Florida.

It is good to see a lot of old friends in the audience, and I look forward to an exciting 3 days. I have been asked to present a historical perspective and, being the old man that I am, perhaps that is appropriate. This symposium reminds me of some of the early meetings in the mid-to-late 1960s on the [133]Xe intracarotid cerebral blood flow (CBF) technique and then, in the early-to-mid 1970s, on the [133]Xe inhalation and intravenous (IV) injection methods. There was a lot of excitement at those meetings. There were new clinical applications and, particularly as the techniques developed, there was an emphasis on methodology and recognition of limitations. Certainly this earlier excitement is paralleled here today. I think it is right to say that the stable xenon/computed tomography (Xe/CT) method has now matured, as evidenced by concerns for methodology and recognition of the limitations as well as the advantages. I congratulate Dr. Yonas for having put together such a comprehensive program.

Although usually identified with [133]Xe techniques, I feel that I have made some small contribution to the stable Xe/CT method. In 1978, Burton Drayer approached me with the suggestion that perhaps the convolution integral might be applied to stable xenon in a manner similar to the way we used it with [133]Xe inhalation. Previous studies had employed stable xenon semi-quantitatively for CT enhancement (1), but Drayer et al. (2) desired a more quantitative CBF method. Their 1980 paper is one of the early efforts to achieve such quantification. This was followed by the systematic and thorough development of the methodology by David Gur and his group at the University of Pittsburgh (3), with whom I served as a consultant. During this time, my colleagues and I performed a few stable xenon studies at the University of Pennsylvania. We provided computer programs to John Meyer, one of the pioneers in the field. Hiro Segawa, who was with us at that time, realized the potential of the technique and, upon returning to Japan, did some of the very early work in that country. Thus I have had some involvement with the method, albeit a minor role.

In 1945, Kety and Schmidt (4,5) introduced the nitrous oxide method for the quantitative measurement of CBF in humans. This pioneer technique is based on the principle that the rate of uptake and clearance of an inert diffusible gas is proportional to blood flow in the tissue, which is the same principle underlying the subsequent radioactive and stable xenon methods. Global estimates of blood flow were obtained by measuring concentrations of the inhaled $N_2O$ gas in arterial and jugular venous blood. When this value was combined with measurement of the arterio-jugular venous difference for oxygen or glucose, global estimates of cerebral metabolic rate also were obtained.

The nitrous oxide method enjoyed wide popularity in the 1950s and 1960s, when it provided a wealth of new information on CBF in both health and disease as well as insight into blood flow regulatory mechanisms (6). Investigations were conducted on a variety of neurological and psychiatric disorders; on the effects of altering blood pressure, arterial $pO_2$, and $pCO_2$; and on normal aging and dementia. This method has served as the gold standard in the subsequent development of other CBF techniques and is still the method of choice for determination of global CBF and metabolism.

In 1961, Lassen and Ingvar (7,8) became the first to use a radioactive gas for the quantitative assessment of regional CBF. Following injection of $^{133}$Xe into an internal carotid artery, tissue clearance was monitored directly by multiple external detectors over the involved hemisphere, thus providing CBF measurements for particular brain regions. In addition to confirming earlier work with the global nitrous oxide technique, this method permitted correlations with focal neurologic and anatomic findings.

Perhaps the greatest contribution of the intracarotid $^{133}$Xe technique is the research on acute pathophysiology in humans (9). Regional variations and regulatory disturbances in CBF were investigated in a variety of brain disorders, including acute stroke and head injury. In fact, hyperemia ("luxury perfusion") was first described by this method. Studies on regional differences in dementia and on changes during functional brain activation (i.e., focal CBF responses to sensorimotor and cognitive stimulation) were also of particular interest. Although invasive, and therefore not widely used today, the intracarotid technique remains the method of choice for accurate topographic measurements of cortical blood flow.

In an effort to avoid the invasiveness of carotid injection, Mallett and Veall (10,11) in 1963 proposed inhalation of $^{133}$Xe, which in a few years was followed by the comparable IV injection technique. Introducing the isotope into the systemic circulation, however, resulted in both a prolonged input and appreciable recirculation, making it necessary to employ a complex mathematical model. Using end-tidal $^{133}$Xe concentration as an estimate of arterial input, Obrist et al. (12) performed a two-compartment deconvolution of the clearance curves. Although a small amount of extracerebral (scalp) contamination occurred, the computed values agreed well with the intracarotid technique.

Because of its noninvasiveness and relatively low radiation dose, the inhalation/

IV injection method has permitted acquisition of extensive normal control data and has been used widely in longitudinal studies (9). It is especially suited for assessment of therapeutic intervention and, with portable instrumentation, can be performed in the intensive care and operating room environments. The first reported observations of impaired cerebrovascular reserve in occlusive vascular disease were made with this method. Studies on cognitive CBF activation, wherein bilateral differences are readily observed, were of particular interest. Although not as accurate as the intracarotid technique, the ease of acquiring data repeatedly and at bedside has made $^{133}$Xe inhalation/IV injection the method of choice for natural history, intensive care, and psychological investigations.

The several $^{133}$Xe techniques, employing fixed external detectors, suffer from an inability to localize CBF changes in subcortical structures. This limitation is primarily due to the "look-through" phenomenon. An advantage of the stable xenon technique is tomographic reconstruction, which permits direct anatomic correlation with the CT image. This certainly will become evident in the papers presented here over the next few days. Attention also will be paid to the limitations of the technique (problems of signal-to-noise ratio, subanesthetic effects, vaso-reactivity), which, together with the method's clear advantages, should place this new technology in proper perspective.

## REFERENCES

1. Winkler SS, Sackett JF, Holden JE, et al. Xenon inhalation as an adjunct to computerized tomography of the brain: preliminary study. *Invest Radiol* 1977;12:15–18.
2. Drayer BP, Gur D, Wolfson SK, Cook EE. Experimental xenon enhancement with CT imaging: cerebral applications. *AJR* 1980;134:39–44.
3. Gur D, Yonas H, Good WF. Local cerebral blood flow by xenon-enhanced CT: current status, potential improvements, and future directions. *Cerebrovasc Brain Metab Rev* 1989;1:68–86.
4. Kety SS, Schmidt CF. The determination of cerebral blood flow in man by the use of nitrous oxide in low concentrations. *Am J Physiol* 1945;143:53–66.
5. Kety SS, Schmidt CF. The nitrous oxide method for the quantitative determination of cerebral blood flow in man: theory, procedure, and normal values. *J Clin Invest* 1948;27:476–483.
6. Sokoloff L. The action of drugs on the cerebral circulation. *Pharmacol Rev* 1959;11:1–85.
7. Lassen NA, Ingvar DH. The blood flow of the cerebral cortex determined by radioactive krypton. *Experientia* 1961;17:42–43.
8. Lassen NA, Ingvar DH. Radioisotopic assessment of regional cerebral blood flow. *Prog Nucl Med* 1972;1:376–409.
9. Obrist WD, Wilkinson WE. Regional cerebral blood flow measurement in humans by xenon-133 clearance. *Cerebrovasc Brain Metab Rev* 1990;2:283–327.
10. Mallett BL, Veall N. Investigation of cerebral blood flow in hypertension, using radioactive-xenon inhalation and extracranial recording. *Lancet* 1963;1:1081–1082.
11. Veall N, Mallett BL. Regional cerebral blood flow determination by $^{133}$Xe inhalation and external recording: the effect of arterial recirculation. *Clin Sci* 1966;30:353–369.
12. Obrist WD, Thompson HK, Wang HS, Wilkinson WE. Regional cerebral blood flow estimated by $^{133}$xenon inhalation. *Stroke* 1975;6:245–256.

*Cerebral Blood Flow Measurement with Stable Xenon-Enhanced Computed Tomography,* edited by Howard Yonas. Raven Press, Ltd., New York © 1992.

# Technical Aspects

Walter F. Good, David Gur, and *Howard Yonas

*Departments of Diagnostic Radiology and Radiation Health and *Neurological Surgery, University of Pittsburgh, Pittsburgh, Pennsylvania 15261*

Although introduced as a morphologic technique, rapid sequential computed tomography (CT) has been used in conjunction with injected and inhaled radiodense contrast agents to derive in vivo physiologic information that traditionally was the sole domain of radionuclide studies (1–4). The use of rapid CT scanning before, during, and after iodine injection was proposed for this purpose in the early 1980s.

One promising application of CT lies in its ability to demonstrate, qualitatively and quantitatively, time-dependent changes on serial images of the brain after intravenous iodine injection or nonradioactive xenon inhalation (5–8). Iodine-enhanced CT exhibits a high degree of image enhancement and, with delayed scanning, has the ability to provide qualitative diagnostic information on defects in blood-brain barrier permeability (9). Nevertheless, there are difficulties in obtaining meaningful absolute flow values and in correlating such data with tissue perfusion. Additionally, only one brain level usually can be studied at a time (10,11).

In 1977, Winkler et al. (12) found that the radiodensity of xenon could be used for imaging by transmission CT. Thereafter, a number of groups began to explore the possible use of stable xenon as a tracer of cerebral blood flow (CBF). With an atomic number of 54 (close to that of iodine), xenon is radiodense, and its use as a blood-flow tracer had been well established with its radioisotope, $^{133}$Xe, when work with the stable gas began. Since then, several groups have undertaken a major investigation of the technical issues associated with the derivation of CBF maps using stable xenon-enhanced CT (Xe/CT) (13–19). In addition, several studies published in recent years have addressed the application of Xe/CT CBF imaging to a spectrum of clinical disorders (20–27).

In 1984, we worked with researchers from the General Electric Company to integrate the Xe/CT CBF technology into the GE 9800 CT scanner. Most major CT-scanner manufacturers now offer comparable clinical systems as an accessory. This chapter reviews the current status of Xe/CT CBF measurement, including advantages, limitations, potential improvements, and possible future directions for its use. Most of the illustrations used are from our own files, but we have tried to include observations and information from other investigators.

## THEORY AND REDUCTION TO PRACTICE

### Methodological Assumptions

Blood flow estimates derived from time-dependent concentration measurements of diffusible indicator in tissue are based on the Fick principle, which states that tissue uptake of an indicator is equal to the amount supplied by the arterial blood less the amount drained or carried away by the venous blood. Kety used this principle to determine the relationship between CBF and the concentrations of indicator in tissue ($C_t$) and blood ($C_a$).

$$C_t(t) = \sum_i w_i f_i \int_0^t C_a(u)e^{-k_i(t-u)}du \qquad [1]$$

In this equation, $i$ represents the various compartments to be considered (fast, slow), and $w_i$ is the fraction of tissue in each of these compartments. If instantaneous equilibrium exists between arterial blood and the surrounding tissue, the flow ($f$) is given by $f_i = \lambda_i k_i$. When such equilibrium cannot be assumed, $f_i = \lambda_i k_i/m$, where $m$ is a number between 0 and 1 that measures the effectiveness of achieving equilibrium (at equilibrium $m = 1$) (28). Despite some challenge to the validity of this assumption in tissue with high flow (29), most measurements based on diffusible-indicator techniques have assumed instantaneous equilibrium ($m = 1$).

These theoretical considerations and the assumption of instantaneous equilibration were used for many years in [133]Xe CBF measurements, which require low indicator concentrations, before being extended to the nonradioactive Xe/CT method. The validity and implications of absolute flow values in situations in which this assumption may break down are discussed elsewhere (16).

### Estimation of Xenon in Arterial Blood

Several direct and indirect methods have been used to monitor time-dependent xenon concentrations in arterial blood. The methods that have been described for direct measurements (30,31) are either somewhat invasive or significantly complicate the procedure. In the indirect methods, end-tidal gas is monitored for time-dependent xenon concentrations, which are assumed to be in equilibrium with arterial blood. This assumption has been validated in several studies, although it does not hold in the case of severely impaired gas exchange in the lung (32). There are three accepted ways to measure the end-tidal xenon concentration in expired gas: to add trace amounts of radioactive xenon to the inhaled nonradioactive gas and monitor the radio-emissions of expired gas, to monitor thermal conductivity changes in the expired gas, or to use mass spectrometry to directly measure the xenon concentration in expired gas (33,34). All three indirect methods require that the estimated concentration in arterial blood be converted to the equivalent enhancement in CT units [$\Delta CT(t)$]. This can be done easily if the hematocrit is known and a technique-dependent (kVp) conversion factor is established for CT enhancement as a function of the amount of xenon dissolved in blood (17,34).

### Preprocessing of the Data

The noise inherent in the CT scanning process has a critical impact on the noise in, and therefore the accuracy of, Xe/CT CBF images. Applying a smoothing filter to the relevant CT images can reduce the noise on the enhancement sequences for the voxels of one level of a flow study. However, this reduction in noise will be offset by a loss of resolution in the flow image. Therefore, the degree of smoothing must be based on both the noise level of the particular CT scanner and the resolution required for the study. Various algorithms have been developed and tested for filtering enhancement data. These filters are all implemented as convolutions having square kernels of odd dimensions from $3 \times 3$ to $9 \times 9$ pixels, with either gaussian or uniform weighting.

CT scanners represent pixel values as integers in Hounsfield units (HU); the maximum enhancement we expect during a flow study is on the order of only 10 HU. Therefore, we always maintain processed CT data in tenths of a HU (CT number multiplied by 10). This allows us to preserve one additional significant figure in pixel values after averaging or smoothing operations have been performed, while still enabling us to represent enhancement values as 1-byte integers (0–255) in our computer system.

Aside from this detail, the initial subtraction step required in the data analysis has been implemented in a straightforward manner. If multiple baseline (unenhanced) images are collected, these are averaged first. The baseline or averaged baseline image then is subtracted pixel by pixel from each enhanced image, producing a sequence of raw enhancement images.

### Flow Calculation

To derive flow and partition coefficient estimates for a voxel of tissue, the series of enhancement values for the voxel must be fitted by some form of equation 1. More specifically, the Kety–Schmidt equation can be written as

$$C(t, k, \lambda) = \lambda k \int_0^t C_a(u) \, e^{-k(t-u)} du \qquad [1']$$

to show the dependence of tissue concentration (enhancement) on time as well as on the two parameters $k$ and $\lambda$. Several approaches can be taken to obtain a least-squares fit to equation 1 (15,35). The following procedure is a somewhat different, yet very efficient, computation.

A sum-of-squares measure of the distance of the enhancement data $E(t_i)$, $t = 1, 2, \ldots$ from equation 1' can be defined as

$$S(k, \lambda) = \sum_i [E(t_i) - C(t_i, k, \lambda)]^2 \qquad [2]$$

where $t_i$ represents the times when the enhancement measurements (CT scans) are made. The problem is to find the values for $k$ and $\lambda$ that minimize $S(k, \lambda)$.

We adopted an approach based on the separability of $S(k, \lambda)$ (36). At a local minimum of $S(k, \lambda)$, $\lambda$ and $k$ must satisfy the simultaneous equations

$$0 = \frac{\partial S(k, \lambda)}{\partial \lambda} = -2k \sum_i [E(t_i)A(t_i, k) - \lambda k A^2(t_i, k)] \qquad [3]$$

and

$$0 = \frac{\partial S(k, \lambda)}{\partial k} = -2\lambda \sum_i [E(t_i)B(t_i, k) - \lambda k A(t_i, k)B(t_i, k)] \qquad [4]$$

where, for simplicity of notation, $A(t_i, k)$ and $B(t_i, k)$ have been defined, respectively, as

$$A(t, k) = \int_0^t C_a(u)\, e^{-k(t-u)} du$$

and

$$B(t, k) = \int_0^t C_a(u)(1 - kt + ku)\, e^{-k(t-u)} du$$

Solving both equation 3 and 4 for $\lambda$, we obtain

$$\lambda = \frac{\displaystyle\sum_i E(t_i)A(t_i, k)}{k \displaystyle\sum_i A^2(t_i, k)} \qquad [5]$$

and

$$\lambda = \frac{\displaystyle\sum_i E(t_i)B(t_i, k)}{k \displaystyle\sum_i A(t_i, k)B(t_i, k)} \qquad [6]$$

Subtracting 5 from 6 gives

$$0 = \frac{\displaystyle\sum_i E(t_i)B(t_i, k)}{k \displaystyle\sum_i A(t_i, k)B(t_i, k)} - \frac{\displaystyle\sum_i E(t_i)A(t_i, k)}{k \displaystyle\sum_i A^2(t_i, k)} \qquad [7]$$

which depends only on $k$. In other words, at a local minimum of $S(k, \lambda)$, $k$ must be a zero of equation 7. Finding zeros of equation 7 is computationally more efficient and more stable than directly minimizing equation 2 using general-purpose optimization techniques. The specific algorithm we use for finding zeros is an adaptation of the routine "zeroin" presented by Forsythe et al. (37).

Once $k$ has been determined, $\lambda$ can be calculated from either equation 5 or 6, and the CBF corresponding to the measured data then can be found from $F = \lambda k$. After flow estimates are derived for each voxel by any computational method, a flow image (map) is generated in which each pixel value represents voxel flow.

### Postprocessing the Flow Image

Postprocessing can improve the appearance and possibly the clinical utility of the raw flow image produced by the least-squares fitting process. Two postprocessing techniques, artifact removal and smoothing, have been developed.

In a least-squares fitting procedure, the minimum "sum of squares" at each voxel is a measure of the degree to which the data points have been fitted by the regression equation. The larger this sum of squares, the lower the confidence in the parameters derived by the fitting process. Because these sums of squares are available at each voxel in which the flow calculation is performed, an "error" image corresponding to the flow image can be constructed by assigning each pixel the appropriate sum of squares divided by $N - 2$, where $N$ is the number of scans in the procedure. Because it coincides with the creation of the flow image, the creation of this error image should be considered a part of the calculation phase rather than part of the postprocessing phase. Nevertheless, the error image can be used during postprocessing to identify questionable points in the flow image.

Higher values in the error image correspond to less reliable flow estimates in the flow image. The error image is itself of value, because viewing it along with the flow image enables an observer to interpret the reliability of regions in the flow image. In using the error image to identify and remove artifacts from a flow image, a threshold can be set for the error image; pixels with errors that fall above the threshold are assumed to correspond to unreliable flow values.

Unreliable flow values can be dealt with in two ways. The simplest is to replace them by zero values under the rationale that large errors usually occur only in areas of severe artifact, on the boundaries between bone and soft tissue, or in extremely low-flow areas where the signal-to-noise ratio (SNR) is poorest. A more sophisticated approach involves replacing a questionable flow value with the average of the more reliable values in the surrounding areas. A $3 \times 3$-pixel region around each questionable pixel is considered. If at least half the pixels in this region are below the error threshold, the questionable flow value is replaced by the average of the "good" values in the region. After the entire flow image is processed using this $3 \times 3$ region averaging, the procedure is repeated with $5 \times$

5-, 7 × 7-, and 9 × 9-pixel regions, respectively. This process generally corrects the values for all questionable pixels, but any that remain are set to zero.

Once artifacts have been removed from the flow image, it is generally desirable to smooth the flow image to remove some of the graininess caused by the rather large variance in flow values that characterize this CBF technique. The filters used for this purpose are identical to those used to smooth the enhancement data. During postprocessing, however, smoothing does not alter mean flow values, whereas smoothing the enhancement images before the flow calculation introduces a bias to the flow estimates.

## Technical Advantages

The Xe/CT method has several distinct advantages over most other CBF-measuring techniques. As an add-on procedure to CT, it is widely accessible. Also, studies can be performed completely noninvasively. Furthermore, Xe/CT studies can be easily repeated in the same tissue of interest after activations or challenges to flow reserve (e.g., $CO_2$, acetazolamide) (38). The direct correlation to anatomy on the baseline CT images enables easy recognition of the specific tissue being studied and permits appreciation of regions with morphologic abnormalities such as increased atrophy. It also allows close comparison of the same tissue or region of interest (ROI) in subsequent studies.

Another advantage of the Xe/CT method is that it computes tissue-specific partition coefficients. Although the partition coefficient has not been used directly in many clinical applications, some have attempted to infer valuable clinical information from partition-coefficient maps in support of the flow information (39). The main advantage of a derived tissue-specific partition coefficient is that errors associated with this parameter directly propagate to derived flow values and may significantly affect the resulting flow maps. Therefore, it is more appropriate to use the tissue-specific partition coefficient than the standard ($\lambda$) values used by other methods.

## LIMITATIONS, PROBLEMS, AND CONCERNS

### System and Computational Errors

The accuracy of Xe/CT-measured regional CBF values can be affected by CT noise, tissue heterogeneity, errors in estimating arterial xenon concentration, and uncertainty about xenon arrival time. The effects of these factors have been evaluated by computer simulation and confirmed through a series of in vivo and phantom experiments. The recently published results of these studies (40–42) indicate that approximating the arterial data by a single exponential introduces relatively small errors (42). On the other hand, CT noise, tissue heterogeneity, and inaccuracies in estimating the xenon-delivery starting time relative to sequential scanning times caused significant errors (40,42). The overall errors of the system in estimating CBF by this technique depend on many factors and can be significant. Using current technology, it is not unlikely that the estimated flow value in a single pixel can have errors exceeding 100%. Such errors for a typical study (excluding patient motion) are detailed elsewhere (43).

These findings clearly demonstrate that the Xe/CT technique cannot produce an accurate and reproducible absolute flow value in tissue volumes corresponding to a single pixel in the flow map ($\sim 1 \times 1 \times 5$ mm$^3$). The system's error depends on the flow value and size of the ROI evaluated. Although the accuracy of absolute flow values is flow and volume (ROI) dependent, errors can be kept at an acceptable level ($\leq 20\%$) in tissue with high- and low-flow values when the ROI exceeds $8 \times 8 \times 10$ mm$^3$ (43).

## Concerns

In addition to the advantages discussed earlier, the Xe/CT CBF method has several distinct limitations. Its use as a clinical diagnostic tool makes safety a primary concern. Several anecdotal reports of respiratory problems and increased intracranial pressure during the inhalation of xenon in high concentrations have slowed the acceptance of this technique as a routine diagnostic procedure (44,45). All systematic studies of patient reactions, however, indicate that only minor transient effects from inhalation have been recorded and that intracranial pressure does not reach levels dangerous to subjects undergoing the studies (46–48). In fact, the reaction rate to inhaled xenon has been lower than that normally recorded with iodinated contrast media, and patient tolerance has been quite acceptable (47).

Furthermore, the Xe/CT CBF method as now performed allows measurements of CBF at two or three brain levels, limiting each study to a volume that is only 20% to 25% of the total brain. Although many territories of the brain can be examined during a single three-level study, flow abnormalities cannot be excluded in regions that are not studied. Another limitation is the likelihood that CT artifacts reduce the ability to acquire high-quality flow information in the lower posterior and anterior regions of the brain.

Patient motion is probably the most difficult technical problem associated with data acquisition in deriving consistent high-quality flow maps, because these maps are developed from a series of subtracted images. A successful high-quality Xe/CT CBF study requires that the patient does not move for approximately 7 to 9 minutes. Special head holders, in combination with different fixation techniques, have proven very useful in limiting motion (a success rate of >90% can be achieved), but improvements in this area are still desirable (38).

Several investigators have examined the effect of xenon on blood flow itself (49–51). One group suggested that in the rat there was a significant differential elevation of only the neocortical flows (50). Others have not observed the same extent or pattern of flow augmentation. Radiolabeled microsphere studies in nonhuman primates have demonstrated either no flow alteration (51) or up to a 17% homogeneous increase of flow in all brain regions (52). A [133]Xe study of CBF changes in normal volunteers during 4 to 5 minutes of xenon inhalation identified a more variable degree of flow enhancement, averaging 30% (53). Because Xe/CT-derived CBF values do not appear to deviate from established norms of flow as much as [133]Xe-derived values do (34,54,55), the true significance of measurements with radioactive xenon is yet to be defined. Our impression after performing more than 2,500 CBF studies in humans and animals is that an increase of flow, to whatever extent it may influence flow calculation, is acceptable and even may be clinically useful, serving as a challenge to flow reserves similar to that obtained during the inhalation of added $CO_2$. Moreover, the elevation of CBF during xenon inhalation can serve only to increase measured flow values; under these conditions, low flow values would be of even greater clinical relevance. A recent report on the potential effects of flow activation on the computational accuracy of the Xe/CT method (56) conflicts with several other investigations on the subject, and this topic is discussed elsewhere in this volume.

### Radiation Exposure

Radiation exposure also must be considered when undertaking a Xe/CT study. Depending on exposure factors, the dose of radiation per CT image can range from 2 to 3.5 cGy. A flow study delivers 8 to 28 cGy to each level examined, depending on the total number of scans obtained (baseline and enhanced). Although these are believed to be clinically acceptable levels and are comparable to other radiographic procedures such as cerebral angiography, they constitute a considerable dose of radiation. However, the radiation field is highly collimated, and contiguous scans are avoided to prevent an overlapping tissue band from receiving even higher radiation. Slice selection minimizes exposure of the lens of the eye. Because the brain is considered less radiosensitive than other organ systems, the risk with even the highest possible exposure delivered by a single- or multiple-level Xe/CT CBF study is relatively low (57). Nevertheless, the known radiation risk to brain tissue has increased during the last decade, a trend likely to continue as we better understand the effects of radiation exposure on different organs (58).

Direct measurements indicate that the radiation dose to the lens of the eye during a typical study is not likely to exceed 0.2 cGy. Adding a scout view will increase this exposure by approximately 0.05 cGy. The average dose to the brain from a typical study of an adult is in the range of 3.5 to 10 cGy, depending on the protocol used. Because of the radiation levels associated with this technique, repeated studies in normal adults and investigational studies in children are not recommended without careful consideration of the potential risks and benefits.

### Other Issues

Obtaining accurate CBF measurements in sequential Xe/CT studies requires xenon clearance from tissue with low flow and, consequently, a delay of 15 to 25 minutes between xenon inhalations. The lower the patient's blood flow, the longer the inhalation period required for high-quality studies and the longer the delay necessary between studies.

Finally, this technique can provide information only on tissue perfusion and the partition coefficient. Metabolic information such as that provided by PET or SPECT, often important to the understanding of disease processes, cannot be obtained with the current Xe/CT CBF method.

## RECENT ADVANCES, POTENTIAL IMPROVEMENTS, AND FUTURE DIRECTIONS

The rapid improvement in computational power in recent years has led to several advances in Xe/CT CBF technology, and others are being investigated. Some of these advances have facilitated the clinical use of the technology, whereas others have resulted in computational improvements. The use of xenon wash-in and wash-out (clearance) enables the acquisition of more data points, particularly during the phase of rapid change, and thereby increases the accuracy of estimated flow values. Arterial concentration has been estimated by double exponentials to improve the input function for the solution of the Kety–Schmidt equation, and attempts have been made at completely eliminating curve fitting of the arterial build-up. The use of look-up tables rather than iterative least-squares computation enables very rapid determination of flow values in each voxel of interest, significantly reducing the time required to obtain and display flow maps. Also, most manufacturers have developed rebreathing systems to reduce the amount of xenon gas used in each study.

The two most important factors in increasing the likelihood for reliable, high-quality studies, however, remain lack of patient motion and an increase in the SNR ratio per unit radiation dose. As previously noted, the first of these problems is being addressed in part through the development of better head holders specifically designed for this application. The SNR of current CT scanners consistently is being improved upon through new detection schemes, more stable x-ray tubes, and better signal-collecting electronics. Unfortunately, progress in this area has been limited, mainly due to physics considerations. There is no doubt that improvements in the SNR per unit dose will directly increase the quality of the blood flow images while providing the option to reduce either the radiation dose or the inhaled xenon concentration currently associated with this technique.

In the future, high-heat-loading x-ray tubes will enable investigation of more than three brain levels during a single Xe/CT study. In addition, simple modifications of current protocols are likely to reduce bone artifacts, thus permitting better measurements of CBF in the low posterior and anterior regions of the brain (e.g., frontal lobes). Certainly other improvements are possible and forthcoming. The use of the Xe/CT method in both clinical and laboratory settings remains to be fully explored. As long as we believe that most acute and many chronic cerebral abnormalities are tissue-perfusion driven, the most important chapter on this tissue-specific, clinically accessible, and anatomically correlatable method is yet to be written.

## ACKNOWLEDGMENTS

The authors appreciate the assistance and interest of the General Electric Medical Systems Division in these studies. This work was supported in part by Grant No. HL27208 from the National Institutes of Health. Dr. Gur is the recipient of an Established Investigator Award from the American Heart Association, and funds are provided by the American Heart Association Pennsylvania Affiliate.

Major portions of this chapter appeared in Gur D, Yonas H, Good WF, "Local Cerebral Blood Flow by Xenon-Enhanced CT: Current Status, Potential Improvements, and Future Directions," *Cerebrovascular and Brain Metabolism Reviews* (Raven Press) 1989;1:68–86. Permission to reprint those portions was granted by Raven Press and the authors.

## REFERENCES

1. Kety SS, Schmidt CF. The nitrous oxide method for the quantitative determination of cerebral blood flow in man: theory, procedure and normal values. *J Clin Invest* 1948;27:476–483.
2. Kuhl DE, Barrio JR, Huang S-C, et al. Quantifying local cerebral blood flow by N-isopropyl-p[$^{123}$I]iodoamphetamine (IMP) tomography. *J Nucl Med* 1982;23:196–203.
3. Lassen N, Ingvar DH, Skinhoj E. Brain function and blood flow. Changes in the amount of blood flowing in areas of the human cerebral cortex, reflecting changes in the activity of those areas, are graphically revealed with the aid of radioactive isotope. *Sci Am* 1978;239:62–71.
4. Obrist WD, Thompson HK, Wang HS, Wilkinson WE. Regional cerebral blood flow estimated by xenon-133 inhalation. *Stroke* 1975;6:245–256.
5. Axel L. Exploring dynamic CT. *Diagn Imaging* 1980;2:4–7.
6. Hayman LA, Sakai F, Meyer JS, Armstrong D, Hinck VC. Iodine-enhanced CT patterns after cerebral arterial embolization in baboons. *AJNR* 1980;1:233–238.
7. Norman D, Stevens EA, Wing SD, Levin V, Newton TH. Quantitative aspects of contrast enhancement in cranial computed tomography. *Radiology* 1978;129:683–688.
8. Traupe H, Heiss WD, Hoeffken W, Zulch KJ. Perfusion patterns in CT transit studies. *Neuroradiology* 1980;19:181–191.
9. Heinz ER, Dubois P, Osborne D, Drayer B, Barrett W. Dynamic computed tomography study of the brain. *J Comput Assist Tomogr* 1979;3:641–649.
10. Gur D, Yonas H, Wolfson SK Jr, et al. Xenon and iodine enhanced cerebral CT: a closer look. *Stroke* 1981;12:573-578.
11. Norman D, Axel L, Berninger WH, et al. Dynamic computed tomography of the brain: techniques, data analysis, and applications. *AJR* 1981;136:759–770.

12. Winkler S, Sackett J, Holden J, et al. Xenon inhalation as an adjunct to computerized tomography of the brain: preliminary study. *Invest Radiol* 1977;12:15–18.
13. Drayer BP, Wolfson SK, Reinmuth OM, Dujovny M, Boehnke M, Cook EE. Xenon enhanced CT for analysis of cerebral integrity, perfusion, and blood flow. *Stroke* 1978;9:123–130.
14. Gur D, Yonas H, Herbert D, et al. Xenon enhanced dynamic computed tomography: multilevel cerebral blood flow studies. *J Comput Assist Tomogr* 1981;5:334–340.
15. Gur D, Good WF, Wolfson SK Jr, Yonas H, Shabason L. In vivo mapping of local cerebral blood flow by xenon-enhanced computed tomography. *Science* 1982;215:1267–1268.
16. Gur D, Wolfson SK Jr, Yonas H, et al. Progress in cerebrovascular disease: local cerebral blood flow by xenon enhanced CT. *Stroke* 1982;13:750–758.
17. Kelcz F, Hilal SK, Hartwell P, Joseph PM. Computed tomographic measurement of the xenon brain-blood partition coefficient and implications for regional cerebral blood flow: a preliminary report. *Radiology* 1978;127:385–392.
18. Meyer JS, Hayman LA, Sakai F, Yamamoto M, Nakajima S, Armstrong D. High-resolution three-dimensional measurement of localized cerebral blood flow by CT scanning and stable xenon clearance: effect of cerebral infarction and ischemia. *Trans Am Neurol Assoc* 1979;104: 85–89.
19. Segawa H, Susumu W, Tamura A, Yoshimasu N, Nakamura O, Ohta M. Computed tomographic measurement of local cerebral blood flow by xenon enhancement. *Stroke* 1983;14:356–362.
20. Darby JM, Yonas H, Gur D, Latchaw RE. Xenon-enhanced computed tomography in brain death. *Arch Neurol* 1987;44:551–554.
21. Darby JM, Yonas H, Marion DW, Latchaw RE. Local "inverse steal" induced by hyperventilation in head injury. *Neurosurgery* 1988;23:84–88.
22. Meyer JS, Nakajima S, Dkabe T, et al. Redistribution of cerebral blood flow following STA-MCA bypass in patients with hemispheric ischemia. *Stroke* 1982;13:774–784.
23. Segawa H, Wakai S, Tamura A, Sano K, Ueda Y, Ohshima M. CBF study by CT with Xe enhancement: experience in 30 cases. *J Cereb Blood Flow Metab* 1981;1:52–53.
24. Tachibana H, Meyer J, Kitagawa Y, Tanahashi N, Kandula P, Rogers RL. Xenon contrast CT-CBF measurements in parkinsonism and normal aging. *J Am Geriatr Soc* 1985;33:413–421.
25. Wozney P, Yonas H, Latchaw RE, Gur D, Good W. Central herniation revealed by focal decrease in blood flow without elevation in ICP: a case report. *Neurosurgery* 1985;17:641–644.
26. Yonas H, Good WF, Gur D, et al. Mapping cerebral blood flow by xenon-enhanced computed tomography: clinical experience. *Radiology* 1984;152:425–442.
27. Yonas H, Gur D, Good BC, et al. Stable xenon/CT blood flow mapping in the evaluation of patients before and after extracranial/intracranial bypass surgery. *J Neurosurg* 1985;62:324–333.
28. Kety SS. Measurement of local blood flow by the exchange of an inert, diffusible substance. In: Bruner HB, ed. *Methods in medical research.* Chicago: Year Book, 1960:228–236.
29. Tomita M, Gotoh F. Local cerebral blood flow values as estimated with diffusible tracers: validity of assumptions in normal and ischemic tissue. *J Cereb Blood Flow Metab* 1981;1:403–411.
30. Drayer BP, Gur D, Wolfson SK, Cook EE. Experimental xenon enhancement with CT imaging: cerebral applications. *AJR* 1980;134:39–44.
31. Wolfson SK Jr, Drayer BP, Boehnke M, Dujovny M, Cook EE. Regional cerebral blood flow by xenon enhanced computed tomography. *Proceedings of the annual meeting of the American Association of Neurological Surgeons,* 1978:1–3.
32. Obrist WD, Thompson HK Jr, King CH, Wang HS. Determination of regional cerebral blood flow by inhalation of xenon-133. *Circ Res* 1967;20:124–135.
33. Dhawan V, Conti J, Rottenberg DA. Mass spectrometric measurement of end-tidal xenon concentration for clinical xenon/CT cerebral blood flow studies. *Proceedings of the Radiological Society of North America annual meeting,* Chicago: RSNA Publications, 1981:176.
34. Meyer JS, Hayman LA, Yamomoto M, Sakai F, Nakajima S. Local cerebral blood flow measured by CT after stable xenon inhalation. *AJNR* 1980;1:213–215.
35. Thaler HT, Baglivo JA, Lu HC, Rottenberg DA. Repeated least squares analysis of simulated xenon computed tomographic measurements of regional cerebral blood flow. *J Cereb Blood Flow Metab* 1982;2:408–414.
36. DeFontane DL, Ross DK, Ternai B. A fast nonlinear least squares method for the calculation of relaxation times. *J Magn Reson* 1975;18:276–281.
37. Forsythe GE, Malcolm AM, Moler CB. *Computer methods for mathematical computation.* Englewood Cliffs, NJ: Prentice-Hall, 1977.

38. Yonas H, Latchaw RE, Johnson DW, Gur D. Xenon-enhanced CT: evaluating cerebral blood flow. *Diagn Imaging* 1988;10:88–94.
39. Moossy J, Martinez J, Hanin I, Rao G, Yonas H, Boller F. Thalamic and subcortical gliosis with dementia. *Arch Neurol* 1987;44:510–513.
40. Good WF, Gur D. The effect of computed tomography noise and tissue heterogeneity on cerebral blood flow determination by xenon-enhanced computed tomography. *Med Phys* 1987;14:557–561.
41. Good WF, Gur D, Herron JM, Kennedy WH. The development of a xenon/computed tomography cerebral blood flow quality assurance phantom. *Med Phys* 1987;14:867–869.
42. Good WF, Gur D, Yonas H, Herron JM. Errors in cerebral blood flow determinations by xenon-enhanced computed tomography due to the estimation of arterial xenon concentrations. *Med Phys* 1987;14:377–381.
43. Gur D, Yonas H, Good WF. Local cerebral blood flow by xenon-enhanced CT: current status, potential improvements, and future directions. *Cerebrovascular and Brain Metabolism Reviews* 1989;1:68–86.
44. Harrington TR, Manwaring K, Hodak J. Local basal ganglia and brainstem blood flow in the head injured patient using stable xenon-enhanced CT scanning. In: Miller JD, Teasdale GM, Rowan JV, Galbraith SL, Mendelow AD, eds. *Intracranial pressure*. New York: Springer-Verlag; 1986.
45. Winkler S, Turski P. Potential hazards of xenon inhalation. *AJNR* 1985;6:974–975.
46. Darby JM, Yonas H, Pentheny S, Marion D. Intracranial pressure response to stable xenon inhalation in patients with head injury. *Surg Neurol* 1989;32:343–345.
47. Latchaw RE, Yonas H, Pentheny S, Gur D. Adverse reactions to xenon-enhanced CT cerebral blood flow determination. *Radiology* 1987;163:251–254.
48. Yonas H, Snyder JV, Gur D, et al. Local cerebral blood flow alterations (Xe-CT method) in an accident victim: a case report. *J Comput Assist Tomogr* 1984;8:990–991.
49. Gur D, Yonas H, Jackson DL, et al. Simultaneous measurements of cerebral blood flow by the xenon/CT method and the microsphere method: a comparison. *Invest Radiol* 1985;20:672–677.
50. Junck L, Dhawan V, Thaler HT, Rottenberg DA. Effects of xenon and krypton on regional cerebral blood flow in the rat. *J Cereb Blood Flow Metab* 1985;5:126–132.
51. Panos PP, Fatouros R, Kishore PRS, et al. Comparison of improved stable xenon/CT method for cerebral blood flow measurements with radiolabeled microspheres technique. *Radiology* 1985;158:334.
52. Gur D, Yonas H, Jackson DL, et al. Measurements of cerebral blood flow during xenon inhalation as measured by the microsphere method. *Stroke* 1985;16:871–874.
53. Obrist WD, Jaggi JL, Harel D, Smith DS. Effect of stable xenon inhalation on human CBF. *J Cereb Blood Flow Metab* 1985;5:S557–558.
54. Drayer BP, Gur D, Yonas H, Wolfson SK Jr, Cook EE. Abnormality of the xenon brain-blood partition coefficient and blood flow cerebral infarction: an in vivo assessment using transmission computed tomography. *Radiology* 1980;135:349–354.
55. Segawa H. Tomographic cerebral blood flow measurement using xenon inhalation and serial CT scanning: normal values and its validity. *Neurosurg Rev* 1985;8:27–33.
56. Giller CA, Purdy P, Lindstrom WW. Effects of inhaled stable xenon on cerebral blood flow velocity. *AJNR* 1990;11:177–182.
57. ICRP. Radiation protection. Recommendations of the International Commission on Radiological Protection. ICRP #26, Oxford, England: Pergamon Press, 1977.
58. Committee on the Biological Effects of Ionizing Radiations. National Research Council, Health Effects of Exposure to Low Levels of Ionizing Radiation, BEIR V. Washington, DC: National Academy Press, 1990.

*Cerebral Blood Flow Measurement with Stable Xenon-Enhanced Computed Tomography,* edited by Howard Yonas. Raven Press, Ltd., New York © 1992.

# Patient Care Considerations

## Susan L. Pentheny

*Department of Radiology, University of Pittsburgh, Presbyterian University Hospital, DeSoto at O'Hara Streets, Pittsburgh, Pennsylvania 15213*

From the patient-care perspective, a team approach is a basic requirement for acquiring safe and technically adequate xenon-enhanced computed tomographic cerebral blood flow (Xe/CT CBF) studies. These studies demand not only the complete attention of the radiology technologist, but also the direct involvement of a nurse, physician assistant, or physician whose primary focus is on patient management. Working together ensures that no time is wasted once patient preparation has begun. Moreover, although the xenon-delivery system includes many safety features to protect the patient against an inadequate supply of xenon or oxygen, it is not a patient monitor and should not be relied upon as such. Like angiography, Xe/CT studies always should be regarded as a special procedure that demands the full attention, cooperation, coordination, and commitment of all personnel involved.

## PREPARATION

Appropriate preparation of the xenon-delivery system varies with the system being used. Although the observations in this chapter specifically apply to the General Electric Xe/CT CBF system, most are not restricted to particular equipment. All systems need to be maintained with clean tubing and resterilizable or disposable non-rebreathing valves for each study. Additionally, the xenon/oxygen concentration must be verified prior to administration.

Once the equipment and xenon source have been checked, the person caring for the patient should allow adequate time to obtain a medical history and to explain the procedure. Talking with the patient to establish rapport from the outset is vital. Any procedural explanation should include clinical indications, anticipated length of study, and possible side effects. Patients thus should be told beforehand that they may experience some very unusual sensations during xenon inhalation. The most common of these is euphoria. Because of its anesthetic properties, however, xenon also may produce brief periods of unresponsiveness or dysphoria, which some patients have described as a frightening sense of impending doom. Patients must realize that such sensations are transient and that

*16*

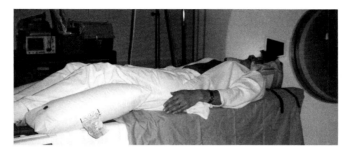

**FIG. 1.** Placement of a wedge under the patient's knees can alleviate some discomfort during the examination.

the clinician will be nearby and monitoring them constantly throughout the examination.

This examination requires prolonged maintenance of an uncomfortable position. Thus when positioning the patient, efforts should be made to provide as much comfort as possible. For example, placing a wedge under the patient's knees can alleviate lower-back or lower-extremity discomfort (Fig. 1).

The greatest challenge in obtaining technically adequate imaging is the prevention of head motion. Because movement as small as a few millimeters in any plane can cause significant misregistration, no motion between images can be tolerated during the acquisition of baseline and enhanced scans. Several head-immobilization techniques are effective, including a custom head holder that lies directly on the CT table for added stabilization (Fig. 2). Additionally, we use a vacuum-activated "bean bag." (An appendix to this chapter lists information on this and other equipment used for Xe/CT studies at the University of Pittsburgh.) With the vacuum released, this device is soft and pliable, molding easily to the contour of the head. Upon vacuum application, it becomes firm, further enhancing head immobilization (Fig. 3).

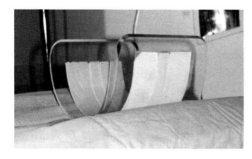

**FIG. 2.** Custom head holder helps prevent patient motion.

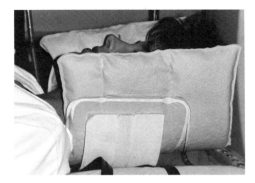

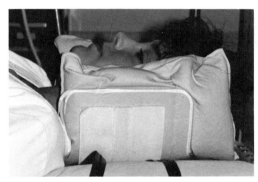
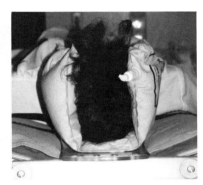

**FIG. 3.** A vacuum-activated "bean bag" molds to the contour of the patient's head to enhance immobilization.

The location of the area to be studied also must be considered in positioning the patient. If the focus is hemispheric, a neutral or slightly flexed head position is ideal. Posterior fossa imaging can best be accomplished with the head maximally flexed, if it is safe to do so. Once the patient is positioned appropriately and comfortably, scanning is initiated. We obtain 7 to 10 images from which to choose levels of interest. Because CT artifact significantly degrades the blood flow information, CT angles are selected to minimize such artifact. Scan planes that include the eyes also are avoided to minimize radiation to the lens.

## XENON DELIVERY

Xenon is administered through either a mouthpiece with the nostrils clipped or a mask that fits snugly over the nose and mouth. Various mask sizes are available (Fig. 4). If a mouthpiece is used, a humidifier should be placed between it and the non-rebreather valve to minimize drying of the mouth.

During inhalation, monitoring should ensure that the patient's breathing is comfortable and unrestricted and that the connections between the xenon-delivery system and the patient are intact. Maintaining verbal contact with the patient throughout the study is crucial. The patient can respond by using pre-

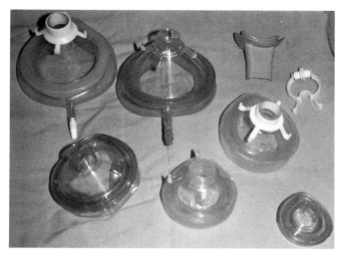

**FIG. 4.** Various mask sizes are available for xenon inhalation.

determined signals such as toe wiggling. Blood pressure, heart rate, oxygen saturation, end-tidal $CO_2$, and end-tidal xenon concentration should be monitored continually throughout the study.

Upon completion of xenon inhalation, the patient should be instructed to take four or five deep breaths to aid in xenon clearance. Then the mask or mouthpiece is removed, and the patient is observed until alert and responding normally. If a second study is planned (e.g., to evaluate the patient's physiologic response to acetazolamide, $pCO_2$ manipulation, blood pressure manipulation, or carotid balloon test occlusion), 15 to 20 minutes must be allowed for xenon clearance.

## POTENTIAL PROBLEMS

Despite head-immobilization techniques, motion continues to be the most frequent problem in Xe/CT CBF studies (see Kalender et al. in this volume). Continuing a study after obvious motion will yield no useful information. Judgment should be exercised regarding sedation; in some situations, small doses of a short-acting narcotic such as fentanyl are effective.

Rarely is it necessary to abort a study due to excess breath delays; most patients will respond to commands to take a breath. If excess breath delays persist, however, it may be necessary to stop the study and check the patient.

Laughing and crying are responses to xenon that patients may be unable to control and often result in head motion. Reassurance may be sufficient to stem these reactions, but sedation also may need to be considered.

Although an infrequent effect of xenon inhalation, vomiting can compromise patient safety, especially when using a mask. We therefore recommend that, whenever possible, the patient be limited to a clear liquid diet for 6 hours prior to the study.

Air leaks during a study usually result in dilution of the xenon concentration. Leaks are most common around the mask. Therefore, the fit of the mask should be checked if the xenon concentration fails to increase at the expected rate. If using a mouthpiece, the patient should be told to keep the mouth tightly closed around it. Early detection and correction of an air leak often saves a study.

Finally, fluctuations in end-tidal $CO_2$ can be avoided by coaching the patient to breathe normally, thus maintaining a fairly constant $CO_2$ level throughout the study.

## SPECIAL PATIENT SITUATIONS

Certain patients may require special measures. For instance, before positioning a hearing-impaired patient, a two-way nonverbal method of communication should be arranged. The overhead lights might be switched off and on as a signal for the patient to respond with toe wiggling.

The edentulous person may have difficulty holding a mouthpiece. This problem can be addressed by using a mask, which will mold to facial contours. For bearded patients, on the other hand, a mouthpiece should be used when possible. If it is necessary to use a mask, an effective seal can be created with a layer of petroleum jelly between the mask and beard. This technique is also effective to seal the area where a nasogastric tube exits the mask.

The patient with a tracheostomy may be stimulated to cough if the non-rebreathing apparatus is attached directly to the tracheostomy tube. This problem can be remedied easily by using a short, flexible tracheostomy tube connected to the valve by a universal adapter.

It is sometimes necessary to study patients with healed laryngectomy stomas. In this situation, inhalation is most effectively accomplished by placing a small pediatric mask, sealed with strips of stoma adhesive, directly over the stoma. The use of petroleum jelly to create a seal is contraindicated because of the close proximity to an unprotected airway.

Patients maintained on mechanical ventilators also can be studied safely and successfully. To do so, it is important to remember to add supplemental oxygen to the system during baseline scanning. Moreover, the monitoring (e.g., vital signs, oxygen saturation, end-tidal $CO_2$) of these critically ill patients must be particularly vigilant. When sedation and neuromuscular blocking agents are in-dicated for the safe and adequate examination of these patients, critical care, anesthesia, and respiratory therapy staff need to be directly involved in the studies.

Overall, the initial step in the acquisition of blood flow data requires a co-operative effort, consideration of the patient, and attention to details. Because of the numerous clinical applications of Xe/CT CBF studies, some subjects may require special care. Thoughtful regard for both general and specific patient needs can increase the likelihood of safe and successful studies.

## APPENDIX

The following equipment is used in conjunction with Xe/CT CBF studies at the University of Pittsburgh.

**Head Immobilizer**
Olympic Vac-Pac
Surgical Positioning Sets
(Size 20) Rectangular 20.8 × 11 cm
Catalogue #51620
Available from:
Olympic Medical
4400 Seventh South
Seattle, Washington 98108
Telephone: 1-800-426-0353
**LP 6 Compact Volume Ventilator**
Life Products
Aequitron Medical Inc.
14800 28th Avenue North
Minneapolis, Minnesota 55447
Telephone: 612-557-9200
**Non-Conductive Single-Use Face Mask**
Vital Signs, Inc.
20 Campus Road
Totowa, New Jersey 07512
Telephone: 1-800-932-0760

*Cerebral Blood Flow Measurement with Stable Xenon-Enhanced Computed Tomography,* edited by Howard Yonas. Raven Press, Ltd., New York © 1992.

# Development, Validation, and Use of Stable Xenon-Enhanced Computed Tomography at the Medical College of Virginia

Panos P. Fatouros, Abund O. Wist, *Anthony Marmarou, *Douglas S. DeWitt, **Richard L. Keenan, and Pulla R.S. Kishore

*Departments of Radiology, *Neurosurgery, and **Anesthesiology, Medical College of Virginia, Virginia Commonwealth University, Box 72, MCV Station, Richmond, Virginia 23298*

Originated in the early 1960s by Ingvar and Lassen (1), the radioactive $^{133}$Xe method of blood flow measurement was developed by Obrist et al. (2) as a noninvasive inhalation method. Such studies can be performed at the bedside and are highly accurate because of the high number of data points. Difficulties arise, however, from poor spatial resolution, the presence of extracerebral activity, and the need to assume the partition coefficient for calculation of the blood flow. Therefore, many investigators have turned to methods that use stable xenon and computed tomography (CT).

This chapter describes the development, validation, and use of the Xe/CT method for evaluating head-injured patients at the Medical College of Virginia (3–6). The noninvasive stable Xe/CT method provides high spatial resolution, good anatomic correlation, and, because the partition coefficient can be determined for each pixel, a more precise flow calculation. Furthermore, since all head-injured patients undergo a CT scan, it can be easily performed on a routine basis. Even so, the technique is affected by head motion; the inhalation of xenon at high concentrations and for prolonged periods might be intolerable to the patient; and the use of x-rays entails a certain amount of risk.

We conducted a three-phase investigation of our Xe/CT technique. Phase 1 involved preliminary tests and mathematical formulation; phase 2, technique validation and baboon studies (normocapnic, hypocapnic, hypercapnic); and phase 3, clinical studies. During the first phase, we made some preliminary measurements in baboons to demonstrate the feasibility of the technique in our hands. We also undertook a detailed mathematical formulation and established parameters for the technique (3). In the second phase, we conducted extensive studies in the baboon and validated the range of the technique against the radiolabeled microsphere standard. These measurements were made under a variety of physiological and technique conditions. In the final stage, we applied the method in the evaluation of several head-injured patients.

## METHODS AND RESULTS

### Mathematical Formulation

The Kety equation for the calculation of the tissue blood flow was used in its normalized form, eliminating the need to interrelate the variables derived from the CT scanner and the gas monitors (3):

$$\Delta H_{br}(T)/\Delta H_{br}(\text{Sat}) = k \cdot \int_0^T [C_a(t)/C_a(\text{Sat})] \cdot \exp(-k \cdot (T - t))dt \qquad [1]$$

where $k$ = the flow rate constant, $\Delta H_{br}(t)$ = CT enhancement in Hounsfield units at time $t$, $\Delta H_{br}(\text{Sat})$ = CT enhancement in Hounsfield units at saturation, $C_a(t)$ = arterial xenon concentration at time $t$, and $T$ = xenon inhalation time.

### Principal Features of the Method

Each patient was scanned for 5.1 seconds with a Picker 1200SX CT scanner at 120 kVp, 80 mA, a 5-mm slice thickness, and a 256 × 256 matrix. Before the blood flow measurement, patients were given 100% oxygen. The following features characterize our method.

A. Xenon arterial concentration
   1. Continuous monitoring of $PaCO_2$ and $PaO_2$
   2. Automatic collection and processing of end-tidal data
   3. Determination of xenon concentration by the subtraction method
   4. Data fitted to a double exponential function
   5. Correction for transit time of xenon
B. Continuous monitoring of intracranial pressure
C. Xenon brain enhancement
   1. 10-minute enhancement
   2. 35% xenon concentration (Linde XeScan stable xenon in oxygen USP, Union Carbide Rare Gases, Specialty Medical Products, Danbury, CT)
D. Cerebral blood flow (CBF) calculation/display
   1. CBF maps:
      a. Method of calculation (separability of $k$ and $\lambda$)
      b. Blood vessel correction
   2. $\lambda$ maps
   3. Region of high-flow/low-flow areas superimposed on CT images

The features listed in A through C enable the generation of highly accurate CBF and $\lambda$ maps as well as images that combine anatomic and flow information.

### Setup for the Measurement

The CBF measurement setup consists of three separate, functionally integrated blocks: the microcomputer-based data collection and processing system, the gas-handling system, and the CT computer. The end-tidal curve is monitored continually by means of the $O_2$ and $CO_2$ analyzers. The concentration of inhaled xenon gas is computed by subtracting the concentrations of $O_2$, $CO_2$, and water from 100. The data points of the exhaled xenon concentration are fitted by an unweighted least-squares routine to a double exponential function (3):

$$C_a(t)/C_a(\text{Sat}) = 1 - a_1 \cdot \exp(-b_1 \cdot t) - a_2 \cdot \exp(-b_2 \cdot t) \qquad [2]$$

Use of a double exponential function to approximate the end-tidal data achieves an excellent fit (7).

There is a delay between the moment the xenon gas is turned on and its arrival at the brain. By extrapolating the enhanced CT numbers to the time axis and averaging this value for many examinations, we determined that this delay is about 10 seconds (4).

### Calculation of Blood Flow

We calculated the blood flow by fitting the enhanced CT numbers, on a pixel-by-pixel basis, with a two-parameter ($k$, $\lambda$) Marquardt nonlinear regression method. To increase the speed of this calculation, we eliminated one parameter analytically from the two equations, thus generating one equation with one variable (8). Comparison of these methods showed that they are completely equivalent.

### Correction of Tissue Flow Maps

Flow in the vessels contributes substantially to the flow values in the tissue flow map, especially near large arteries. We developed a method to generate vessel maps and deduct the vessel flows to produce corrected tissue flow maps (9).

### Validation of the Stable Xe/Ct Method

We validated our stable Xe/CT CBF method by comparing values obtained with this method to those derived with radiolabeled microspheres in baboons (4,6). In the first series of baboons, we demonstrated that the stable Xe/CT technique, when applied with all the features outlined here, shows a high degree of correlation and reasonable numeric agreement with the well-established microsphere technique over the whole range of normal CBF values. In the second

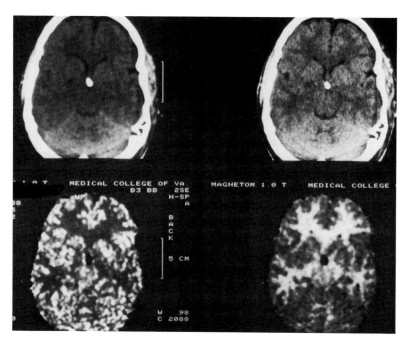

**FIG. 1.** Composite image of baseline CT (*upper left*), 5-minute xenon/CT (*upper right*), flow map (*lower left*), and λ map (*lower right*).

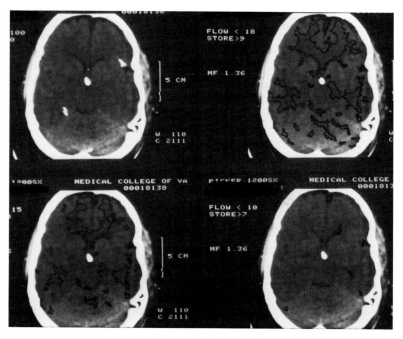

**FIG. 2.** Composite image of the baseline CT with superimposed areas of high flow, >100 ml/100 g/min (*upper left*), and low flow: <18 ml/100 g/min (*upper right*), <15 ml/100 g/min (*lower left*), and <10 ml/100 g/min (*lower right*).

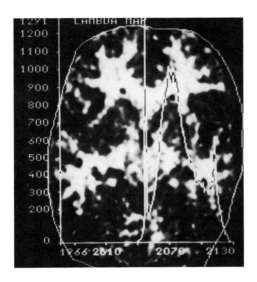

**FIG. 3.** Lambda map with overlaid histogram. The peak at extreme right corresponds to the white matter (λ around 1.4), and the middle peak corresponds to the gray matter (λ around 0.8).

series of experiments, we tested the technique against radioactive microspheres over a wide range of CBF rates (10–300 ml/100 g/min) under conditions of normocapnia, hypocapnia, and hypercapnia. Again, there was a high correlation between the values obtained by the two techniques. Because these measurements were performed under "ideal" conditions of extended inhalation at higher concentrations, we examined whether Xe/CT CBF values calculated from five scans during the first 5 minutes differed from those calculated from the entire series of scans. Our analysis indicates a good correlation between the extended and time-limited measurements (6). Figures 1 to 3 show baseline images, flow maps, and λ maps from the clinical application of this technique.

## CONCLUSION

The technique developed at our institution has a high correlation with the radiolabeled microsphere method and is comparably accurate. Moreover, it offers several innovations that enhance accuracy and clinical utility.

## REFERENCES

1. Ingvar DH, Lassen NA. Cerebral function, metabolism and blood flow. News and trends from the VIIIth International CBF Symposium in Copenhagen, June 1, 1977. *Acta Neurol Scand* 1978;57: 262–269.
2. Obrist WD, Thompson HK, King CH, Wans HS. Determination of regional cerebral blood flow by inhalation of xenon. *Circ Res* 1967;20:124–135.
3. Kishore PRS, Rao GU, Fernandez RE, et al. Regional cerebral blood flow measurements using stable xenon enhanced computed tomography: a theoretical and experimental evaluation. *J Comput Assist Tomogr* 1984;8:619–630.

4. Fatouros PP, Wist AO, Kishore PRS, et al. Xenon/computed tomography cerebral blood flow measurements: methods and accuracy. *Invest Radiol* 1987;22:705–712.
5. Wist AO, Fatouros PP, Kishore PRS, et al. Methods for determining blood flow in the brain. Part II. Stable xenon/CT method. *J Clin Engin* 1987;12:213–220.
6. DeWitt DS, Fatouros PP, Wist AO, et al. Stable xenon versus radiolabeled microsphere cerebral blood flow measurements in baboons. *Stroke* 1989;20:1716–1723.
7. Wist AO, Fatouros PP, DeWitt DS, et al. A new approach to modeling the increase of xenon concentration in arterial blood for cerebral flow determinations. *Modeling and Simulation* 1985;16: 1837–1841.
8. Wist AO, Rao G, Arora G. A non–invasive method for the determination of blood flow in the brain. *Proceedings of AAMSI Congress* 1984;463–466.
9. Wist AO, Cothran SJ, Fatouros PP, et al. An investigation to measure velocity, flow, and pressure in vessels of the brain using the stable xenon/CT method. *Modeling and Simulation* 1989;20: 1743–1748.

*Cerebral Blood Flow Measurement with Stable Xenon-Enhanced Computed Tomography,* edited by Howard Yonas. Raven Press, Ltd., New York © 1992.

# Current Status of Stable Xenon-Enhanced Computed Tomography in Japan and Our Future Strategies

Ryuta Suzuki and Kimiyoshi Hirakawa

*Department of Neurosurgery, Tokyo Medical and Dental University, 1-5-45 Yushima Bunkyo-ku, Tokyo 113, Japan*

The Japanese life span is being prolonged. In 1988, the average expectancy was 75.5 years for men and 81.3 years for women, the longest life expectancies in the world (1). This increase in the number of the elderly raises several serious sociomedical issues, including the treatment of senile dementia, strokes, and similar illnesses affecting the aged.

Although stroke has been the third leading cause of death since 1985 (2), the number of deaths caused by a stroke has been decreasing. This is mainly because of lowered mortality from intracerebral hemorrhage. Among the elderly, however, the incidence of stroke has been growing, especially those caused by cerebral infarction. Among other generations, deaths resulting from traffic accidents have been increasing in Japan, reaching 13,600 in 1988 (1), and a not negligible number of survivors, many still young, have been left with serious neurological deficits. Thus, the number of patients with neurological problems is rising, and proper sociomedical care is needed.

Because of a growing demand to better understand the functions of the brain and the pathophysiologies of neurological diseases, many sophisticated machines are now part of the equipment at Japanese hospitals (Table 1). More than 5,000 computed tomography (CT) scanners are currently in use; magnetic resonance imaging units now number 500 and can be expected to reach 1,000 in the near future. These modern machines are found throughout the country, and their ready availability is superb. Even so, although these modern tools can assist in morphological examinations, they cannot provide information about a patient's neurologic function. A reliable cerebral blood flow (CBF) measurement is needed for proper diagnosis and treatment.

As shown in Table 1, distributed throughout Japan are 15 positron-emission tomography (PET) units, 70 ring-type single-photon-emission CT (SPECT) units, and 90 xenon inhalators for stable xenon/CT (Xe/CT) CBF evaluations. Yet few institutions are using these machines clinically to perform CBF studies on

**TABLE 1.** *Modern neuroimaging devices in Japan (1989)* [a]

| Device | Number |
|---|---|
| X-ray CT | 5000 |
| Magnetic resonance imaging | 500 |
| Single-photon-emission CT (ring-type) | 70 |
| Positron-emission tomography | 15 |
| Xenon inhalators | 90 |

[a] These devices service a population of 124 million. Related resources include 720 neurosurgical units, 80 university-based and another 139 in large teaching hospitals, and 2,749 board-certified neurosurgeons.

patients. Based on a survey of peer-reviewed articles published in Japan, the majority of CBF measurements are being done to compile data used in research. CBF studies on patients should be pursued as a matter of clinical routine, especially in critical cases, with the results forming part of the decision-making data that govern the mode of treatment.

In conducting CBF studies, the PET, SPECT, and Xe/CT methods each have their advantages and their drawbacks (Table 2). For routine clinical use, Xe/CT would appear to be the preferred method, because CT scanners are readily available almost everywhere, the studies can be used in cases of emergency, and the images provide superior anatomical resolution. In spite of these advantages, however, only some 20 to 30 institutions have used Xe/CT for CBF measurements, and even fewer have used this method to conduct CBF studies as a clinical routine.

There are various reasons why the Xe/CT method has yet to receive full acceptance. One major problem is the limited supply of xenon gas, a result of the gas not yet being listed among pharmaceutical drugs in Japan. In addition, Xe/CT is thought by many to be too invasive a procedure for clinical use.

**TABLE 2.** *Comparison of cerebral blood flow measurement methods*

| | Xe/CT | SPECT (IMP, HMPAO) | PET |
|---|---|---|---|
| Spatial resolution | ⊙ | × | △ |
| Anatomical correlation | ⊙ | × | △ |
| Quantitative | ○ | × | ○ |
| Adverse effect | anesthetic | none | |
| Noninvasiveness | △ | △ | × |
| Emergent availability | ⊙ | × | × |
| Repeatability | ⊙ | × | ○ |
| Simplicity | △ | ○ | × |
| Tracer availability | × | ○ | × |
| Facility's availability | ⊙ | ○ | × |
| Information other than CBF | × | ○ | ⊙ |
| Capital cost | low | medium | high |
| Cost of a test | $150 | $300 | high |

⊙ very good, ○ good, △ fair, × poor

The first Japanese reports discussing the clinical use of Xe/CT to measure CBF began appearing in the early 1980s (3,4), after which several algorithms and patient protocols were introduced (5,6). Most authors have used the long-inhalation method to obtain accurate partition coefficients. One report discusses a Xe/CT study performed under general anesthesia, and another discusses the use of this method when continuous arterial blood scanning was required. These reports have tended to stress the difficulties of the procedures, making both doctors and patients unwilling to hazard such examinations. Recently, however, several authors have introduced the use of short-inhalation periods (7–9), thereby minimizing both the invasiveness of the method and the consumption of xenon gas; this may be the better approach for clinical CBF studies.

Our future strategies include devising a simple, noninvasive measurement method with an acceptable degree of accuracy, thus contributing to the further clarification of brain diseases. To achieve this, governmental understanding and the cooperation of CT manufacturers are essential. It will be no easy task to integrate the work of researchers from different fields, but all difficulties encountered should be approached with an unyielding enthusiasm.

## REFERENCES

1. *Asahi yearbook 1990.* Tokyo: Asahi Newspaper Co.
2. *Figures on cancer in Japan.* Tokyo: Foundation for Promotion of Cancer Research, 1987.
3. Ono H, Ono K, Mori K. Mapping of CBF distribution by dynamic Xe-enhanced CT scan method. *J Cereb Blood Flow Metab* 1981;1(Suppl 1):S51–52.
4. Goto F, Ebihara S, Takagi Y, et al. The cerebral blood flow and metabolism in patients with spontaneous occlusion of the circle of Willis [in Japanese]. In: *The annual report of the Research Committee on Spontaneous Occlusion of the Circle of Willis of the Ministry of Health and Welfare, Japan* 1980;65–71.
5. Segawa H, Wakai S, Tamura A, Yoshimasu N, Nakamura O, Ohta M. Computed tomographic measurement of local cerebral blood flow by xenon enhancement. *Stroke* 1983;14:356–362.
6. Kuriyama Y, Karasawa J, Sawada T, et al. rCBF measurement using cold xenon and CT—a "shuttle" method [in Japanese]. *Circulation Science* 1983;3:600–604.
7. Kimura T, Inoue J, Timuzawa I, et al. Regional cerebral blood flow measurement by xenon enhanced CT using a brief inhalation technique [in Japanese]. *Medical Imaging Technology* 1984;2: 106–113.
8. Suzuki R, Hiratsuka H, Matsushima Y, et al. Cerebral blood flow measurement by means of xenon-enhanced CT with brief-xenon-inhalation methods [in Japanese]. *Progress in Computed Tomography* 1986;8:139–144.
9. Touho H, Karasawa J, Nakagawara J, et al. Mapping of local cerebral blood flow with stable xenon-enhanced CT and the curve-fitting method of analysis. *Radiology* 1988;1968:207-212.

*Cerebral Blood Flow Measurement with Stable Xenon-Enhanced Computed Tomography,* edited by Howard Yonas. Raven Press, Ltd., New York © 1992.

# Reproducibility of Xenon-Enhanced Computed Tomography Cerebral Blood Flow Results

## Hiromu Segawa

*Department of Neurosurgery, Fuji Brain Institute and Hospital, 270-12 Sugita, Fujinomiya 418, Japan*

The xenon-enhanced computed tomography cerebral blood flow (Xe/CT CBF) method has proven capable of providing quantitative CBF images with reasonable resolution. To assess the reproducibility and, hence, the reliability of the data obtained with this technique, we conducted double Xe/CT CBF studies in five patients.

## METHODS

The five patients who underwent these studies all had small lesions; one had a pituitary adenoma, two had cerebral infarcts, and two had brain tumors. Each study was performed while the patient inhaled 50% xenon for 25 minutes. We began the second studies 30 to 55 minutes after the first. We then compared the CBF values obtained in anatomically identical regions (eight in gray matter and six in white matter) in each of the two studies. All regions appeared normal on the accompanying CT images.

## RESULTS

The CBF values in the first and second studies corresponded closely. Expressing the correlation ($r$) as $Y = 0.88X - 1.77$ (where $X$ is the value in the first study and $Y$ is that of the second study), $r$ ranged from 0.897 to 0.963 (average: 0.934 ± 0.029) (Fig. 1). Table 1 demonstrates the ratio of the blood flow values in the second study to those in the first study for each subject. The mean values in gray matter obtained in the second study were consistently lower than those in the first, the ratio ranging from 0.77 to 0.96. White-matter values in the second study were also lower (Fig. 2), with one exception: In the patient whose studies were done 45 minutes apart, white-matter flow in the second study was 1.04

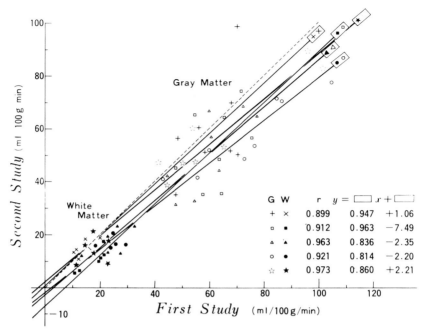

**FIG. 1.** Correlation of the two measurements in each of the five patients. The second study (*y*) was performed 30 to 55 minutes after the first study (*x*). Overall, there was a good correlation (average *r* = 0.934) between the two studies. (G, gray matter; W, white matter.)

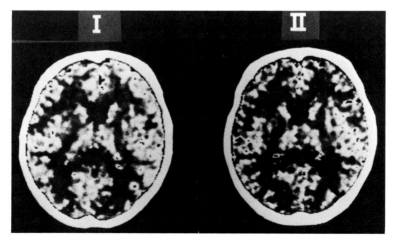

**FIG. 2.** Blood flow maps from the first and second studies in one of the patients. The second study showed slightly lower flow values, especially in white matter.

**TABLE 1.** *Individual second-study flow values as a ratio of first-study values*

| | Interstudy interval | | | | |
|---|---|---|---|---|---|
| | 30 min | 30 min | 35 min | 45 min | 55 min |
| Gray matter | 0.77** | 0.84* | 0.79* | 0.96 | 0.92 |
| White matter | 0.68* | 0.56** | 0.76* | 1.04 | 0.86 |

Decreased significantly at second study, *$P < 0.05$ and **$P < 0.01$.

that of the first. The values obtained in the second study tended to be lowest when there was a shorter interval (i.e., 30 minutes) between the studies.

## DISCUSSION

Two factors could have affected the flow values obtained in the second study: the intracerebral xenon residual from the first study or an anesthetic effect of the xenon. Residual xenon at the time of baseline CT scanning for the second study was estimated to be $0.06 \pm 0.03$ and $0.50 \pm 0.27$ Hounsfield units for gray and white matter, respectively. Such high levels of residual xenon may have significantly distorted the results of the second study. Theoretically, more xenon will remain in white matter than in gray matter at the end of a study, because its solubility in white-matter is 1.5 times higher than in gray matter and because the white-matter "wash-out" rate is slower. The presence of residual xenon also is supported by the fact that in the second study, white-matter blood flow values were reduced more than gray-matter flows in four of five patients (see Table 1). It is less likely that a xenon-induced anesthetic effect would have reduced blood flow in the second studies, because this effect is short-lived once xenon inhalation has stopped.

The following measures should effectively reduce the residual xenon from the first study. Because the concentration of xenon gas inhaled during an initial study directly affects the concentration of residual xenon, we recommend the use of short inhalation periods and low xenon concentrations. Currently, we conduct studies using 30% xenon inhaled for 5 minutes. In addition, double studies should be sufficiently separated to maximize the clearance of xenon. We favor an interstudy delay of greater than 30 minutes.

## REFERENCES

1. Segawa H, Sano K, Maehara T, et al. Cerebral blood flow study by CT with xenon enhancement. Symposium Abstract. *J Comput Assist Tomogr* 1980;4:710.
2. Segawa H, Wakai S, Tamura K, et al. CBF study by CT with xenon enhancement. Experience in 30 cases. *J Cereb Blood Flow Metab* 1981;1(Suppl 1):52–53.
3. Segawa H, Wakai S, Tamura A, et al. Computed tomographic measurement of local cerebral blood flow by xenon enhancement. *Stroke* 1983;14:356–362.
4. Ueda Y, Kimura K, Nagai M, et al. rCBF measurement by CT and its imaging. *J Cereb Blood Flow Metab* 1981;1(Suppl 1)1:54–55.

*Cerebral Blood Flow Measurement with Stable Xenon-Enhanced Computed Tomography,* edited by Howard Yonas. Raven Press, Ltd., New York © 1992.

# Conserving Xenon and Other Gases in Ventilator-Controlled Systems

Abund O. Wist, Panos P. Fatouros, *Richard L. Keenan, and **Anthony Marmarou

*Departments of Radiology, *Anesthesiology, and **Neurosurgery, Medical College of Virginia, Virginia Commonwealth University, Box 72, MCV Station, Richmond, Virginia 23298*

Several years ago, we compared our modified stable xenon/computed tomography (CT) method (1–4) with the radiolabeled microsphere method. We noticed that in the initial series of studies, the end-tidal $CO_2$ tension varied greatly (Fig. 1). Because such changes in $CO_2$ concentrations will substantially affect the measurement of blood flow, in the next series of studies we kept the $CO_2$ tension constant by continual manual variation of ventilator function (Fig. 2) and by administering a muscle relaxant drug. Nevertheless, we found that using manual control to change the $CO_2$ tension from 40 to 20 mm Hg might take an hour or longer and frequently would cause an overshoot with values transiently below 20 mm Hg. To achieve faster and more consistent control of the $CO_2$ tension, we investigated the use of an automatic control system. Such a system also would relieve the operator of having to watch the $CO_2$ values continually during a test.

Several systems have been designed and constructed for the automatic maintenance of $CO_2$. Lambertson and Wendel (5) developed a $CO_2$ controller based mainly on mechanical components. Later, several other automatic ventilating systems were developed that included the use of analog devices, analog computers, and minicomputers. Ohlson et al. (6) and Giard et al. (7,8) were the first to use microcomputers for the automatic control of ventilators and for the recirculation of $CO_2$ and $O_2$. To achieve a short response time (5 minutes), Giard et al. used a highly sophisticated algorithm together with a fairly complex mechanical ventilating system. In a study of an earlier manual recirculation system designed by Bracken et al. (9), a test of the anesthetic effect of xenon showed that xenon had no toxic effect in rabbits, even when it was applied for 48 hours at a concentration of 80%.

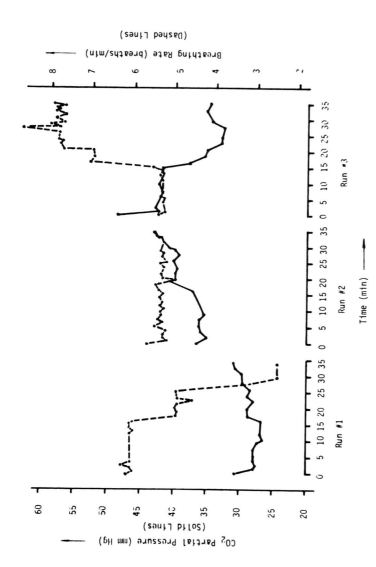

**FIG. 1.** Time dependence of the $CO_2$ tension (*solid lines*) and breathing rate (*dashed lines*) for three consecutive test runs using baboons. Notice the wide deviations of $PaCO_2$ from the set value of 40 mm Hg due to lack of continuous ventilator adjustment.

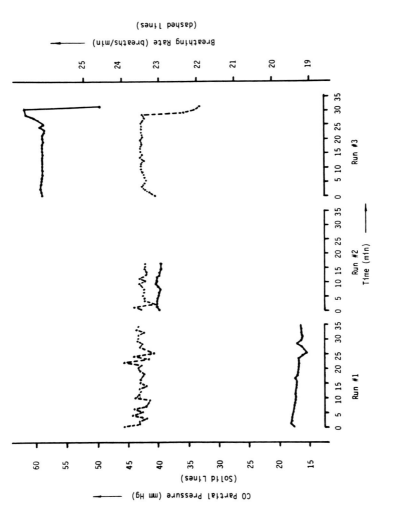

**FIG. 2.** Time dependence of the $CO_2$ tension (*solid lines*) and breathing rate (*dashed lines*) for three consecutive animal test runs. $CO_2$ tension is continuously regulated by manipulating the breathing rate and maintained at 20, 40, and 60 mm Hg during runs #1 and #3 respectively.

## METHOD

Because our Xe/CT system already contains the required major components, such as gas sensors, monitors, gas controls, and a microcomputer system, installing an automatic control is fairly straightforward. First, we exchanged the ventilator for one with electronic controls. To send the commands of the microcomputer to the ventilator, we designed and constructed an interface consisting of four components. The first two components transfer the control signals for the minute volume and frequency from the microcomputer to the ventilator using two digital-to-analog converters. The third interface transfers the time when the lung is fully exhaled to the microcomputer. The fourth interface transmits control signals from the microcomputer to a proportional gas valve. Finally, a three-mode control program was written in Pascal to collect the $CO_2$ and $O_2$ values and to automatically adjust the ventilator and the proportional valve (10,11).

## RESULTS

We tested the automatic $CO_2$ controller with an artificial lung. Figure 3 shows the response of the automatic system when the $CO_2$ concentration in the artificial lung was increased by a factor of two and then, in another test, divided in half. In the three-mode control (second graph from bottom), when the $CO_2$ tension was halved—simulating a reduction from 40 to 20 mm Hg $CO_2$ tension—it returned to the preset value with a time constant of about 2½ minutes. The overshoot was around 25%. If the overshoot is too large, it can be reduced by gradually approaching the preset value using an additional program. A similar overshoot occurs when the tension is doubled.

All of these experiments were conducted with a nonrecirculating system. Because of the high expense of the xenon gas, we performed an additional investigation to determine whether the controller described above also could be used to recirculate xenon. Such a system requires microcomputer-controlled valves, and we designed and built an interface for a proportional valve. Tests showed that the gas flow could be controlled quickly and accurately.

Next, we set up an experimental rebreathing system. Although tests showed our system to be functional, its air resistance and the air volume might be too large for some patients and certainly for small animals such as mice or rats. Therefore, we are modifying the system to reduce its air resistance and volume. Basically, we intend to use an air bag that can be compressed by a controller. Proportional valves will be used to inject appropriate gas mixtures into the bag. A microcomputer will time the operation of the bag and valves. The advantages of such a system include very low air resistance, low dead volume, and fast response. It also can be cleaned easily and is very safe (11).

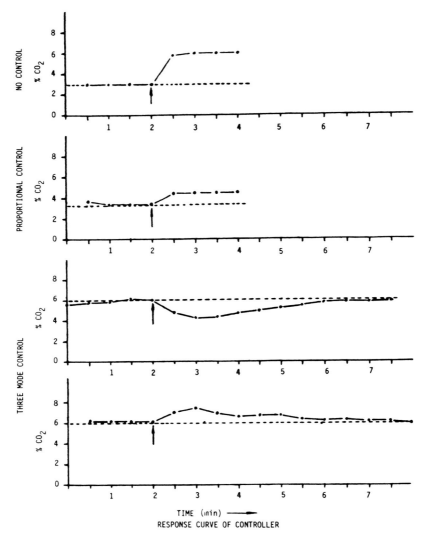

**FIG. 3.** Response curves of automatic $CO_2$ controller to changes in $CO_2$ tension using a test lung. Top curve: no control. Second curve: proportional control. Third curve: three-mode control for reduced $CO_2$ tension. Bottom curve: three-mode control for increased $CO_2$ tension.

## CONCLUSION

Our investigation shows that it is possible to design a relatively inexpensive automatic ventilator for the accurate, safe, and rapid control of all gases that may be used in clinical studies. Further developments are necessary to adapt it to a recirculating system that has a minimum air resistance and air volume and that can be operated with different modes of ventilation. Such a system can be valuable for patients having breathing difficulties and for small animals in the laboratory.

## REFERENCES

1. Kishore PRS, Rao GU, Fernandez RE, et al. Regional cerebral blood flow measurements using stable xenon enhanced computed tomography: a theoretical and experimental evaluation. *J Comput Assist Tomogr* 1984;8:619–630.
2. Fatouros PP, Wist AO, Kishore PRS, et al. Xenon/computed tomography cerebral blood flow measurements: methods and accuracy. *Invest Radiol* 1987;22:705–712.
3. Wist AO, Fatouros PP, Kishore PRS, et al. Methods for determining blood flow in the brain. Part II. Stable xenon/CT method. *J Clin Engin* 1987;12:213–220.
4. DeWitt DS, Fatouros PP, Wist AO, et al. Stable xenon versus radiolabeled microsphere cerebral blood flow measurements in baboons. *Stroke* 1989;20:1716–1723.
5. Lambertson CJ, Wendel H. An alveolar $pCO_2$ control system: its use to magnify respiratory depression by meperidine. *J Appl Physiol* 1960;15:43–48.
6. Ohlson KB, Westenskow DR, Jordan WS. A microprocessor based feedback controller for mechanical ventilation. *Ann Biomed Eng* 1982;10:35–48.
7. Giard MH, Perrin F, Bouchet P, et al. EOLE: un system de controle automatique de $pO_2$ et de $pCO_2$ en ventilation assiste. *Med Biol Eng Comput* 1983;21:503–508.
8. Giard MH, Perrin F, Bertrand O, et al. An algorithm for the automatic control of $O_2$ and $CO_2$ in artificial ventilation. *IEEE Trans Biomed Eng* 1985;32:658–667.
9. Bracken A, Burns THS, Newland DS. A trial of xenon as a non-explosive anesthetic. *Anesthesia* 1956;11:40–49.
10. Wist AO, Fatouros PP, Keenan RL, Stewart M, Marmarou A, Kishore PRS. Development of an automatic system to control carbon dioxide concentration in ventilator controlled systems. In: Saha S, ed. *Biomedical engineering V: recent developments*. New York: Pergamon Press; 1986;415–420.
11. Wist AO, Fatouros PP, Keenan RL, Kishore PRS. Investigation of a new method to control xenon and other gases in mechanical ventilators used in the stable xenon/CT technique. In: Krause W, ed. *Digest of papers, Sixth Southern Biomechanical Engineering Conference*, Dallas, 1987;31–33.

*Cerebral Blood Flow Measurement with Stable Xenon-Enhanced Computed Tomography,* edited by Howard Yonas. Raven Press, Ltd., New York © 1992.

# Optimization of the Inhalation Protocol

Shigeki Nakano, Tetsuo Yamashita, Shiro Kashiwagi, Masaaki Hayashi, Teiichi Takasago, and Haruhide Ito

*Department of Neurosurgery, Yamaguchi University School of Medicine, 1144 Kogushi Ube, Yamaguchi 755, Japan*

In stable xenon/computed tomography cerebral blood flow (Xe/CT CBF) monitoring, a short period of inhalation using low-concentration xenon seems advisable, because the anesthetic effect of xenon induces motion artifacts and activation of CBF. However, low concentrations and short inhalation periods can lead to inaccurately estimated values, due to the low signal-to-noise ratio and fewer data points. Therefore, it is important to find an efficient way to acquire data under these conditions. To determine the most efficient technique, we compared the flow and λ values and the resolution in flow and λ images obtained with five different inhalation methods.

## SUBJECTS AND METHODS

Our subjects were five normal volunteers, 23 to 36 years of age (mean: 27.5 years). The following are the five inhalation methods we used and the number of CT scans ($n$) each involves:

1. Three-minute wash-in/5-minute wash-out (3-in/5-out): xenon inhalation for 3 minutes and desaturation for 5 minutes; CT scans at 1-minute intervals ($n = 8$).
2. Three-minute wash-in (3-in): xenon inhalation for 3 minutes; CT scans at 1-minute intervals ($n = 3$).
3. Six-minute wash-in (6-in): xenon inhalation for 6 minutes; CT scans at 1-minute intervals ($n = 6$).
4. Ten-minute wash-in (10-in): xenon inhalation for 10 minutes; CT scans at 1-minute intervals for 6 minutes and another scan at 10 minutes ($n = 7$).
5. Twenty-five-minute wash-in (25-in): xenon inhalation for 25 minutes; CT scans at 1-minute intervals for 6 minutes and additional scans at 10, 15, and 25 minutes ($n = 9$).

In one additional subject (a 37-year-old man), we performed both the 3-in/5-out and the 8-in to compare the two methods with the same number of scans (8 scans). In all methods, subjects inhaled the same gas mixture: 30% Xe, 30% $O_2$, and 40% $N_2$. Our Xe/CT system consisted of a Somatom DR3 CT scanner with Evax CBF evaluation software (Siemens Medical Systems) and a Xetron III xenon inhalator (Anzai Sogyo Co. Ltd.) Details of our technique are reported elsewhere (1). We calculated flow and λ values in the thalamus and the frontal white matter in both hemispheres.

## RESULTS

### Flow Images and Values

Figure 1 shows flow images for the five different methods. The resolution improved in both the white matter and gray matter as the inhalation time lengthened in the wash-in-only methods (#2–5). The resolution with the 3-in/5-out method was as good as that in the 25-in. Changes in flow values with each method are shown in Fig. 2.

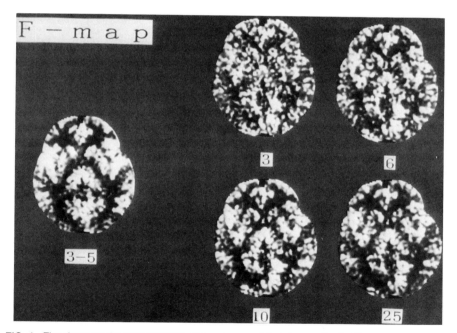

**FIG. 1.** Flow images obtained with five different xenon inhalation methods. The image on the left is from the 3-minute wash-in/5-minute wash-out method. Top right, images from the 3- and 6-minute wash-in methods. Bottom right, images from the 10- and 25-minute wash-in methods.

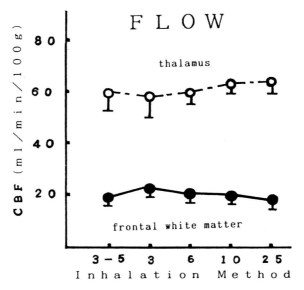

**FIG. 2.** Flow values obtained with five different xenon inhalation methods.

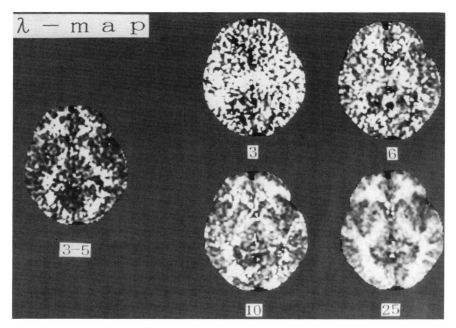

**FIG. 3.** Lambda images from five different xenon inhalation methods. Left, from the 3-minute wash-in/5-minute wash-out method; top right, the 3- and 6-minute wash-in methods; bottom right, the 10- and 25-minute wash-in methods.

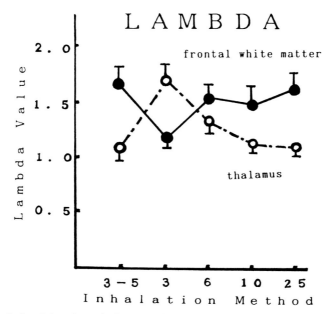

**FIG. 4.** Lambda values obtained with five different xenon inhalation methods.

### Lambda Images and Values

Figure 3 shows λ images for the five different methods. Here again, we found that the resolution in both white and gray matter improved with longer inhalation times in the wash-in-only protocols, and that the resolution with the 3-in/5-out method was as good as that with the 25-in. In both the thalamus and frontal white matter, λ values from the 3-in/5-out method were almost the same as those obtained with the 25-in (Fig. 4).

### Comparison of the 3-in/5-out and the 8-in Methods

Table 1 lists the flow and λ values obtained in the subject who underwent both the 3-in/5-out and the 8-in methods.

**TABLE 1.** *Comparison of flow and λ values in the 3-minute wash-in/5-minute wash-out and 8-minute wash-in methods in a normal adult*

| Method | Thalamus | | Frontal white matter | |
|---|---|---|---|---|
| | Flow[a] | λ | Flow[a] | λ |
| 3-in/5-out | 58.9 | 1.11 | 20.4 | 1.70 |
| 8-in | 57.0 | 1.35 | 20.5 | 1.57 |

[a] ml/100 g/min

## DISCUSSION

This study showed that the 3-in/5-out method produced an image resolution and value accuracy equivalent to that achieved with long wash-in methods such as the 25-in. Flow values obtained with the 3-in/5-out method were consistent with those measured by positron-emission tomography (2,3). The λ values from this method also agreed with those reported previously for Xe/CT CBF studies using longer inhalation periods (4,5) and were close to the theoretical values calculated from the Ostwald solubility coefficients (6).

In clinical studies, we have found that λ values calculated with the data of the 3-in method were higher in the thalamus than in the frontal white matter. This is quite improbable given the physiological characteristics of the tissues and indicates unsatisfactory estimation of the parameters with that method. However, when data acquisition was added during the 5-minute wash-out phase after the 3-minute wash-in phase (method #1), the λ values appeared to be far more physiological and approached those obtained with longer inhalation. Compared with the 8-in method, which has the same number of data points and should have better signal-to-noise ratio, the flow and λ values and the image quality of the 3-in/5-out method were at least as reliable.

Theoretically, one problem associated with the wash-in/wash-out method (#1) is the possible difference in CBF during wash-in and wash-out phases resulting from xenon's effect on CBF. If such a difference exists, it undermines the basic assumption of the Kety-Schmidt equation: the constancy of the flow during data acquisition. The activation of CBF appears to be inevitable with the use of xenon in any method, and it is important to minimize this effect. With 3-minute inhalation of 30% xenon, any CBF activation should be minimal.

From a practical standpoint, the 3-in/5-out method is more cost-effective than the conventional 6- to 8-minute wash-in method. We have used the 3-in/5-out method in 50 clinical studies over the last 6 months. The study was nondiagnostic, due to head motion, in only one case. In addition, none of these studies caused respiratory problems.

The 3-minute wash-in/5-minute wash-out method is a useful modification of the Xe/CT CBF technique. It improves the rate of successful examinations by reducing the anesthetic effects of xenon while preserving the data accuracy and image quality of techniques that involve longer inhalation.

## REFERENCES

1. Kashiwagi S, Yamashita T, Abiko S, et al. Measurement and imaging of cerebral blood flow with stable xenon and computed tomography (Xe-CT). *Electromedica* 1986;54:136–144.
2. Baron JC, Steinling M, Tanaka T, Cavalheiro E, Soussaline F, Collard P. Quantitative measurement of CBF, oxygen extraction fraction (OEF) and $CMRO_2$ with $^{15}O$ continuous inhalation techniques and positron computed tomography (PET): experimental evidence and normal values in man. *J Cereb Blood Flow Metab* 1981;Suppl 1:5–6.

3. Yamamoto YL, Thompson CJ, Meyer E, Robertson JS, Feindel W. Dynamic positron emission tomography for study of cerebral hemodynamics in a cross section of the head using positron-emitting $^{68}$Ga-EDTA and $^{77}$Kr. *J Comput Assist Tomogr* 1977;1:43–56.
4. Sakai F, Gotoh F, Ebihara S, et al. Xenon enhanced CT method for the measurement of local cerebral blood flow in man. *J Cereb Blood Flow Metab* 1981;Suppl 1:29–30.
5. Segawa H, Susum W, Tamura A, Yoshimasu N, Nakamura O, Ohta M. Computed tomographic measurement of local cerebral blood flow by xenon enhancement. *Stroke* 1983;14:356–362.
6. Steward A, Allott PR, Cowles AL, Mapleson WW. Solubility coefficients for inhaled anaesthetics for water, oil, and biological media. *Br J Anaesth* 1973;45:282–292.

*Cerebral Blood Flow Measurement with Stable Xenon-Enhanced Computed Tomography,* edited by Howard Yonas. Raven Press, Ltd., New York © 1992.

# Modification of Xenon-Enhanced Computed Tomography for Assessing Regional Cerebral Blood Flow in Newborns

Janet R. Emery, Joyce L. Peabody, Stephen Ashwal, Assaad Assaad, Wes Brown, and *Joseph Thompson

*Departments of Pediatrics and *Radiation Sciences, Loma Linda University Medical Center, Loma Linda, California 92350*

Sick prematurely born infants are at particular risk for cerebral hemorrhagic and ischemic injury because of the immaturity of their cerebral vasculature (1,2) and the many fluctuations in cerebral blood flow resulting from the intensive care they require (3,4). Yet routine quantitative measurement of regional cerebral blood flow (rCBF) in these infants has not been possible. Despite the successful use of stable xenon-enhanced computed tomography (Xe/CT) in adults, this technique has not been used to measure rCBF in sick infants because of their unique characteristics. This prompted us to ask, can the technique for Xe/CT imaging be modified to provide a method for measuring rCBF in sick premature infants?

## TECHNIQUE MODIFICATIONS

Table 1 lists the characteristics of premature infants that necessitate changes in the Xe/CT rCBF technique using the GE 9800 CT system. The respiratory circuit for the GE 9800 Xe/CT system was designed for spontaneously breathing adults who have respiratory minute volumes of 6 L (500 ml/breath and 12 to 13 breaths/minute). In contrast, premature infants (weighing, 0.5–2.5 kg) have tidal volumes of 3 to 15 ml/breath and respiratory rates of 35 to 45 breaths/minute, resulting in a minute volume of 100 to 680 ml. In addition, these infants usually are treated with continuous-flow mechanical ventilators.

To modify the GE 9800 system for the study of such infants, the respiratory circuit had to be adapted to meet the differences in ventilation. To adjust for the smaller tidal volumes, we used smaller-caliber tubing between the patient port and the xenon analyzer to reduce the volume of gas sampled. This narrower tubing has higher resistance to gas flow and thus samples a smaller volume of gas when the flow rate and sampling time are held constant. The sample volume

**TABLE 1.** *Characteristics of premature infants requiring modification of the GE 9800 Xe/CT system*

| Characteristic (versus adults) | Modification |
| --- | --- |
| Minute volume reduced<br>  a. Tidal volumes, 6 cc/breath<br>    (versus 500 cc/breath)<br>  b. Respiratory frequency, 35–45 breaths/minute<br>    (versus 12–13 breaths/minute) | Smaller gas sample |
| Treated with continuous-flow ventilators | Change in timing of gas sampling from inspiration to expiration |
| Immature brain tissue, heightening concern about effects of radiation | Fewer scans |

was decreased further by reducing the flow rate (rheostat adjusted to 67% of adult setting) on the xenon pump.

To make the system compatible with continuous-flow respirator circuitry, we changed the timing of gas sampling from inspiration, as used in the adult system, to exhalation. The exhaled gas was sampled by a technique commonly used in neonatal pulmonary physiology for measuring end-tidal carbon dioxide concentrations (5,6). With this technique, expiratory gases are aspirated only during exhalation from a 26-gauge gas catheter inserted directly into the endotracheal tube. After positive-pressure inflation of the chest during inhalation, the net flow of exhaled gases is from the patient's chest to the ventilator circuit. To change the sampling time from inspiration to expiration, we also had to devise a way for the neonatal ventilator to signal the xenon pump. In the adult system, inspiration depolarizes a capacitor, which then signals the xenon pump to begin. For the infant system, the release of the inspiratory-pressure valve produces an electrical signal. This signal depolarizes the capacitor and thus activates the xenon pump.

In addition to the differences between adult and infant ventilation, the heightened concern over the effects of radiation on immature brain tissue required some modifications in technique. To minimize the number of xenon-enhanced scans, we performed one baseline and four enhanced scans instead of the standard two baseline and six enhanced scans used in adult studies. This change was accomplished with options already provided by the current software.

## PRELIMINARY TESTING

This modified system has undergone preliminary testing in several infants and in an animal model. Although there are no established normal values for rCBF in preterm infants, the hemispheric CBF values obtained with this system are within the range measured by other investigators using different techniques in smaller groups of infants (Table 2). In addition, the response of the infants' rCBF to changes in carbon dioxide tensions in the blood ($pCO_2$) was similar to the $CO_2$ response reported for adults studied with Xe/CT. Figure 1 shows the Xe/CT images of one infant studied at a normal $pCO_2$ and again at a lower $pCO_2$.

**TABLE 2.** *Hemispheric CBF values reported*

| Technique | Investigator/year | Cerebral blood flow (ml/100 g/min) |
|---|---|---|
| [133]Xe clearance | Greisen 1986 (8) | 5.6–36.8 |
| [133]Xe clearance | Ment 1984 (9) | 21.4–48.4 |
| Positron-emission tomography | Altman 1988 | 4.9–23.0 |
| Stable Xe/CT | | 11.4–36.8 |

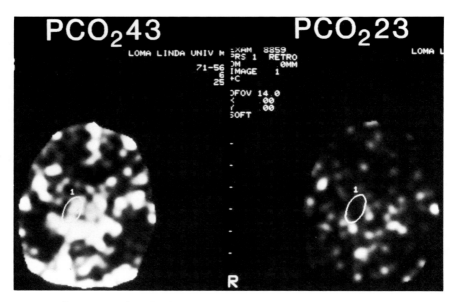

**FIG. 1.** Comparison of Xe/CT CBF images from one infant at two different pCO$_2$ levels.

## LIMITATIONS OF USE IN PREMATURE INFANTS

Although our results suggest that the GE 9800 Xe/CT system can be modified to measure rCBF in sick premature infants, there may be significant limitations to its use as a clinical tool. First, the technique may be inaccurate in patients with serious lung disease. A basic assumption of the technique is that end-expiratory gases are in equilibrium with blood levels and can be used to estimate blood concentrations. This assumption is true only when ventilation and perfusion are equally distributed and well matched. Because many premature infants have lung disease—including respiratory distress syndrome, pneumonia, and pulmonary air leaks—their end-expiratory gas concentrations may not accurately reflect their blood gas concentrations.

Second, pCO$_2$ must be continually monitored during the study. Accurate interpretation of the rCBF values depends on reliable pCO$_2$ measurements. Yet in sick premature infants, $pCO_2$ fluctuates tremendously, and a baseline, steady-state $pCO_2$ value may not be reached or accurately known. In addition, the smaller respiratory tubing used for infants can become plugged with airway secretions. Therefore, it is essential to confirm patency of all tubing and catheters at the beginning of each study.

The small diameter of the infant's head can lead to errors in the measured Xe/CT attenuation (7). This, in turn, can cause errors in the rCBF calculation, which is based on Xe/CT attenuation values. This error in measured attenuation may necessitate a correction of the flow calculations if absolute values of rCBF are to be measured.

Finally, the anatomic distribution of the cerebrovascular bed in the premature infant brain changes as the brain develops. Because of these changes, it can be difficult to interpret rCBF values measured at different times in develpoment. The progressive myelination during postnatal development of the premature infant's brain also will affect flow rates considerably and further complicate interpretation of quantitative measurements.

## CONCLUSIONS

Our experience has shown it possible to modify the GE 9800 Xe/CT system for rCBF measurements in premature sick infants. The potential for clinical and research applications is promising. Nevertheless, there currently remain substantial limitations to its use as a routine clinical tool.

## REFERENCES

1. Hambleton G, Wigglesworth JS. Origin of intraventricular haemorrhage in the preterm infant. *Arch Dis Child* 1976;51:651.
2. Pape KE, Wigglesworth JS. *Haemorrhage, ischaemia, and the perinatal brain*. Philadelphia: JB Lippincott, 1979.
3. Lou HC, Lassen NA, Tweed WA, Johnson G, Jones M, Palahniuk J. Pressure passive cerebral blood flow and breakdown of the blood-brain barrier in experimental fetal asphyxia. *Acta Paediatr Scand* 1979;68:57.
4. Altman DI, Powers WJ, Perlman JM, Herscovitch P, Volpe SL, Volpe JJ. Cerebral blood flow requirements for brain viability in newborn infants is lower than in adults. *Ann Neurol* 1988;24:218–226.
5. Dumpit FM, Brady JP. A simple technique for measuring alveolar $CO_2$ in infants. *J Appl Physiol* 1978;45:648.
6. Strang L. Alveolar gas and anatomical dead-space measurements in normal newborn infants. *Clin Sci* 1961;21:107.
7. Thompson JR, Moore RJ, Hinshaw DB, Hasso AN. Density resolution artifacts encountered when scanning infant heads with x-ray computed tomography (CT). Proceedings of SPIE, The International Society for Optical Engineering, 1982;347:184.
8. Greisen G. Cerebral blood flow in preterm infants during the first week of life. *Acta Paediatr Scand* 1986;75:43–51.
9. Ment LR, Duncan CC, Ehrenkranz RA. Intraventricular hemorrhage in the preterm neonate: timing and cerebral blood flow changes. *J Pediatr* 1984;104:419–425.

*Cerebral Blood Flow Measurement with Stable Xenon-Enhanced Computed Tomography,* edited by Howard Yonas. Raven Press, Ltd., New York © 1992.

# Adequate Rate of Xenon Inhalation in the End-Tidal Gas-Sampling Method

Sadao Suga, Takeshi Kawase, Hideki Koyama, Shigeo Toya, *Hayao Shiga, and **Nobuo Takenaka

*Departments of Neurosurgery and *Diagnostic Radiology, School of Medicine, Keio University, 35 Shinanomachi, Shinjuku-ku, Tokyo 160, Japan; and **Department of Neurosurgery, Ashikaga Red Cross Hospital, 3-2100 Honjou, Ashikaga, Tochigi 326, Japan*

Stable xenon-enhanced computed tomography (Xe/CT) is a useful technique to measure cerebral blood flow (CBF) in patients with clinical evidence of a cerebral lesion (1,2). Calculating the absolute value of CBF with the Xe/CT method requires measurement of the arterial xenon concentration ($Cxe_a$). Rather than sampling arterial blood to obtain this measurement, the less invasive end-tidal gas-sampling (E-T gas) method can be performed (3). In this method, the xenon concentration in end-tidal gas ($Cxe_g$) is substituted for $Cxe_a$ (3). Although studies using radioactive xenon inhalation (3–5) have found a close correspondence between $Cxe_g$ and $Cxe_a$, it is not known if the rate of xenon inhalation influences the relation of these two variables in the E-T gas method. We compared the correlation between $Cxe_a$ and $Cxe_g$ for various rates of xenon gas delivery and evaluated the reliability of the E-T gas method.

## PATIENTS AND METHODS

We conducted our study on 11 patients (three men and eight women) with a mean age of 48 years. Of this group, three patients had cerebral infarctions, three had aneurysmal subarachnoid hemorrhages, three had cerebrovascular anomalies, one had a brain tumor, and one had no intracranial lesion.

We simultaneously performed the E-T gas and the blood-sampling methods. In the E-T gas method, we measured $Cxe_g$ with the newly developed xenon inhalation system (Yufu Seiki, Tokyo) with which the rate of xenon delivery can be controlled. We measured the $Cxe_g$ using the xenon concentration analyzer included in the system and converted it to the increase in Hounsfield units (HU) with the formula for hematocrit correction (6). At the same time, we measured $Cxe_a$ in a modified blood-sampling method. Cannulas were inserted into the patient's brachial artery and vein, and a shunt circuit was introduced through a

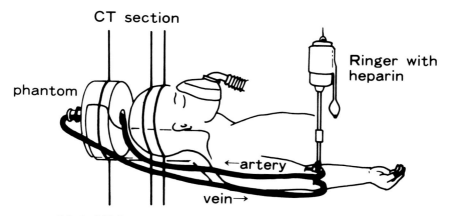

**FIG. 1.** A-V shunt system for use in Xe/CT cerebral blood flow studies.

phantom and placed in the CT gantry (Fig. 1). We called this the "A-V shunt method." In this method, we measured the increase in HU of arterial blood passing through the phantom.

Xenon was delivered to the patients at a rate of 0.6 to 1.2 L/min for 25 minutes during dynamic CT scanning. After scanning, the arterial build-up rate $k$ (arterial $k$), the maximal increase in HU, and the absolute value of hemispheric CBF were calculated for both methods with an on-line program.

## RESULTS

We divided the patients into two groups according to the value of arterial $k$, which represented the inhalation speed of xenon: (a) the slow inhalation group (arterial $k \le 0.2$ in the E-T gas method) and (b) the rapid inhalation group (arterial $k > 0.2$ in the E-T gas method). We then compared the xenon concentration curves obtained with each method. In the slow inhalation group, the curve obtained with the E-T gas method corresponded to that of the A-V shunt method (Fig. 2). In contrast, we found no correlation between the two methods in the rapid inhalation group (Fig. 3).

When we compared the arterial $k$ value calculated by each method, we again found a good correlation in the slow inhalation group (Fig. 4). There was no correlation between arterial $k$ values obtained by each method in the rapid inhalation group (Fig. 5).

The CBF values obtained by each method in the slow inhalation group were in good agreement. In this group, the mean CBF value obtained by the E-T gas method was $95 \pm 10\%$ of those obtained by the A-V shunt method. In the rapid inhalation group, however, the mean CBF value obtained by the E-T gas method was $83.3 \pm 22.5\%$ of those obtained by A-V shunt method.

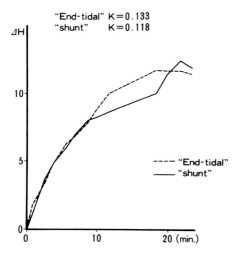

"End-tidal" K=0.133
"shunt"    K=0.118

$\Delta$H

10-

5-

---- "End-tidal"
——— "shunt"

0-

0        10        20 (min.)

FIG. 2. Example of a relatively low arterial k, producing a good correlation between the xenon concentration curves obtained by each method. $\Delta H$ is the increase in Hounsfield units in each method.

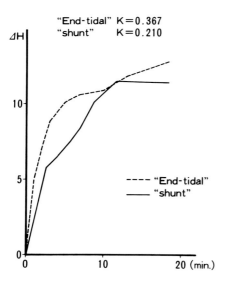

"End-tidal" K=0.367
"shunt"    K=0.210

$\Delta$H

10-

5-

---- "End-tidal"
——— "shunt"

0-

0        10        20 (min.)

FIG. 3. Example of a relatively high arterial k, resulting in a poor correlation between the curves obtained by each method.

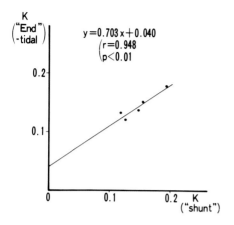

## "End-tidal" K ≤ 0.2

$y = 0.703x + 0.040$
$(r = 0.948$
$(p < 0.01$

**FIG. 4.** In the slow inhalation group, we found good correlation in *k* values obtained by each method.

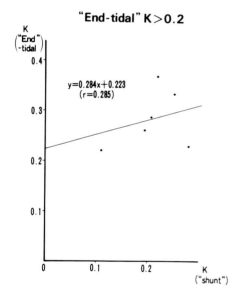

## "End-tidal" K > 0.2

$y = 0.284x + 0.223$
$(r = 0.285)$

**FIG. 5.** No correlation was found in *k* values obtained by each method in the rapid inhalation group.

## DISCUSSION

When arterial $k$ was >0.2 by the E-T gas method, which correlated with the rapid inhalation of xenon, the $k$ values obtained were higher than those with the A-V shunt method, and CBF values were underestimated. However, previous investigators have found a good correlation between $Cxe_g$ and $Cxe_a$ (3–5). This discrepancy may be a result of the difference in dead space in each inhalation system. For example, a mouthpiece was fitted to the patient (3), whereas our patients usually wore a face mask. With a face mask, there is more dead space in the respiratory system, such as the nasal cavity and the space within the mask, than there is with a mouthpiece. We found a close correspondence between the curves for both methods in a tracheostomized patient, who had even less dead space. Therefore, $Cxe_g$ probably was different from $Cxe_a$ in the rapid inhalation group because the sampling gas was a mixture of expiratory gas and inspiratory gas within the dead space. In other words, as xenon gas is rapidly inhaled, expiratory gas and highly concentrated inhaled gas may mix in the dead space if the patient is wearing face mask. As a result, $Cxe_g$ values sampled from a mask may be overestimated compared to $Cxe_a$.

Our findings indicate that xenon should be delivered slowly in the E-T gas method of Xe/CT. Nevertheless, when xenon was inhaled too slowly, we could not always complete the Xe/CT study because of motion artifacts from the gas's anesthetic effect (7). When xenon inhalation became prolonged, excitement commonly occurred when the xenon level remained around 30%. When the $Cxe_g$ was above 40%, patients were calmer for a prolonged period and motionless in a stage of slight anesthesia. In this respect, the inhalation speed should be kept slow with a desired concentration of over 40%. Overall, we found the E-T gas method of Xe/CT CBF monitoring to be a reliable and less invasive technique when xenon is inhaled slowly with an arterial $k < 0.2$.

## REFERENCES

1. Meyer JS, Hayman LA, Amano T, et al. Mapping local blood flow of human brain by CT scanning during stable xenon inhalation. *Stroke* 1981;12:426–436.
2. Okabe T, Meyer JS, Okayasu H, et al. Xenon-enhanced CT CBF measurements in cerebral AVM's before and after resection. *J Neurosurg* 1983;59:21–31.
3. Meyer JS, Hayman LA, Yamamoto M, Sakai F, Nakajima S. Local cerebral blood flow measured by CT after stable xenon inhalation. *AJNR* 1980;1:213–225.
4. Veall N, Mallett BL. Regional cerebral blood flow determination by [133]Xe inhalation and external recording: the effect of arterial recirculation. *Clin Sci* 1966;30:353–369.
5. Obrist WD, Thompson HK Jr, King CH, Wang HS. Determination of regional cerebral blood flow by inhalation of 133-xenon. *Circ Res* 1967;20:124–135.
6. Kelcz F, Sadek KH, Hartwell P, Joseph PM. Computed tomographic measurement of the xenon brain-blood partition coefficient and implications for regional cerebral blood flow: a preliminary report. *Radiology* 1978;127:385–392.
7. Segawa H, Yoshimasu N, Nakamura O, et al. Computed tomographic measurement of regional cerebral blood flow by xenon enhancement. *No To Shinkei* 1982;34:291–297.

*Cerebral Blood Flow Measurement with Stable Xenon-Enhanced Computed Tomography,* edited by Howard Yonas. Raven Press, Ltd., New York © 1992.

# Local Blood-Brain Partition Coefficient (λ) of Xenon Measured in the Normotensive and Hypotensive Brain

Shigeharu Takagi, Yukito Shinohara, Masahiro Yamamoto, Munetaka Haida, Hitoshi Hamano, and Yutaka Kametsu

*Department of Neurology, Tokai University School of Medicine, Bohseidai, Isehara, Kanagawa 259-11, Japan*

One advantage of the stable xenon/computed tomography cerebral blood flow (Xe/CT CBF) method is the ability to measure CBF and the blood-brain partition coefficient (λ) of xenon simultaneously (1). In ischemic or infarcted tissue, low regional λ values have been obtained by the equilibrium method (1–3). Yamamoto et al. (4) reported that the λ value for brain tissue specimens sampled after 24 hours of complete ischemia was 0.8. Because xenon is more lipid-soluble than water-soluble, the λ value for brain tissue cannot be lower than 0.7, the partition coefficient of xenon between blood and water (5). The low λ values (less than 0.7) found in brain tissue in vivo may have resulted from a methodological problem. In a low-flow region such as white matter, equilibrium between blood and brain might not be obtained even after prolonged inhalation of xenon (6).

We conducted a study to establish how accurately the λ values can be measured in a normotensive condition as well as in an induced hypotensive condition in which the CBF might be decreased because the mean arterial blood pressure (MABP) is below the range of cerebrovascular autoregulation. We also wanted to determine whether the λ values during arterial hypotension differ from those in normotension.

## MATERIALS AND METHODS

In seven macacas of either sex, weighing 5 to 8 kg, anesthesia was induced with intramuscular injections of ketamine hydrochloride and maintained with intraperitoneal administration of chloralose-urethan. Respiration was controlled by a respirator (Harvard Model 607E) after the subjects were immobilized with an intravenous injection of alcuronium dichloride. An extracorporeal circuit

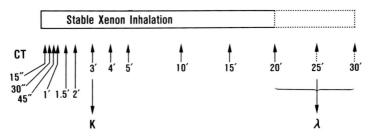

**FIG. 1.** Schedule of stable xenon inhalation and computed tomographic scanning. Xenon was inhaled for 20 to 30 minutes; arrows indicate times at which scans were obtained.

was made from the axillary artery to the femoral vein, and the shunt tubing was placed in the subcutaneous tissue around the skull.

After undergoing baseline CT brain scanning with a Toshiba TCT-80A scanner, the subjects inhaled 39% xenon in oxygen for 20 to 30 minutes. As shown in Fig. 1, we measured time-concentration curves of xenon in the brain and arterial blood by scanning the brain and the extracorporeal circuit simultaneously, every 15 seconds for the first minute, every minute for the next 4 minutes, and every 5 minutes during the rest of the inhalation period. Local λ values were calculated by the equilibrium method from data obtained at least 15 minutes into the inhalation period. Local $k$ values, related to CBF by the expression CBF = $k$ · λ, were calculated by the autoradiographic strategy from the image taken 3 minutes after the start of xenon inhalation, using an NEC PC9801 F personal computer. The same procedures were repeated during hypotension induced by exsanguination or by the administration of trimethaphan camsylate.

We then studied the CBF in defined regions of interest (ROI) measuring 2.1 mm by 2.1 mm in 5-mm-thick CT slices. ROIs were placed at the frontal cortex, thalamus, corpus callosum, and internal capsule. The mean values for the enhancement of each ROI were translated into CBF and λ values.

## RESULTS

### Local λ and $k$ Values in Normotensive and Hypotensive Conditions

Table 1 shows the λ values measured 20 minutes after the start of inhalation and $k$ values from the various regions under normotension and hypotension. The MABP decreased from 113 ± 19 mm Hg (mean ± SD) in normotension to 43 ± 4 mm Hg in the hypotensive condition. The mean λ value in the frontal cortex decreased significantly, from 0.93 to 0.82 ($P < 0.05$). In the thalamus, corpus callosum, and internal capsule, mean λ values decreased slightly, but these differences did not reach statistical significance. The $k$ values decreased

**TABLE 1.** *Local λ and k values in normotensive and hypotensive states*

| | λ at 20 min | | $k$ (min$^{-1}$) | |
|---|---|---|---|---|
| | Normotensive | Hypotensive | Normotensive | Hypotensive |
| Frontal cortex | 0.93 ± 0.07* | 0.82 ± 0.11* | 0.53 ± 0.26 | 0.43 ± 0.13 |
| Thalamus | 1.07 ± 0.14 | 1.05 ± 0.14 | 0.46 ± 0.23 | 0.50 ± 0.27 |
| Corpus callosum | 0.92 ± 0.17 | 0.89 ± 0.15 | 0.22 ± 0.17 | 0.17 ± 0.12 |
| Internal capsule | 1.07 ± 0.12 | 0.96 ± 0.14 | 0.14 ± 0.06 | 0.09 ± 0.08 |

* Statistically significant difference ($P < 0.05$)

slightly with decreasing MABP in all regions studied except the thalamus. Again, these changes were not statistically significant.

## Calculated λ Values at Different Times

Figure 2A shows the local λ values under normotension as measured from the CT images taken 15 and 20 minutes after the start of inhalation. Although the λ values rose slightly in the gray matter such as, thalamus, and frontal cortex, increases were much larger in the internal capsule and corpus callosum. This finding indicates that, in the low-flow areas, equilibrium between the blood and brain is not obtained within 20 minutes after the start of xenon inhalation.

In the hypotensive state with the MABP below the floor of autoregulation, CBF also should be below the normal values. In five animals, we extended the duration of xenon inhalation to 30 minutes. Figure 2B shows the measured local λ values in four regions. These values increased along with the time of xenon inhalation in the white matter, where blood flow was very low. By 30 minutes

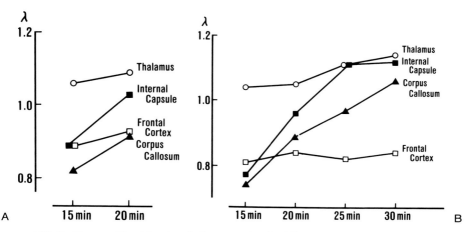

**FIG. 2.** Measured local λ values in the normotensive (A) and hypotensive (B) states.

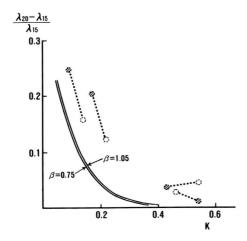

**FIG. 3.** Actual and simulated rates of increase in the local λ values. The percentage change in the λ values is plotted against the k values. Open-dotted circles and hatched circles indicate the rates of increase in the measured λ values under normotension and hypotension, respectively. Solid curve shows the simulated rate of increase against the k values.

of inhalation under induced hypotension, λ values were no longer lower than under normotension, except in the frontal area.

### Rate of Increase in Measured λ Values

The vertical axis in Fig. 3 indicates the rate of increase in measured λ between 15 and 20 minutes after inhalation began. The horizontal axis shows the k value in each region. In the regions with low CBF, the rate of increase in measured λ values was high, indicating that equilibrium was not reached in the low-flow regions. The solid curve shows the expected or theoretical rate of increase in λ between 15 and 20 minutes, calculated by a simulation study. Beta values indicate the growth rate of the arterial curve: $Ca(t)$ = constant $(1 - e^{-\beta t})$. They did not seem to influence the simulated curve. The actual (observed) rate of increase was far higher than the simulated curve (expected rate of increase).

### DISCUSSION

In low-flow areas such as the white matter, our study indicated that equilibrium between the blood and the brain is not reached before 20 minutes of xenon inhalation under normotension or before 30 minutes under hypotension. Thus, the λ values cannot be measured accurately unless inhalation is adequately extended.

The rate of increase in λ values with increasing inhalation time was greater than expected. Possible explanations for this finding include the following: (a) An ROI included more than one compartment, and the "slow" compartment was not equilibrated; (b) the CBF was reduced by the xenon itself; or (c) a high concentration of xenon does not obey the tracer theory. Further experiments are necessary to resolve this problem.

Our results showed that λ values did not change during induced hypotension in the thalamus, corpus callosum, and internal capsule, whereas they decreased in the frontal cortex. Because the wash-in of xenon into the brain was slower than expected, local λ values may not be measured accurately before 20 minutes of continual inhalation or, in the low-flow regions, before 30 minutes.

## REFERENCES

1. Meyer JS, Hayman LA, Nakajima S, Amano T, Lauzon P. Local cerebral blood flow and tissue solubility measured by stable, xenon-enhanced computerized tomography. *Adv Neurol* 1981;30: 73–84.
2. Meyer JS, Hayman LA, Amano T, et al. Mapping local blood flow of human brain by CT scanning during stable xenon inhalation. *Stroke* 1981;12:426–436.
3. Kitagawa Y, Meyer JS, Tachibana H, Mortel KF, Rogers RL. CT-CBF correlations of cognitive deficits in multi-infarct dementia. *Stroke* 1984;15:1000–1009.
4. Yamamoto M, Haida M, Takagi S, et al. The changes in partition coefficient of xenon gas of rat cerebral tissue (λ) after circulatory arrest measured in vitro. *J Cereb Blood Flow Metab* 1987;7(Suppl 1):S568.
5. Kelcz F, Hilal SK, Hartwell P, Joseph PM. Computed tomographic measurement of the xenon brain-blood partition coefficient and implications for regional cerebral blood flow: a preliminary report. *Radiology* 1978;127:385–392.
6. Dhawan V, Haughton VM, Thaler HT, Lu HC, Rottenberg DA. Accuracy of stable xenon/CT measurements of regional cerebral blood flow: effect of extrapolated estimates of brain-blood partition coefficients. *J Comput Assist Tomogr* 1984;8:208–212.

*Cerebral Blood Flow Measurement with Stable Xenon-Enhanced Computed Tomography,* edited by Howard Yonas. Raven Press, Ltd., New York © 1992.

# Dual Concentration Method for Measuring the Local Partition Coefficient

Ryoichi Toshima, Keizo Toyohara, Toshihiro Ebisawa, Sadatomo Shimojo, and Osamu Sakai

*The Second Department of Medicine, Jikei University School of Medicine, 3-25-8 Nishishinbashi, Minato-ku, Tokyo 105, Japan*

The xenon-enhanced computed tomography (Xe/CT) method has the distinctive advantage of simultaneously measuring both local cerebral blood flow (LCBF) and the local partition coefficient value (Lλ). The Lλ value, which decreases with tissue damage or edema, provides important information about cerebral ischemia. Accurate measurement of Lλ, however, requires a long period of xenon inhalation, especially in low-flow tissue such as white matter and ischemic lesions. The resulting anesthetic effect and the cost of massive xenon consumption thus have been the major factors limiting clinical application of Xe/CT studies. To overcome these problems, we devised the dual concentration Xe/CT method.

## METHODS

We used the dual concentration method to obtain Lλ and LCBF values in five normal subjects. Studies were performed with the Siemens Somatom SF x-ray CT scanner (256 × 256 pixels, 10-second scan). After a baseline scan, each subject inhaled a mixture of 50% xenon balanced with oxygen for 2 minutes. Then another CT scan was performed. Immediately thereafter, the gas was switched to a mixture with 25% xenon, and inhalation continued for 6 minutes. Additional CT images were obtained at the end of this period of inhalation. We monitored the xenon concentration in expiratory gas using the thermal conductivity method and converted these data to CT values (Hounsfield units) for arterial xenon enhancement with a correction for the hematocrit.

Kety's equation was used to calculate Lλ and LCBF values (1). Arterial build-up and xenon wash-out were assumed to follow a mono-exponential curve, both having the same rate constant value. We performed simulation studies to verify the effect of this method and to compare it with the conventional method, which was assumed to use continuous inhalation of 35% xenon and the same inhalation period.

We transferred the CT images to the image-processing system and calculated the Lλ and LCBF values for every pixel. A filtering process of 4 × 4 pixels square smoothing was applied to CT images for noise cancellation. Consequently, the Lλ and LCBF maps were derived and displayed on a monitor. We then chose the regions of interest and obtained the mean and standard deviation (SD) of these values.

## RESULTS

Figure 1 shows the xenon-enhancement simulation curves for both this method and the conventional one. The gray-matter enhancement immediately followed the arterial curve, and full saturation was reached at the end of the study in both methods. In contrast, the enhancement in the white matter was markedly delayed. In the conventional method, the enhancement of white matter slowly increased, then ceased abruptly at the end of the study. In the dual concentration method, the white-matter enhancement rapidly increased during initial inhalation of 50% xenon, finally nearing the level of saturation at the end of the study.

Using the dual concentration method with our five subjects, we obtained the following values for mean (and SD) Lλ and LCBF (in ml/100 g/min), respectively:

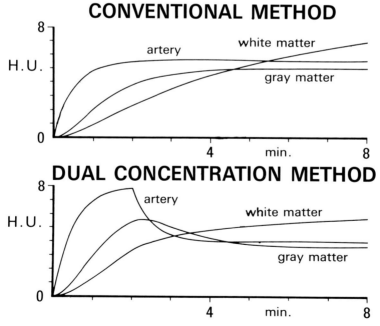

**FIG. 1.** Comparison of the simulation curves for xenon enhancement in the dual concentration and conventional methods. H.U., Hounsfield units.

0.76 (0.10) and 92.2 (11.9) in the frontal cortex, 0.78 (0.08) and 95.9 (8.4) in the temporal cortex, 0.77 (0.11) and 90.7 (11.7) in the occipital cortex, 0.86 (0.06) and 100.2 (13.1) in the caudate nucleus, 1.07 (0.12) and 101.0 (8.9) in the thalamus, and 1.59 (0.09) and 23.6 (2.0) in the cerebral white matter. In all subjects, the anesthetic effects of the studies were found to be minimal.

## DISCUSSION

It is well known that a high concentration of xenon has an anesthetic effect. Previous investigations have detected anesthetic effects when concentrations of more than 50% xenon were administered for longer than 3 minutes (2). It has been documented that inhalation of 35% xenon for more than 5 minutes causes agitation or sedation (3). Moreover, a study in baboons found that 4-minute inhalation of 35% xenon caused a significant increase in CBF (4). Xenon-induced changes in CBF would impair the important assumption in any flow study using diffusible inert gas, namely, that a steady state is maintained.

Because blood flow is calculated as the product of λ and the rate constant, the Lλ value plays an important role in obtaining the correct LCBF value. But reliable measurement of the Lλ value requires a long period of xenon inhalation. Although measurement of Lλ in gray matter requires a minimum of 4 minutes' inhalation, at least 15 minutes is necessary in white matter, even if curve fitting and extrapolation are applied, because it takes about 30 minutes for xenon to saturate white matter (5). Even longer inhalation is needed for xenon saturation in an infarct or edematous tissue, which has low build-up rate constant values.

To measure Lλ reliably in a clinical setting, we developed the dual concentration method, which enabled the xenon concentration to attain near saturation in less time. Thus, even in white matter, Lλ values could be obtained with a relatively short period of xenon inhalation. Moreover, because inhalation of high-concentration xenon was limited to 2 minutes, the anesthetic effect was minimized and gas was conserved. We conclude that the dual concentration Xe/CT method makes it feasible to measure local partition coefficients and correct LCBF values for clinical applications.

## REFERENCES

1. Kety SS. Measurement of local blood flow by the exchange of an inert, diffusible substance. *Methods Med Res* 1960;8:228-236.
2. Meyer JS, Hayman LA, Yamamoto M, Sakai F, Nakajima S. Local cerebral blood flow measured by CT after stable xenon inhalation. *AJNR* 1980;1:213-225.
3. Gur D, Wolfson SK, Yonas H, et al. Progress in cerebrovascular disease: local cerebral blood flow by xenon enhanced CT. *Stroke* 1982;13:750-758.
4. Hartmann A, Wassman H, Czernicki Z, Dettmers C, Schumacher HW, Tsuda Y. Effect of stable xenon in room air on regional cerebral blood flow and electroencephalogram in normal baboons. *Stroke* 1987;18:643-648.
5. Dhawan V, Haughton VM, Thaler HT, Lu HC, Rottenberg DA. Accuracy of stable xenon/CT measurements of regional cerebral blood flow: effect of extrapolated estimates of brain-blood partition coefficients. *J Comput Assist Tomogr* 1984;8:208-212.

Cerebral Blood Flow Measurement with Stable
Xenon-Enhanced Computed Tomography,
edited by Howard Yonas. Raven Press, Ltd.,
New York © 1992.

# A Method to Identify Blood Vessels for Generating Corrected Cerebral Blood Flow Maps

Abund O. Wist, Panos P. Fatouros, and Stafford J. Cothran

*Department of Radiology, Medical College of Virginia, Virginia Commonwealth University, Box 72, MCV Station, Richmond, Virginia 23298*

In the stable xenon/computed tomography (Xe/CT) method, the blood flow in brain tissue is measured by adding xenon to breathing gas and calculating the blood flow from the observed increase in Hounsfield units (HU), using the Kety equation. As the surrounding arteries supply the xenon-infiltrated tissue, they also show an increase in HU. Indeed, these vessels have much higher HU values, both because the arterial flow is much higher than flow in surrounding tissue and because the xenon concentration in the vessel increases much faster. In a flow map, these vascular flows thus appear as spikes (1).

In current Xe/CT blood-flow-monitoring techniques, averaging is used to "smooth" noise and artifacts from the CT scanner and the tissues. But smoothing routines also remove the sharp spikes that represent vessel flows in the flow map. In addition, smoothing artificially increases the blood flow values in the tissues surrounding a vessel, the increase being especially large around the larger arteries. This effect is an important consideration in the investigation of certain pathologic brain conditions such as ischemia.

## METHOD

Because blood flow is known to be much higher in the cerebral vessels than in surrounding tissues, flow values can be used to differentiate between tissue and vessels. We developed additional algorithms to measure the arterial diameter or flow velocity (2).

### Differentiation of Vessels from Tissues

We first calculated the flow values from the original enhanced HU levels. To distinguish tissue from vessels, we then set the threshold flow at three times the average flow in the CT slice. The average flow included the total white-matter and gray-matter flow as well as the vascular flow. The vascular flow in the CT slice should be, on average, of the same magnitude as the combined gray- and white-matter flow. Therefore, even very high gray-matter flows always should be below this threshold. Furthermore, if a vessel stays within a voxel as determined by the pixel area and the thickness of the CT slice, then flow determination is not influenced by the angle at which the vessel intersects the slice. When the angle is large and the vessels bisect the voxel, the determined flow value is decreased by the reduced volume the vessel occupies in the voxel.

Noise or artifacts in the CT image will not produce any flow values; they are not enhanced by xenon and, consequently, no flow can be calculated from them. An exception would occur only if the noise or artifact mimicked xenon enhancement in the successive CT images. This would be a rare event, and flow values generated in this way probably would be similar to the surrounding tissue flow. Therefore, it is extremely unlikely that any noise or artifact in the CT image would be mistakenly calculated as vascular flow.

By combining all vessel locations, a map can be generated (Fig. 1). Because of the numerous vessels in a brain, only those occupying four or more pixels (1 mm or larger) are shown. To better depict the location of the vessels, the flow map is overlaid on the corresponding baseline image.

### Correction of Tissue Flow Map

The tissue-flow map can be corrected by removing all values for the vessel flows and replacing them with those of the surrounding tissue. The corrected flow map is much smoother and less spotty than our standard tissue-flow map. Moreover, the corrected map provides accurate flow values for tissue near large arteries and in low-flow areas.

### Diameter of Vessels

The diameter of all vessels occupying at least four pixels can be calculated from their cross section in the vessel map. If a vessel is smaller than a pixel, diameter can be determined from its saturation value. Measurements show that saturation values are equal for all vessels that completely occupy a pixel. Therefore, if the saturation value of a pixel containing a vessel is lower than the highest saturation value, then the vessel must be smaller than the area of the pixel. The actual area of the vessel then can be estimated from the linear relationship between the vessel area and the difference between the saturation value of the pixel and that of the surrounding tissue. Vessels that are located only partly in a given pixel can be handled in the same way.

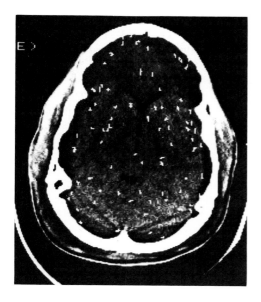

**FIG. 1.** A vessel map overlaid on a baseline CT image.

## Velocity Determination

Once the area or diameter of the vessel has been determined, the average velocity in the vessel can be obtained simply by dividing the flow value by the area. The flow distribution in large vessels can be estimated from the different flow values of the pixels occupied by the vessels.

## Configuration of Vessels

To determine the configuration of vessels and their position in the CT image, we selected small sections of the flow maps and then recorded the saturation and flow value of each pixel in these sections. Again, because the flow and saturation values are much higher in the vessel than in the surrounding tissue, the configuration of the vessel can be found by following the higher numbers, making sure that a flow value is constant along each vessel.

## RESULTS

Using these methods, we calculated the location, configuration, diameters, and velocities of vessels in several patients and animals (Figs. 2–4). Table 1 compares the results in the patient and in the animal depicted in the figures. The pathologically decreased flow values and velocities in the comatose patient

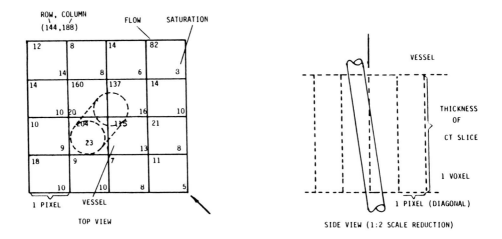

VESSEL #91 IN CT SLICE OF PATIENT #2

**FIG. 2.** A vessel from a comatose patient crosses the CT image at only a slight angle, occupying about three-quarters of a pixel.

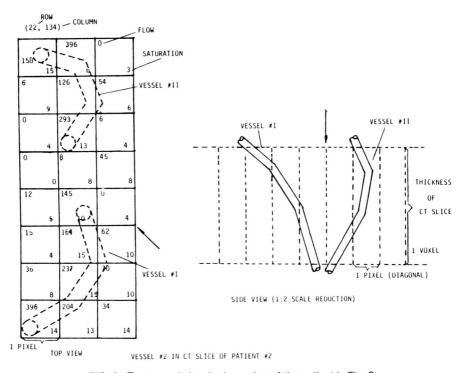

VESSEL #2 IN CT SLICE OF PATIENT #2

**FIG. 3.** Two vessels in a brain section of the patient in Fig. 2.

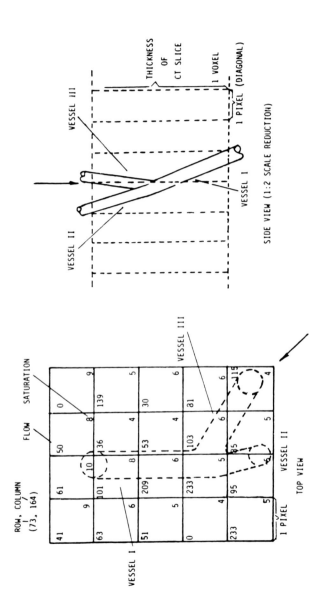

**FIG. 4.** A branching vessel from an animal brain. Note how the two branched vessels are appropriately smaller than the parent vessel.

**TABLE 1.** *Vessel parameters for patient #2 and animal #8*

| No. of local flow map | Coordinates of local flow map[a] | Vessel # in local flow map | Baseline enhanced HU[b] | Flow[c] (ml/100 g/min) | Slope[c] | Saturation enhanced HU[c] | Cross section[d] (mm$^2$) | Velocity[d] (cm/sec) |
|---|---|---|---|---|---|---|---|---|
| *Patient #2* | | | | | | | | |
| 2 | 22/134 | I | 30 | 396 | 7.8 | 13 | 0.09 | 2.8 |
|   |        | II | 40 | 396 | 6.9 | 13 | 0.09 | 2.8 |
| 4 | 25/148 | I | 26 | 3836 | 7.7 | 15 | 0.07 | 8.8 |
| 91 | 144/188 | I | 33 | 616 | 14.0 | 18 | 0.5 | 0.05 |
| 128 | 193/159 | I | 36 | 163 | 8.0 | 16 | 0.07 | 1.0 |
|   |        | II | 41 | 224 | 9.0 | 16 | 0.1 | 0.9 |
|   |        | III | 36 | 366 | 13.0 | 20 | 0.5 | |
| *Animal #8* | | | | | | | | |
| 27 | 73/164 | I | 36 | 262 | 0.5 | 8 | 0.2 | 0.2 |
|   |        | II | 33 | 170 | 1.4 | 5 | 0.2 | 0.10 |
|   |        | III | 34 | 103 | 2.6 | 5 | 0.2 | 0.08 |
| 54 | 102/159 | I | 41 | 521 | 1.7 | 8 | 1.0 | 1.0 |
| 83 | 120/143 | I | 38 | 736 | 1.5 | 10 | 0.9 | 0.5 |
|   |        | II | 40 | 507 | 1.1 | 11 | 0.6 | 0.4 |
|   |        | III | 41 | 262 | 1.0 | 10 | 0.3 | 0.8 |

[a] Row/column (see Figs. 2–4), [b]measured, [c]calculated, [d]estimated.

were higher than those in the normal but anesthetized animal. The diameter of the vessels, on the other hand, appeared to be larger in the animal than in the patient.

## CONCLUSIONS

Our investigation shows that the flow, location, configuration, and diameter of the vessels in the brain can be determined, even if the vessels are smaller than a pixel. These determinations can be used to correct the tissue flow and λ maps, making them more accurate, especially near large arteries. Knowledge of the blood flow in the different vessels also can give the physician additional information on the supply of blood to other areas in the brain. Furthermore, because this technique noninvasively measures the concentration of xenon in the arteries of the brain, it can be used to confirm the calculated values of xenon concentration obtained from exhaled air.

## REFERENCES

1. Wist AO, Cothran SJ, Fatouros PP, et al. An investigation to measure the blood vessel flow in the brain by the stable xenon/CT method. *Modeling and Simulation* 1988;19:1729–1733.
2. Wist AO, Cothran SJ, Fatouros PP, et al. An investigation to measure velocity, flow, and pressure in vessels in the brain using the stable xenon/CT method. *Modeling and Simulation* 1989;20: 1743–1748.

*Cerebral Blood Flow Measurement with Stable Xenon-Enhanced Computed Tomography,* edited by Howard Yonas. Raven Press, Ltd., New York © 1992.

# Discussion

Participants:
Dr. Joseph Darby (Pittsburgh, Pennsylvania, USA)
Dr. Abund O. Wist (Richmond, Virginia, USA)
Dr. Anthony Marmarou (Richmond, Virginia, USA)
Dr. David Gur (Pittsburgh, Pennsylvania, USA)
Dr. Willi Kalender (Erlangen, Germany)
Dr. Panos P. Fatouros (Richmond, Virginia, USA)
Dr. Neils Lassen (Copenhagen, Denmark)
Dr. Walter Good (Pittsburgh, Pennsylvania, USA)
Dr. Walter Lindstrom (Cleveland, Ohio, USA)

In the discussion that followed the first group of presentations, Dr. Darby expressed concern about a system proposed by Dr. Wist that automatically would add $CO_2$ to maintain end-tidal $pCO_2$ values. Dr. Darby noted that end-tidal $CO_2$ values fall during nearly all Xe/CT studies in patients and in animals during fixed volume ventilation. Yet in his experience, arterial $CO_2$ levels do not fall so consistently; therefore, "correcting" for an end-tidal $CO_2$ decrease could lead to falsely high arterial $CO_2$ values. Dr. Wist responded that the decrease in arterial gas levels normally does parallel the drop in end-tidal values and that the system he and his colleagues have developed to measure and correct $CO_2$ every 0.1 seconds could maintain stable end-tidal $pCO_2$ and $PaCO_2$ levels.

(Editor's note: Although end-tidal values in healthy persons may correlate well with arterial values at slow respiration rates, end-tidal sampling becomes progressively less representative of true arterial values with more rapid respiratory rates, lung disorders, or impaired diffusion.)

In reflecting back over several presentations, Dr. Marmarou observed that Xe/CT-derived high-flow values tend to vary more than do CBF values obtained with either microspheres or $^{133}$Xe. He questioned whether this was a methodological problem. In responding, Dr. Gur said that fast flow was less accurately measured with Xe/CT because the abrupt rise in CT enhancement that occurs with fast flow is poorly characterized by the relatively few and widely spaced CT images that can be acquired with current technology. Thus, the rate constant ($k$) would be obtained with less reliability than with those other methods.

Dr. Kalender commented that the arterial curve would best be characterized mathematically by the use of the actual data points, rather than by forcing the data to fit a mono- or multi-exponential variable. Dr. Fatouros agreed that the end-tidal curve is a complex function often requiring multiple exponentials for mathematic characterization. Dr. Gur, however, responded that the use of a single, weighted exponential, though not an ideal approach, can in fact characterize normal physiology nicely. He also noted that this method had been incorporated within the GE system with a high level of technical success.

Dr. Lassen then proposed that a simplified approach to the partition coefficient ($\lambda$) would achieve a far less "noisy" image with less statistical error than possible in trying to measure $\lambda$. He recommended either assigning a "book value" for $\lambda$ or using the CT image to characterize gray- and white-matter regions and then applying compartment-specific $\lambda$ values to calculate CBF. He also cautioned that because the solubility of xenon in tissue varies only between 0.4 and 1.5, CBF values calculated without restraining possible $\lambda$ to these limits would create significant errors in CBF measurements. Dr. Gur responded that calculating CBF without considering $\lambda$ causes a significant error in flow values in tissues altered by disease, and Dr. Good pointed out that although errors in $k$ and $\lambda$ occur independently, they tend to occur in opposite directions. Thus, the calculated flow volume, which is a product of $\lambda$ and $k$, remains very stable. Dr. Lindstrom added that physiologically reasonable $\lambda$ values can be obtained consistently in normal tissue from a 6-minute study. In fact, he had found abnormal $\lambda$ values useful in identifying pathological regions. He cautioned that to forgo the unique ability of Xe/CT to derive $\lambda$ values would be like "throwing out the baby with the bath water."

*Cerebral Blood Flow Measurement with Stable Xenon-Enhanced Computed Tomography,* edited by Howard Yonas. Raven Press, Ltd., New York © 1992.

# Simplified Method for Mapping Local Cerebral Blood Flow

Jun Karasawa, Hajime Touho, and Hisashi Shishido

*Department of Neurosurgery, Osaka Neurological Institute, 2-6-23 Shonai-Takara-machi, Toyonaka, Osaka 561, Japan*

The measurement of cerebral blood flow has important applications in the management of ischemic cerebrovascular diseases and head injuries (1–4). Positron emission tomography undoubtedly provides superior information about cerebral blood flow and metabolism and has been used clinically, but is not readily available (5). On the other hand, computerized tomography (CT) and stable xenon inhalation provide optimal resolution and correct estimates of both local $\lambda$ (L$\lambda$) and local cerebral blood flow (LCBF) values, even in disease states (6–9a).

We previously calculated the arterial build-up range and build-up rate constant with serial sampling of arterial blood. That method, however, is thought to be too invasive (4). We designed the present investigation to evaluate the theoretic and clinical aspects of our new and simple method of measuring LCBF. This method uses the inhalation of low-concentration stable xenon and curve-fitting analysis with continuous monitoring of the end-tidal xenon concentration.

## SUBJECTS AND METHODS

We measured the LCBF in ten control subjects aged 22 to 57 years (mean: 31.6 ± 4.8 years) with minor head trauma in the chronic stage. We also studied 82 experimental patients aged 28 to 82 years (mean: 61.8 ± 11.8 years) with cerebral infarction in the acute ($n = 9$) or chronic stage ($n = 73$); 72 were inpatients at the time of their studies. The cerebral ischemic lesions in these 82 subjects included 78 supratentorial infarctions and 4 infratentorial.

Throughout the LCBF studies, we continually monitored the electrocardiogram, spontaneous carbon dioxide concentration, and spontaneous xenon concentration in both inspiratory and expiratory phases. The xenon concentration was measured with a thermoconductivity gas analyzer.

To decrease the total volume of xenon, we used a cold gas delivery system (AZ-733, Anzai Sogyo, Tokyo). A mixture of oxygen and 30% xenon was prepared beforehand in a spirometer. Patients first inhaled pure oxygen for about 15 minutes, then the gas mixture in the closed respiratory circuit. The xenon level was maintained automatically. We used a CT scanner with a $512 \times 512$ matrix and 10-mm collimation (Quantex RX, Yokogawa Medical Systems, Ltd. Tokyo). Exposure factors included a 3-second scanning time, 120 kVp, and 130 mA, which are thought to minimize the standard deviation (SD) for the scanner data. Although a smoothing process reduces the resolution of the CBF image, we performed preanalysis smoothing routines ($11 \times 11$ pixels) to reduce the pixel-to-pixel variation resulting from our low xenon concentration and an inhalation time as short as 4 minutes.

During wash-in and wash-out periods, we obtained ten serial CT scans, one every 20 seconds for each scan level. We selected two levels for CBF analysis. End-tidal xenon concentrations were continually monitored and recorded, and the arterial build-up rate constant and build-up range were calculated on line according to the following formula (4):

$$ha(t) = Aa[e^{-Ka(t-\tau)} - e^{-Kat}] \qquad [1]$$

$$hi(t) = Ai[g(t - \tau) - g(t)] \qquad [2]$$

where $[e^{-Kit} + Ki(e^{-Kit} - e^{-Kat})/(Ka - Ki)]$ is replaced by $g(t)$. In this formula, $Ai = \lambda i \cdot Aa$, $\tau = t$ for $0 < t < T$, and $\tau = T$ for $t > T$; $ha(t)$ and $hi(t)$ represent the increase in Hounsfield units (HU) in arteries and cerebral tissue, respectively, for xenon. $Ka$ and $Ki$ are the respective build-up rate constants for arteries and cerebral tissue, and $Aa$ and $Ai$ are the corresponding build-up ranges. $\lambda i$ is defined as the partition coefficient for brain tissue. $T$ is the duration of xenon inhalation. Note that, $ha(t)$ shows a linear exponential increase and decrease, and $hi(t)$ shows a bi-exponential increase and decrease.

$Aa$, $Ka$, $Ai$, and $Ki$ were calculated from the time-dependent xenon concentrations in arterial blood and cerebral tissue of interest by applying the least-squares method to equations 1 and 2. Thus,

$$Ea = [ha(Tm) - Aa(e^{-Ka(Tm-\tau)} - e^{-Katm})]^2 \qquad [3]$$

$$Ei = \{hi(Tm) - Ai[g(Tm - \tau) - g(Tm)]\}^2 \qquad [4]$$

where $ha(Tm)$ and $hi(Tm)$ are measured values, and $Aa(e^{-Ka(Tm-\tau)} - e^{KaTm})$ and $Ai [g(Tm - \tau) - g(Tm)]$ are calculated values fitted by equations 1 and 2. Tm is scanning time (m = $1 \sim 6$). The values of $\lambda i(Ai/Aa)$ and $Ki$ can be calculated as both $Ea$ and $Ei$ become minimum with the least-squares method. Finally, $fi = 100 \cdot \lambda i \cdot Ki$ (ml/100 g/min), where $fi$ is LCBF.

## RESULTS

Table 1 shows the LCBF and local partition coefficients ($\lambda$ values) for selected regions of interest in the control group. The $\lambda$ values for the gray matter and deep nucleus ranged from 0.76 to 0.98, whereas those for the white matter were

**TABLE 1.** *Normal local partition coefficient (Lλ) and local cerebral blood flow (LCBF) values in the control subjects*

| Region of interest | Side | Mean LCBF (SD) (ml/100 g/min) | Mean Lλ (SD) |
|---|---|---|---|
| Frontal gray matter | R | 61.2 (3.1) | 0.81 (0.08) |
| | L | 62.6 (3.4) | 0.80 (0.07) |
| Frontal white matter | R | 32.4 (2.0) | 1.20 (0.11) |
| | L | 33.1 (1.9) | 1.28 (0.15) |
| Caudate nucleus | R | 78.2 (4.0) | 0.82 (0.08) |
| | L | 77.6 (3.8) | 0.81 (0.07) |
| Lentiform nucleus | R | 68.9 (3.6) | 0.78 (0.10) |
| | L | 67.2 (3.2) | 0.76 (0.11) |
| Internal capsule | R | 31.0 (2.2) | 1.26 (0.10) |
| | L | 33.1 (2.4) | 1.29 (0.09) |
| Thalamus | R | 83.6 (3.9) | 0.98 (0.10) |
| | L | 81.4 (3.7) | 0.94 (0.08) |
| Occipital gray matter | R | 62.4 (2.8) | 0.83 (0.10) |
| | L | 61.8 (2.6) | 0.82 (0.08) |
| Pons | R | 31.6 (1.8) | 1.26 (0.10) |
| | L | 30.8 (2.1) | 1.24 (0.11) |
| Brachium pontis | R | 31.9 (2.4) | 1.28 (0.10) |
| | L | 32.1 (2.0) | 1.27 (0.09) |
| Cerebellar cortex | R | 50.8 (2.8) | 0.83 (0.07) |
| | L | 51.2 (3.0) | 0.82 (0.07) |

R, right; L, left; SD, standard deviation.

more than 1.0. The corresponding values for LCBF were 61.8 to 80.4 ml/100 g/min and 28.6 to 34.0 ml/100 g/min. In the cerebellar cortex, LCBF was about 10 ml/100 g/min lower than in the cerebral gray matter. In the brainstem and cerebellar peduncle, LCBF values were nearly equivalent to those in the supratentorial white matter. In the control group, the SD of the gray and white matter averages ranged from 2.6 to 3.4 and from 1.9 to 2.4, respectively. An increase or decrease in LCBF of 10% or more was considered significant in this study.

## Illustrative Cases

Case 1: A 28-year-old man sustained a cerebral concussion but was alert and free of neurologic deficits. A CT scan revealed no abnormalities (Fig. 1). His LCBF, measured 28 days after the accident, was higher in the gray matter than in the white matter or the internal capsule. The local λ of the gray matter was lower than that of the white matter or the internal capsule.

Case 2: A 34-year-old man with a cerebral concussion was admitted to our hospital. He was well oriented and had no neurologic deficits. A Xe/CT CBF study of the posterior circulation was performed 1 month after the accident (Fig. 2). The maps demonstrated that λ was higher, and LCBF lower, in the internal capsule, brainstem, cerebellar peduncle, and cerebellar white matter than in the

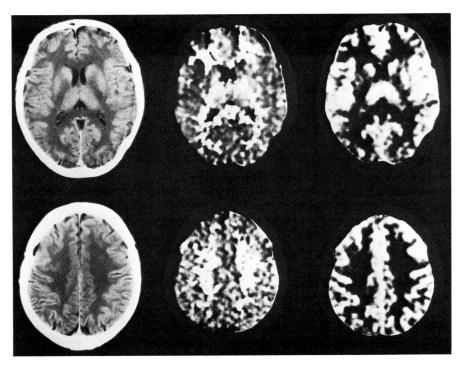

**FIG. 1.** Plain CT (*left*), λ maps (*middle*), and cerebral blood flow maps (*right*) in a 28-year-old man (control).

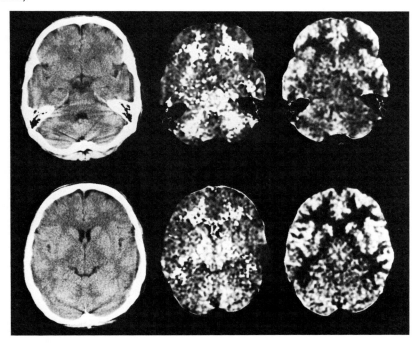

**FIG. 2.** Plain CT (*left*), λ maps (*center*), and cerebral blood flow maps (*right*) in a 34-year-old man with cerebral concussion in the chronic stage. The λ and CBF maps of the posterior circulation are normal.

cerebellar cortex. The LCBF in the cerebellar cortex was slightly lower than in the cerebral cortex.

## DISCUSSION

Several attributes make the Xe/CT CBF method a valuable and accurate technique for measuring LCBF. Its local blood flow images provide optimal resolution and are correlated with the anatomical structures on plain CT images. Also, the flow information derived from these maps corresponded to the neurologic conditions of our patients. Moreover, other than the exposure of a limited brain volume to repeated CT scanning, the method is safe.

Stable xenon has been used successfully as a contrast agent during CT scanning of the brain, and its anesthetic pharmacology and clinical safety have been studied extensively (10–14). Prolonged inhalation of high concentrations has anesthetic effects and can be used for light surgical anesthesia. These anesthetic effects can be minimized if lower concentrations are inhaled for briefer intervals. After inhalation, stable xenon is freely diffusible through all tissues, particularly cerebral tissue, because of its high lipid solubility (15). Using 30% xenon, inhaled as reported by Yonas et al. (16), we had no significant difficulties in measuring LCBF.

Our study employed a method for the three-dimensional measurement of LCBF and Lλ with xenon-enhanced CT. The λ value can be calculated with a double integration method, which takes about 15–20 minutes. In contrast, the saturation method requires more than 20 minutes to calculate λ. The build-up rate constant is calculated with the autoradiographic method or integration method (17,18). With our technique, the build-up range and build-up rate constant for arteries and cerebral tissue can be calculated simultaneously, as both $Ea$ and $Ei$ become minimum with the least-squares method ($\delta Ea/\delta Aa = \delta Ea/\delta Ka = 0$, $\delta Ei/\delta Ai = \delta Ei/\delta Ki = 0$).

In this series, the average SD of our CT scanner was less than 1.8 HU ($\Delta H$), and xenon caused a maximum increase of more than 4.0 HU in the brain. Because the xenon-induced change in HU in the brain was more than $2\Delta H$, our flow measurements can be considered reliable.

Our results support the clinical usefulness of the present method for several reasons. First, the Lλ and LCBF can be measured and mapped simultaneously. In addition, the volume of xenon consumed in a single study can be decreased to less than 1000 ml. Finally, the entire time required for the study is only about 20 minutes.

## REFERENCES

1. Fieshi C, Battistini N, Beduschi A, Boselli L, Rassanda M. Regional cerebral blood flow and intraventricular pressure in acute head injuries. *J Neurol Neurosurg Psychiatry* 1974;37:1378–1388.

2. Overgaard J, Jweed WA. Cerebral circulation after head injury. I. Cerebral blood flow and its regulation after closed head injury with emphasis on clinical correlation. *J Neurosurg* 1974;41: 531–541.

3. Ingvar DH, Lassen HN. Cerebral function, metabolism and blood flow. *Acta Neurol Scand* 1978;57:262–269.

4. Touho H, Karasawa J, Nakagawara J, et al. Mapping of local cerebral blood flow with stable xenon-enhanced CT and the curve-fitting method of analysis. *Radiology* 1988;168:207-212.

5. Baron JC, Bousser MG, Rey A, Guillard A, Comar D, Castaigne P. Reversal of local "misery-perfusion syndrome" by extra-intracranial arterial bypass in hemodynamic cerebral ischemia. A case study with $^{15}O$ positron emission tomography. *Stroke* 1981;12:454–459.

6. Drayer BP, Gur D, Wolfson SK Jr, Cook EE. Experimental xenon enhancement with CT imaging: cerebral applications. *AJR* 1980;134:39–44.

7. Gur D, Wolfson SK Jr, Yonas H, et al. Progress in cerebrovascular diseases: local cerebral blood flow by xenon enhanced CT. *Stroke* 1982;13:750–758.

8. Meyer JS, Hayman LA, Yamamoto M, Sakai F, Nakajima S. Local cerebral blood flow measured by CT scan after stable xenon inhalation. *AJNR* 1980;1:213–225.

9. Kelcz F, Hilal SK, Hartwell P, Joseph PM. Computed tomographic measurement of the xenon brain-blood partition coefficient and implications for regional cerebral blood flow: a preliminary report. *Radiology* 1978;127:385–392.

9a. Karasawa J, Kuriyama Y, Kikuchi H, et al. Simultaneous measurement of multi-level l-CBF by using xenon and a CT scanner—development of the shuttle method. *CT Kenkyu* 1983; 5:37–44 (abst).

10. Drayer BP, Wolfson SK, Rosenbaum AE, Dujovny M, Boehnke M, Cook EE. Comparative cranial CT enhancement in the normal primate. *Invest Radiol* 1979;14:88–96.

11. Cullen SC, Gross EG. The anesthetic properties of xenon in animals and human beings, with additional observations on krypton. *Science* 1951;113:580–582.

12. Foley WD, Haughton VM, Schmidt J, Wilson CR. Xenon contrast enhancement in computed body tomography. *Radiology* 1978;129:219–220.

13. Morris LE, Knott JR, Pittinger CB. Electroencephalographic and blood gas observations in human surgical patients during xenon anesthesia. *Anesthesiology* 1955;16:312–319.

14. Pittinger CB, Moyers J, Cohen SC, Featherstone RM, Gross EG. Clinicopathologic studies associated with xenon anesthesia. *Anesthesiology* 1953;14:10–17.

15. Pittinger CB, Featherstone RM. Xenon concentration in brain and other body tissue. *J Pharmacol Exp Ther* 1954;70:110–118.

16. Yonas H, Good WF, Gur D, et al. Mapping cerebral blood flow by xenon-enhanced computed tomography: clinical experience. *Radiology* 1984;152:428–442.

17. Rottenberg DA, Lu HC, Kearfott KJ. The in vivo autoradiographic measurement of regional cerebral blood flow using stable xenon computerized tomography noise. *J Cereb Blood Flow Metab* 1982;2:173–178.

18. Suzuki R, Hiratsuka H, Ohno K, Inaba Y, Kimura T, Inoue J. Topographic mapping of regional cerebral blood flow by xenon-enhanced CT: introducing a simplified method as a routine examination. *No To Shinkei* 1985;37:73–80 (abst).

*Cerebral Blood Flow Measurement with Stable Xenon-Enhanced Computed Tomography,*
edited by Howard Yonas. Raven Press, Ltd.,
New York © 1992.

# Experience in 450 Patients

Shiro Kashiwagi, Tetsuo Yamashita, Shigeki Nakano,
Masaaki Hayashi, Teiichi Takasago, Haruhide Ito,
*Willi Kalender, and **Kazuo Mulakami

*Department of Neurosurgery, Yamaguchi University School of Medicine, 1144 Kogushi
Ube, Yamaguchi 755, Japan; *Siemens Medical Systems, Henkestr. 127,
8520 Erlangen, Germany; and **Anzai Medical Co. Ltd., 2-3-4 Higashigotanda,
Shinagawa, Tokyo 141, Japan*

The stable xenon/computed tomography (Xe/CT) method has been recognized both as a valuable research tool and as a useful clinical examination for topographic evaluation of cerebral blood flow (CBF). Although its theoretical basis and methodological principles have been established, refinements in the xenon delivery system, computational process, and inhalation protocol can advance the routine clinical use of this technology. We will describe several such improvements in our stable Xe/CT CBF system and our accumulated clinical experience with this technique.

## SUBJECTS AND METHODS

Over the last 5 years at our institution, Xe/CT CBF studies have been conducted in 450 subjects (348 men and 102 women) with ages ranging from 1 to 75 years (average: $51.8 \pm 15.4$ years). Of this total, 400 were patients with various intracranial diseases: 290 with ischemic cerebrovascular disease, 23 with brain tumors, 6 with aneurysms, 30 with Moya Moya disease, 28 with arteriovenous malformations, 10 with intracerebral hemorrhage, and 13 others. The other 50 subjects were normal volunteers.

The stable Xe/CT CBF studies were performed with a Somatom DR3 CT scanner with software for CBF imaging (Siemens Medical Systems). We used a Xetron III closed-circuit inhalator (Anzai Medical Co. Ltd.) to deliver the xenon gas. The theoretical background, validity, and clinical applications of the stable Xe/CT CBF method have been reported previously (1–6). In brief, our technique is as follows. After two baseline CT scans, the patient inhales a mixture of 30% xenon, 40% oxygen, and 30% nitrogen through a face mask for 6 minutes while a series of CT scans are obtained at 1-minute intervals. Our scan parameters are 96 kVp, 680 mA-s, a 7-second scan time, and an 8-mm slice thickness. We measure the end-tidal xenon concentration with an AZ-723-XS xenon monitor

(Anzai Medical Co. Ltd.). The inhalator is equipped with an interface that provides automated transfer of the end-tidal xenon data. It also synchronizes the clocks within the xenon inhalator and the CT scanner. At the end of CT scanning, the end-tidal xenon concentration data, stored in a microcomputer, are transferred automatically to the CT host computer. There, combined with the hematocrit levels, these values are converted to arterial xenon enhancement data.

To calculate flow and λ maps, we used the two-parameter optimization method described by Koeppe et al. (7). This method consists of a modified algorithm that performs a series of linear least-squares calculations instead of a single iterative, nonlinear least-squares calculation. The general solution for tissues consisting of different flow compartments is given by Kety's equation:

$$C(t) = W_i \cdot f_i \int_0^t Ca(u)e^{-Ki(t-u)}du$$

$$f_i = k_i \cdot \lambda_i$$

where $i = 1, 2, \ldots, n$ is an index for the different compartments and $W_i$ is the weighting factor for each of the compartments. $C(t)$ and $Ca(t)$ represent the concentration of tracer in tissue and arterial blood, respectively. The flow, $f_i$ for compartment $i$, can be expressed as the product of the flow-rate parameter $k_i$ and the tissue parameter $\lambda_i$.

The exponentials of the arterial xenon concentration and the CT "build-up" then are used to calculate CBF, assuming an expected range of $k$ values. The parameter optimization is performed with a grid search technique to fit the value $k$ and a conventional least-squares fit for the flow, $f$. Then λ is derived simply by dividing $f$ by $k$.

## RESULTS

The average time for one study was 15 to 20 minutes. Used on a PDP 11/44 computer with a floating point processor, our evaluation software enables calculation of three 128 × 128-matrix parameter images and 12 enhanced images in less than 2 minutes. Less than 3 L of 100% xenon gas were required for a study. We estimated the total radiation dose to the center of the brain to be approximately 20 cGy. The signal-to-noise ratio per unit dose was approximately 30% higher at 96 kVp than for routine scan conditions at 125 kVp on the Somatom DR3 scanner.

Studies were successful in 435 subjects (96.7%). In 12 cases (2.67%), images were disturbed by head motion, leading to nondiagnostic studies. In three cases (0.63%), the procedure could not be completed because of the subject's anxiety or claustrophobia.

In most of the patients with cerebral disease, the CBF values and images provided information useful in their clinical management. Recent application of a Diamox (acetazolamide) test to the Xe/CT CBF examination demonstrated cerebral hemodynamic reserve in the ischemic brain (see Yamashita et al. in this volume).

## DISCUSSION

The newly developed xenon delivery system, a closed-circuit rebreathing xenon inhalator with a high-quality xenon sensor, reduces the amount of xenon required. It also improves efficiency through automatic data transfer by means of an on-line data link between the microcomputer in the inhalator and CT host computer.

To calculate the blood flow data, we have eliminated curve fitting of the arterial build-up to solve the Kety-Schmidt equation. We use look-up tables rather than iterative least-squares computation, enabling extremely rapid derivation of flow values in each voxel of interest and reducing computational time significantly. The values we measured in normal subjects and the CBF changes in the patients with cerebrovascular disease agreed with those reported in the literature (3,5,6).

The anesthetic effect of xenon and activation of CBF are of concern when inhalation time exceeds 4 to 5 minutes, even when relatively low concentrations (27% to 35%) of xenon are used (1,8–11,12). We are currently investigating the use of the desaturation (wash-out) phase in addition to the saturation (wash-in) phase to acquire more data points, thereby increasing the accuracy of estimated flow values with a shorter period of inhalation. Our preliminary results showed that measurements and image quality with the 3-minute wash-in/5-minute wash-out protocol (xenon inhalation for 3 minutes) are at least equivalent to those with the 8-minute wash-in protocol (8-minute xenon inhalation). (Details of the wash-in/wash-out protocol and the preliminary results are described in this volume by Nakano et al.). This modification may solve some of the practical drawbacks related to longer xenon inhalation, such as motion artifacts and minor respiratory problems, and facilitate routine use of the stable Xe/CT CBF technique.

## REFERENCES

1.  Gur D, Yonas H, Jackson DL, et al. Measurement of cerebral blood flow during xenon inhalation as measured by the microspheres method. *Stroke* 1985;16:871–874.
2.  Kashiwagi S, Yamashita T, Abiko S, et al. Measurement and imaging of cerebral blood flow with stable xenon and computed tomography (Xe/CT). *Electromedica* 1986;54:136–144.
3.  Meyer JS, Hayman LA, Amano T, et al. Mapping local blood flow of human brain by CT scanning during stable xenon inhalation. *Stroke* 1981;12:426–436.
4.  Yamashita T, Abiko S, Kashiwagi S, Aoki H. Evaluation of cerebral revascularization with xenon enhanced CT CBF study. In: Gagliardi R, Benvenuti L, eds. *Controversies in EIAB for cerebral ischemia*. Bologna: Monduzzi Editore; 1986:149–154.
5.  Yonas H, Good WF, Gur D, et al. Mapping cerebral blood flow by xenon-enhanced computed tomography: clinical experience. *Radiology* 1984;152:435–442.
6.  Yonas H, Wolfson SK, Gur D, et al. Clinical experience with the use of xenon-enhanced CT blood flow mapping in cerebral vascular disease. *Stroke* 1984;15:443–450.
7.  Koeppe RA, Holden JE, Ip WR. Performance comparison of parameter estimation techniques for the quantitation of local cerebral blood flow by dynamic positron computed tomography. *J Cereb Blood Flow Metab* 1985;5:224–234.

8. Dettmers C, Hartmann A, Tsuda Y, et al. Stable xenon effects on regional cerebral blood flow and electroencephalography in normal baboons and volunteers. In: Wullenweber R, Klinger M, Brock M, eds. *Advances in neurosurgery*, vol 15. Berlin: Springer-Verlag; 1987:67–71.

9. Giller CA, Purdy P, Lindstrom WW. Effects of inhaled stable xenon on cerebral blood flow velocity. *AJNR* 1990;11:177–182.

10. Obrist WD, Jaggi JL, Smith DS. Effect of stable xenon inhalation on human CBF. *J Cereb Blood Flow Metab* 1985;5(Suppl 1):S557–558.

11. Yonas H, Grundy B, Gur D, Shabason L, Wolfson S, Cook E. Side effect of xenon inhalation. *J Comput Assist Tomogr* 1981;5:591–592.

12. Cullen SC, Gross EG. The anesthetic properties of xenon in animals and human beings, with additional observations on krypton. *Science* 1951;113:580–582.

*Cerebral Blood Flow Measurement with Stable Xenon-Enhanced Computed Tomography,* edited by Howard Yonas. Raven Press, Ltd., New York © 1992.

# Estimated Values in Normal Subjects

Christian Dettmers, Karl Broich, Alexander Hartmann, *Laszlo Solymosi, Andreas Jacobs, and **Willi Kalender

*Departments of Neurology and *Neuroradiology, University of Bonn, Sigmund Freud Str. 25, D-5300 Bonn 1, Germany; and **Siemens Medical Systems, Henkestr. 127, 8520 Erlangen, Germany*

To facilitate the evaluation of normal and pathological cerebral blood flow (CBF) conditions in patients, we studied the CBF in 17 normal subjects using the xenon-enhanced computed tomography (Xe/CT) technique.

## SUBJECTS AND METHODS

Twenty-four normal volunteers with no history of cerebrovascular disease participated in the investigation. Their ages ranged from 19 to 45 years (mean: $28.8 \pm 7.4$ years). The study was performed with a Siemens Somatom DR H CT scanner at 96 kVp and 540 mA-s. An Ansai Xetron 3 inhalator was used to deliver a 28% xenon concentration mixed with 30% oxygen and room air. We limited the study to one standard level of the brain: 2 cm above, and parallel to, the orbitomeatal line. We obtained two baseline scans, followed by eight to ten enhanced scans during a 10-minute inhalation period. We calculated the CBF and the partition coefficient, $\lambda$, using the single-compartment model and applied a motion-correction algorithm if necessary (see Kalender et al. in this volume). Regions of interest corresponding to the anatomical structures listed in Table 1 were defined on the computer monitor for each subject, and mean CBF and $\lambda$ values calculated for these regions.

## RESULTS

Of the 24 participants, one stopped inhalation after 3 minutes because of anxiety. In two subjects, the study was aborted because of extensive movement. We also had to exclude the results of four other studies because of major motion artifacts that could not be corrected. We observed no other major side effects. Tolerable side effects included dizziness and reduced consciousness at the end of inhalation. Irregularities in the frequency of ventilation without systematic change in end-expiratory $PaCO_2$ occurred often.

**TABLE 1.** *Local blood flow and partition coefficient (λ) measured with the Xe/CT method in 17 normal subjects*

| Territory | Blood flow (ml/100 g/min) | | λ | |
|---|---|---|---|---|
| | Mean | SD | Mean | SD |
| Hemisphere | 44.4 | 5.7 | 1.18 | 0.06 |
| Anterior cerebral artery | 43.7 | 8.5 | 1.23 | 0.15 |
| Middle cerebral artery | 48.0 | 6.5 | 1.17 | 0.09 |
| Posterior cerebral artery | 44.6 | 7.3 | 1.04 | 0.09 |
| Thalamus | 74.2 | 11.5 | 1.08 | 0.07 |
| Internal capsule | 29.4 | 5.5 | 1.53 | 0.11 |
| Corpus callosum | 18.9 | 3.7 | 1.52 | 0.19 |
| White matter | 16.1 | 2.9 | 1.65 | 0.16 |
| Gray matter | 53.1 | 7.3 | 1.12 | 0.10 |

Seventeen subjects completed the 10-minute inhalation. The average time of the last scan was $9.1 \pm 1.0$ minutes after inhalation began. The mean hemispheric CBF value was $44.4 \pm 5.7$ ml/100 g/min. The regional CBF and λ values for the group are listed in Table 1.

### DISCUSSION

We used a relatively low concentration of xenon because we believed that the dizziness, motion, and reduced consciousness would be more tolerable with 28% xenon than with 35% or 40%. However, the low concentration demanded a longer inhalation period. We chose to calculate λ for each subject instead of using a fixed value because it seemed a more accurate method, especially if CBF was measured under pathological circumstances. The λ values for gray and white matter were higher than those originally measured in vitro by Veall and Mallett (1). This issue needs further clarification.

**TABLE 2.** *Xe/CT-derived mean local cerebral blood flow values from the literature*

| Author | Year | Subjects | | Mean (SD) local flow (ml/100 g/min) | | |
|---|---|---|---|---|---|---|
| | | Mean age (yrs) | n | Frontal cortex | Thalamus | White matter |
| Meyer et al. (2) | 1981 | 38 | 30 | 82.3 (8.5) | 85.8 (8.0) | 29.2 (5.9) |
| Meyer et al. (3) | 1981 | 41 | 33 | 81.3 (9.9) | 84.3 (16.8) | 42.4 (8.3) |
| Amano et al. (4) | 1982 | 64 | 7 | 67.6 (8.8) | 63.5 (7.5) | 24.7 (4.8) |
| Meyer et al. (5) | 1984 | 52 | 20 | 75.4 (13.8) | | 26.5 (4.5) |
| Tachibana et al. (6) | 1985 | 70 | 11 | 67.3 (7.7) | 65.9 (7.0) | 22.8 (4.1) |
| Tachibana et al. (7) | 1985 | 66 | 15 | 68.9 (8.9) | 68.3 (8.9) | 24.9 (4.3) |
| Meyer (8) | 1985 | 49 | 13 | 75.5 (11.9) | 70.7 (11.6) | 27.1 (5.7) |
| Kashiwagi et al. (9) | 1986 | 56 | 7 | 67.7 (9.6) | 81.8 (18.7) | 24.7 (2.0) |
| Dettmers | 1991 | 29 | 17 | 53.1 (7.3) | 74.2 (11.5) | 16.1 (2.9) |

Cortical gray-matter CBF was below the values estimated by most authors, especially those using methods different from ours. This variation was probably due to the partial volume effect, indicating that CT spatial resolution limits the ability to measure the distinct enhancement of pure gray matter within the cortex. Blood flow in the thalamus was well within the range reported by others (Table 2). In the white matter, though, CBF was somewhat low compared to values in other reports and increased less than expected during xenon inhalation (see chapters by Dettmers and by Broich in this volume).

Overall, we believe that the Xe/CT technique facilitates quantitative estimation of local CBF with relatively little technical effort. The major problem in the practical performance of the measurement is motion artifact. Investigations are under way to assess whether additional scans during the wash-out period might improve the statistics.

## REFERENCES

1. Veall N, Mallett BL. The partition of tracer amounts of xenon between human blood flow and brain tissue at 37° C. *J Phys Med Biol* 1965;10:375–380.
2. Meyer JS, Hayman LA, Amano T, et al. Mapping local blood flow of human brain by CT-scanning during stable xenon inhalation. *Stroke* 1981;12:426–436.
3. Meyer JS, Hayman LA, Nakajima S, Amano T, Lauzon P. Local cerebral blood flow and tissue solubility measured by stable, xenon-enhanced computerized tomography. In: Carney AL, Anderson EM, eds. *Advances in neurology: diagnosis and treatment of brain ischemia*, vol 30. New York: Raven Press, 1981.
4. Amano T, Meyer JS, Okabe T, Shaw T, Mortel KF. Stable xenon CT cerebral blood flow measurements computed by a single compartment—double integration model in normal aging and dementia. *J Comput Assist Tomogr* 1982;6:923–932.
5. Meyer JS, Okayasu H, Tachibana H, Okabe T. Stable xenon CT CBF measurements in prevalent cerebrovascular disorders (stroke). *Stroke* 1984;15:80–90.
6. Tachibana H, Meyer JS, Kitagawa Y, Tanahashi N, Kandula P, Rogers RL. Xenon contrast CT-CBF measurements in parkinsonism and normal aging. *J Am Geriatr Soc* 1985;33:413–421.
7. Tachibana H, Meyer JS, Okayasu H, Shaw TG, Kandula P, Rogers RL. Xenon-contrast CT-CBF scanning of the brain differentiates normal age-related changes from multi-infarct dementia and senile dementia of Alzheimer type. *J Gerontol* 1984;39:415–423.
8. Meyer JS. Measurement of cerebral blood flow by stable xenon contrast computerized tomography. In: Hartmann A, Hoyer S. Cerebral blood flow and metabolism. Berlin: Springer, 1985;315–327.
9. Kashiwagi S, Yamashita T, Abiko S, et al. Messung und bildliche Darstellung des Hirnblutflusses mit stabilem Xenon und Computer-tomographie (Xe-CT). *Electromedica* 1986;54:136–144.

*Cerebral Blood Flow Measurement with Stable Xenon-Enhanced Computed Tomography,* edited by Howard Yonas. Raven Press, Ltd., New York © 1992.

# Regional Cerebral Blood Flow and Partition Coefficient Values in Neurologically Normal Patients

## Hiromu Segawa

*Department of Neurosurgery, Fuji Brain Institute and Hospital, 270–12 Sugita, Fujinomiya 418, Japan*

There have been several reports on local blood flow values in the normal human brain. Many of these concern flow values estimated by positron-emission tomographic (PET) scanning. Yet this methodology is controversial, especially because of the tracer used. In contrast, the xenon-enhanced computed tomography cerebral blood flow (Xe/CT CBF) method uses a well-understood diffusible CBF tracer and yields quantitative flow values that appear to be sensitive to local changes in tissue composition and that can be directly correlated with CT-defined anatomy.

## SUBJECTS AND METHODS

We obtained regional CBF values in seven patients aged 22 to 56 years (mean: 33.9 years). At the time of the study, the patients, were free of neurologic signs referable to their primary disease, which included pituitary adenoma and aneurysm. These subjects inhaled 50% xenon mixed with oxygen for 25 minutes through a face mask connected to a closed rebreathing ventilation system. We obtained serial CT scans every 3 to 5 minutes at five levels. The arterial build-up rate $(k)$, partition coefficient $(\lambda)$, flow values, and flow images were displayed on a monitor (1–4). Average values were obtained for $4 \times 4$-mm$^2$ (64 pixels) regions of interest. We used an error map to confirm the reliability of the blood flow values, especially those in the posterior fossa, which frequently contained CT artifacts.

## RESULTS

### Regional Blood Flow Values

In the basal ganglia, the highest blood flow values were in the caudate nucleus, followed by the putamen, then the thalamus (Table 1, Fig. 1). The highest cortical flow was in the frontal region, with values in the temporal cortex and the occipital cortex succeeding in that order. Although blood flow in the basal ganglia was higher than in the cerebral cortex (Fig. 2), the difference was not statistically significant. Mean cerebral white-matter flow values ranged from 17 to 24 ml/100 g/min. Blood flow in the infratentorial areas (Fig. 3) was significantly lower than in the supratentorial gray matter. Blood flow for the cerebellar cortex ($n =$ 5) was $47 \pm 8$ ml/100 g/min (mean $\pm$ 50), or 62% of mean cerebral cortical flow. At $59 \pm 16$ ml/100, pontine flow ($n = 4$) was unexpectedly higher than cerebellar blood flow. Midbrain blood flow ($n = 5$) was lowest.

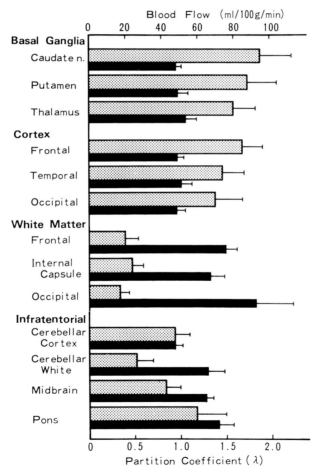

**FIG. 1.** Regional blood flow (*shaded bars*) and λ values (*solid bars*) in the seven neurologically normal subjects. These values were fairly constant in the supratentorial gray and white matter. Values in the infratentorial structures were between gray-matter and white-matter norms.

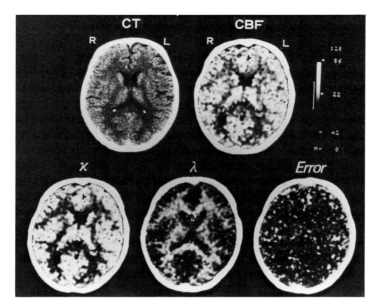

**FIG. 2**. Images in this subject demonstrate that local CBF can be correlated directly with CT-defined anatomy. Blood flow was higher in the basal ganglia than in the cortex. Frontal blood flow was also increased. $K$, build-up rate; λ, partition coefficient.

**TABLE 1**. *Regional blood flow and partition coefficient (λ) values in neurologically normal subjects*

| Region | Mean flow (SD) (ml/100 g/min) | Mean λ (SD) |
|---|---|---|
| Basal ganglia | | |
|   Caudate nucleus | 95 (7) | 0.97 (0.05) |
|   Putamen | 88 (16) | 0.98 (0.12) |
|   Thalamus | 80 (12) | 1.07 (0.12) |
| Cortex | | |
|   Frontal | 85 (11) | 0.98 (0.07) |
|   Temporal | 74 (12) | 1.02 (0.12) |
|   Occipital | 70 (15) | 0.97 (0.10) |
| White matter | | |
|   Internal capsule | 24 (6) | 1.34 (0.15) |
|   Frontal | 20 (7) | 1.51 (0.12) |
|   Occipital | 17 (5) | 1.84 (0.40) |
| Infratentorial | | |
|   Pons | 59 (16) | 1.42 (0.16) |
|   Cerebellar cortex | 47 (8) | 0.94 (0.08) |
|   Midbrain | 42 (8) | 1.28 (0.08) |
|   Cerebellar white | 26 (9) | 1.30 (0.18) |

SD, standard deviation.

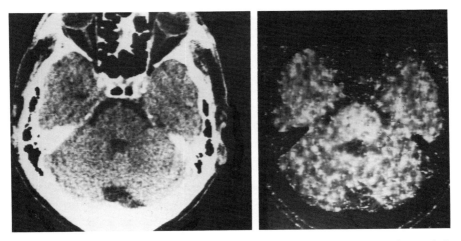

**FIG. 3.** Infratentorial blood flow. Blood flow in the pons was higher than that in the cerebellar cortex.

### Regional Partition Coefficient

The partition coefficients (λ) for the cerebral cortex and the basal ganglia were quite consistent, ranging from 0.97 to 1.07. In the cerebral white matter, however, they varied between 1.34 and 1.84. The low mean value in the internal capsule ($1.34 \pm 0.15$) can be attributed to the partial volume effect involving the adjacent basal ganglia. The high value obtained for the occipital white matter is less reliable because of the relatively poor xenon enhancement in that region. The mean λ value in the cerebellar cortex was $0.94 \pm 0.08$, close to that in the cerebral cortex. Average λ values in the midbrain ($1.28 \pm 0.08$, $n = 5$) and pons ($1.42 \pm 0.16$, $n = 4$) were between those for normal gray and white matter. This can be explained by the mixture of lower-flow gray matter and higher-flow white matter in that region.

### DISCUSSION

The regional blood flow values we measured are not in close agreement with those obtained using PET (5). The discrepancies may be partly the result of a difference in each method's spatial resolution and, thus, a difference in the size of the area surveyed. The full-width half-maximum resolution of the PET method is 12 to 14 mm, whereas our method can provide a resolution of 4 to 5 mm. Using a lower-resolution method, high flow values in the cortex, which is approximately 5 mm thick, would be averaged with the low flow values in the neighboring white matter. Flow in cortical areas would tend to be artificially high.

Blood flow in the frontal region appeared to be higher than in the occipital region, with greater values in the caudate nucleus and putamen than in the thalamus. This is consistent with the tendency toward higher flows in the frontal lobes reported by Wilkinson et al. (6) and Ingvar (7) using the $^{133}$Xe method.

Studies using the PET method have found mean flow values in the cerebellar cortex to be approximately 40% higher than mean values in the cerebral cortex (5). In contrast, our data showed that cerebellar blood flow values were 62% of cerebral cortical flow values. Numerous reports can be found concerning regional blood flow and glucose metabolism in various animals, but none has demonstrated that flow in the cerebellar cortex is higher than in the cerebral cortex (8–11). Furthermore, Mazziotta et al. (12) found in humans that the metabolic rate of glucose for the posterior fossa structures was 63% that for the cerebrum. Therefore, it seems unlikely that cerebellar blood flow is higher than cerebral blood flow. Although $^{15}$O is considered the most reliable tracer among positron emitters, blood-flow studies using this agent may still have methodological problems that require further investigation.

## REFERENCES

1. Segawa H, Sano K, Maehara T, et al. Cerebral blood flow study by CT with xenon enhancement. *J Comput Assist Tomogr* 1980;4:710 (abst).
2. Segawa H, Wakai S, Tamura K, et al. CBF study by CT with xenon enhancement. Experience in 30 cases. *J Cereb Blood Flow Metab* 1981;1(Suppl 1):52–53.
3. Segawa H, Wakai S, Tamura A, et al. Computed tomographic measurement of local cerebral blood flow by xenon enhancement. *Stroke* 1983;14:356–362.
4. Ueda Y, Kimura K, Nagai M, et al. rCBF measurement by CT and its imaging. *J Cereb Blood Flow Metab* 1981;1(Suppl 1):54–55.
5. Frackowiak RS, Lenzi GL, Jones T, et al. Quantitative measurement of regional cerebral blood flow and oxygen metabolism in man using $^{15}$O and positron emission tomography: theory, procedure and normal values. *J Comput Assist Tomogr* 1980;4:727–736.
6. Wilkinson IMS, Bull JWD, du Boulay GH, et al. Regional blood flow in the normal cerebral hemispheres. *J Neurol Neurosurg Psychiatry* 1969;32:367.
7. Ingvar DH. "Hyperfrontal" distribution of the cerebral gray matter flow in resting wakefulness: on the functional anatomy of the conscious state. *Acta Neurol Scand* 1979;60:12–25.
8. Landau WM, Freygang WH, Rowland LP, et al. The local circulation of the living brain: values in the unanesthetized and anesthetized cat. *Trans Am Neurol Assoc* 1955;80:125–129.
9. Sakurada O, Kennedy C, Jehle J, et al. Measurement of local cerebral blood flow with iodo($^{14}$C)antipyrine. *Am J Physiol* 1987;234:1159–1166.
10. van Uitert RL, Levy DE. Regional brain blood flow in the conscious gerbil. *Stroke* 1978;9:67.
11. Sokoloff L, Reivich M, Kennedy C, et al. The ($^{14}$C)deoxyglucose method for the measurement of local cerebral glucose utilization: theory, procedure and normal values in the conscious and anesthetized albino rat. *J Neurochem* 1977;28:897–916.
12. Mazziotta JC, Phelps ME, Miller J, et al. Tomographic mapping of human cerebral metabolism: normal unstimulated state. *Neurology* 1981;31:503–516.

*Cerebral Blood Flow Measurement with Stable Xenon-Enhanced Computed Tomography,* edited by Howard Yonas. Raven Press, Ltd., New York © 1992.

# Local Cerebral Blood Flow and Local Lambda Values Change with Normal Advancing Age

John S. Meyer, Akira Imai, Makoto Ichijo, Masahiro Kobari, and Yasuo Terayama

*Cerebral Blood Flow Laboratory, Veterans Affairs Medical Center, 2002 Holcombe Boulevard, Houston, Texas 77211 and Department of Neurology, Baylor College of Medicine, One Baylor Plaza, Houston, Texas 77030*

During the past 40 years, several investigators using various $^{133}$Xe cerebral blood flow (CBF) monitoring methods have reported declines in CBF with advancing age. Working under the assumption that local $\lambda$ values remain fixed during normal aging, these investigators assigned arbitrary values for xenon brain-blood partition coefficients ($\lambda$ values) in both gray and white matter. Local $\lambda$ values can change with advancing age, however, and are known to be altered by many neurological disorders. For these reasons, local CBF values derived from the products of local $\lambda$ values and local flow rate constants may be in error. Thus, methods that measure local $\lambda$ values before computing local CBF values are desirable for measuring changes in cerebral perfusion that accompany normal aging. Our chapter reports the successful achievement of this objective and presents results of xenon contrast measurements of local CBF and local $\lambda$ values that occur during normal aging.

## SUBJECTS

Our subjects were 32 normal volunteers (17 men and 15 women) aged 20 to 88 years. All subjects underwent neurological examination, neuropsychological examination including the Cognitive Capacity Screening Examination (CCSE), brain computed tomography (CT) scanning, and clinical and laboratory tests. Criteria for admission to this study were normal neurological findings; normal cognitive function indicated by CCSE scores of 27 or above; absence of a history of stroke or any neurological or psychiatric disorder; and exclusion by CT and magnetic resonance imaging of cerebral infarction, mass lesion, hydrocephalus, or any other abnormality of the brain other than cerebral atrophy. Risk factors for stroke were identified in 19 persons (hypertension in 10, diabetes mellitus in 2, hyperlipidemia in 11, and heart disease in 3).

## METHODS

We measured local CBF using our modification of the Xe/CT CBF monitoring method, details of which have been reported elsewhere (1). Subjects first underwent two control noncontrasted CT scans. We then obtained seven serial CT scans at 1-minute intervals between the second and eighth minutes of inhalation of 27% xenon gas (Linde XeScan stable xenon in oxygen USP, Union Carbide Rare Gases, Specialty Medical Products, Danbury, CT). The xenon was administered with a specially designed gas delivery system (Enhancer 3000, Diversified Diagnostic Products, Inc.), and scanning was performed with a high-resolution, rapid CT scanner (Somatom DR version H, Siemens Medical Systems, Inc.). We obtained the CBF measurements in a quiet room with ambient low-level lighting; subjects were in the relaxed, dorsal decubitus position with their eyes closed and ears unplugged. We monitored the end-tidal partial pressures of xenon gas and carbon dioxide on a polygraph during CBF measurements. Local values of λ and CBF were calculated and displayed as color-coded images superimposed directly on the brain slices using a desk-top computer program. The two control scans served as baselines, and the seven enhanced scans were used to define the local tissue xenon saturation curves according to Kety's formula.

## RESULTS

Figure 1 shows the relationships between age and local CBF values for cortical gray matter, subcortical gray matter, and white matter among these normal volunteers. Cortical and subcortical CBF decreased significantly with advancing

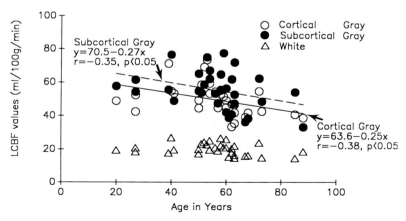

**FIG.1.** Age-related declines in mean local cerebral blood flow (LCBF) values for white matter and cortical and subcortical gray matter. Lines of regression for cortical and subcortical gray matter are statistically significant.

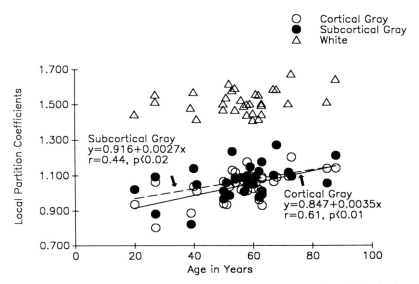

**FIG. 2.** Age-related changes in mean local λ values for white matter and cortical and subcortical gray matter in normal volunteers. With advancing age, significant increases occurred in local λ values for cortical and subcortical gray matter.

age. White matter values also showed trends of age-related declines, but these did not reach a significant level.

Results of cross-sectional analysis of the relationships between advancing age and mean local partition coefficient values for cortical gray matter, subcortical gray matter, and white matter are shown in Fig. 2. The local λ values for cortical and subcortical gray matter showed significant increases with advancing age.

We measured the following values (mean ± SD) for pooled local CBF (in ml/ 100 g/min) and local λ, respectively, among 22 neurologically normal volunteers between 50 and 68 years of age: frontal cortex, 52.8 (10.9) and 1.04 (0.11); temporal cortex, 49.4 (11.8) and 1.09 (0.08); occipital cortex, 45.8 (12.0) and 1.01 (0.07); caudate nucleus, 55.1 (15.5) and 1.03 (0.10); putamen, 53.7 (15.7) and 1.07 (0.13); thalamus, 57.7 (15.2) and 1.14 (0.10); frontal white matter, 15.8 (3.3) and 1.55 (0.10); occipital white matter, 18.9 (4.0) and 1.47 (0.12); and internal capsule, 26.4 (5.5) and 1.52 (0.10). We found local CBF values to be relatively higher in the frontal cortex than in other regions of cortical gray matter.

## DISCUSSION

Using the Xe/CT CBF method, our study confirmed declines of cortical gray-matter blood flow with advancing age, as reported previously by investigators using the [133]Xe inhalation method. In addition, we demonstrated age-related decreases in local CBF values for subcortical gray matter. These results are compatible with reported declines in local CBF obtained by previous [133]Xe and stable Xe/CT measurements as well as by positron-emission tomography (2–4).

Concerning the relationship between age and local λ values, we found that gradual increases in local λ values for cortical and subcortical gray matter occurred with advancing age. The accumulation of lipofuscin in neurons and the relative compacting of gray matter that accompany the aging process are believed to cause these age-related increases.

## ACKNOWLEDGMENTS

This work was supported by the Department of Veterans Affairs, Washington, D.C., and Siemens, Inc., Iselin, New Jersey.

## REFERENCES

1. Meyer JS, Shinohara T, Imai A, et al. Imaging local cerebral blood flow by xenon-enhanced computed tomography. Technical optimization procedures. *Neuroradiology* 1988;20:283–292.
2. Meyer JS, Ishihara N, Deshmukh VD, et al. Improved method for noninvasive measurement of regional cerebral blood flow by [133]Xe inhalation. Part 1. Description of method and normal values obtained in healthy volunteers. *Stroke* 1978;9:195–205.
3. Naritomi H, Meyer JS, Sakai F, Yamaguchi F, Shaw T. Effects of advancing age on regional cerebral blood flow: studies in normal subjects and subjects with risk factors for atherothrombotic stroke. *Arch Neurol* 1979;36:410–416.
4. Lenzi GL, Frackowiak RSJ, Jones T, et al. $CMRO_2$ and CBF by the oxygen-15 inhalation technique: results in normal volunteers and cerebrovascular patients. *Eur Neurol* 1981;20:285–290.

*Cerebral Blood Flow Measurement with Stable
Xenon-Enhanced Computed Tomography,*
edited by Howard Yonas. Raven Press, Ltd.,
New York © 1992.

# Xenon-Enhanced Computed Tomography Display Capabilities to Correlate Brain Anatomy with Blood Flow and Lambda

## Lois M. Gruenauer and Walter W. Lindstrom

*Picker International, Inc., 595 Miner Road, Highland Heights, Ohio 44143*

Stable xenon-enhanced computed tomographic cerebral blood flow (Xe/CT CBF) measurements have been shown to aid in the clinical diagnosis and treatment of many forms of cerebrovascular disease (1–3). Quantifying blood perfusion in brain tissue can yield information on the functional status of the brain. That the use of this technology in the United States has grown slowly may be partly due to the difficult and complex data analysis and the long study and calculation times often required. Better methods of data analysis thus may improve the use of clinical information from Xe/CT CBF studies. Most current techniques require the painstaking drawing of regions of interest (ROI) to calculate average flow values and rely on the eye to separate gray matter from white. Another method, thresholding, uses a very narrow window and various window-level settings to view a flow map essentially as black (below the flow threshold) and white (above the flow threshold). This technique can be used to obtain an overview of the full flow map and make gross side-to-side comparisons.

The data available for analysis after a Xe/CT procedure are the CT image, flow map, $\lambda$ map, and confidence map. Lambda, defined as the partition coefficient of xenon in brain tissue, has been under-utilized in data analysis. In some systems, the $\lambda$ map is not even displayed. Yet $\lambda$ can supply valuable information on tissue type and health. Integrating information from the flow and $\lambda$ maps would be an ideal way to optimize clinical data analysis. With this in mind, a technique was developed to plot the pixels within any ROI using an interactive histogram display along with displays of the CT, flow, and $\lambda$ maps. Combined with short study and calculation times, this method uses the power of the computer to improve the utility of the Xe/CT CBF procedure.

Measuring CBF with stable Xe/CT studies can provide physicians with valuable information about an array of cerebrovascular diseases and conditions. With improved Xe/CT display and data analysis capabilities, these studies can be even more clinically useful. This chapter describes the histogram and includes a few examples of clinical applications for this unique method of analysis.

## METHODS

The Xe/CT procedure and data analysis capabilities described herein are an option on the Picker 1200 CT scanner (Picker International, Highland Heights, OH). This option consists of a xenon delivery system and operating software. A xenon protocol within the standard operating system controls the gas delivery system and timing of the procedure.

The study begins with a pilot scan to select the position of the desired number of slices (one to seven brain levels). Two background scans per level are taken while the patient breathes room air. The patient then begins inhaling xenon (20–35% xenon and 25–70% oxygen; Linde XeScan stable xenon in oxygen USP, Union Carbide Rare Gases, Specialty Medical Products, Danbury, CT) for either 5 or 7 minutes. CT scans are taken at each chosen level after 1.5, 3, 5, and 7 (if applicable) minutes of xenon inhalation. The baseline-subtracted

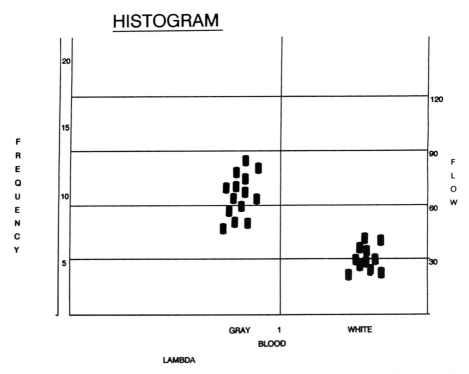

**FIG. 1.** Flow/λ histogram. Each pixel within a region of interest is plotted by its λ value on the horizontal axis and by its flow value (ml/100 g/min) on the right-hand vertical axis; 1 is the λ value of blood. The point distribution below 1 represents pixels with gray-matter λ values and flows of 50–80 ml/100 g/min. The point distribution above 1 represents pixels with white-matter λ values and flows of 20–40 ml/100 g/min. Clearly in this instance, average gray-matter flow would be significantly greater than average white-matter flow.

enhanced images then are displayed, and the images to be used in the flow/λ calculation can be selected. Calculation of the flow and λ maps for each level is completed within 16 seconds.

Our standard display shows the CT image and the flow, λ, and confidence maps for each level selected. A gray-scale ring around the flow, λ, and confidence maps provides a quick reference. The window width and level for each quadrant can be set individually to optimize each image. A desired ROI, when activated, will appear simultaneously on the CT image and all three maps. The height, width, tilt, and position of the ROI can be set as desired. This simultaneous ROI display capability enables easier correlation between anatomy and CBF values.

Creating a histogram of flow and λ values within an ROI, enables the computer to plot (display) each pixel by its λ and flow values while continuing to display the CT, flow, and λ maps. The histogram plots each pixel within a selected ROI as a function of its λ value on the horizontal axis and its flow value (ml/100 g/min) on the right vertical axis (Fig. 1).

Each point on the histogram also is plotted as a function of its frequency of occurrence. This is indicated by the intensity of the point on the display, with a brighter point indicating more λ/flow pairs of the same value. The gray-scale vertical strip to the left of the histogram acts as a reference for the number of λ/flow pairs. The display updates each time the ROI is moved, and the average flow and λ values for the ROI are updated and printed as required. It is also possible to interact with the display via the keyboard, entering upper and lower limits for λ to calculate and display the average flow and λ within the selected boundaries. A similar selection procedure using upper and lower limits for flow can be performed as well.

Figures 2 through 5 illustrate some display capabilities of the histogram and its advantages in analyzing the data. Figures 2 and 3 show the same ROI and histogram, but the upper and lower λ boundaries have been selected to determine averages for gray and white matter, respectively. Figure 4 illustrates that the Xe/CT CBF method can be used to measure zero flow and that the histogram can be set up to calculate the percentage of zero flow within an ROI. Figure 5 demonstrates the value of integrating λ into the analysis of the blood flow map.

## RESULTS

In these examples, upper and lower boundaries of λ were set to determine the average flow of either gray or white matter, even when the ROI contained both. The selected region on the histogram was highlighted with a box, and the average flow and λ values were displayed. Because λ values are tissue specific, the histogram will show flow distributions for normal and abnormal gray and white matter. Typical λ values for healthy gray matter are 0.8 to 0.95. Because xenon is more soluble in fat, white-matter λ values normally range from 1.2 to 1.35.

For the entire ROI shown in Figs. 2 and 3, the flow averaged 38.4 ml/100 g/min; λ averaged 1.063. After the lower and upper λ boundaries were set to

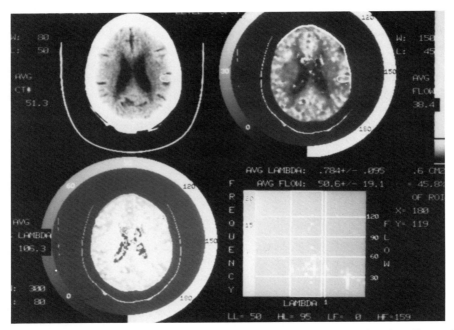

**FIG. 2.** Flow/λ display showing CT image, flow and λ maps, and histogram. A region of interest (ROI) is shown on the CT image and flow and λ maps. In this example, the upper and lower λ boundaries are set at 0.5 and 0.95, respectively, to identify gray matter. A box is shown around this region on the histogram. Directly above the histogram, the average λ and flow of the selected region are displayed.

identify gray matter (Fig. 2), we found that the average flow of the gray matter within the ROI was 50.6 ± 19.1 ml/100 g/min and that the average λ was 0.784 ± 0.095. Gray matter constituted 45.8% of the ROI. When the boundaries were set to identify white matter (Fig. 3), which represented 47.7% of the ROI, the average flow of the white matter within this ROI was 26 ± 12.6 ml/100 g/min and the average λ was 1.339 ± 0.043.

Figure 4 shows an ROI drawn around a small infarction and neighboring brain tissue. Flow within the whole ROI averaged 20 ml/100 g/min; λ, 1.039. When the lower λ boundary was set to 0 and the upper boundary to 0.1, the histogram showed that average flow and λ were 0 in 9.7% of the ROI.

The CT image in Fig. 5 shows extensive atrophy, especially evident in the region on the left side of the brain highlighted by the ROI. The flow map demonstrates unusually high flows in this region. The histogram distribution shows that the λ values of these high-flow areas are centered around 1, the λ value of blood. With the lower λ boundary set at 0.95 and the upper boundary at 1.2, the average flow was 110.6 ± 21.3 ml/100 g/min, and average λ was 1.105 ± 0.049.

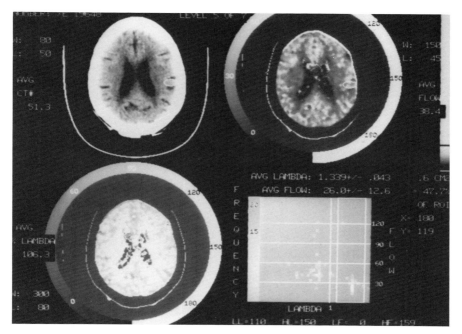

**FIG. 3.** Same flow/λ display shown in Fig. 2 but with the lower and upper λ boundaries set to measure white-matter values. The lower limit is set at 1.1, and the upper at 1.5, as shown by the box around this region.

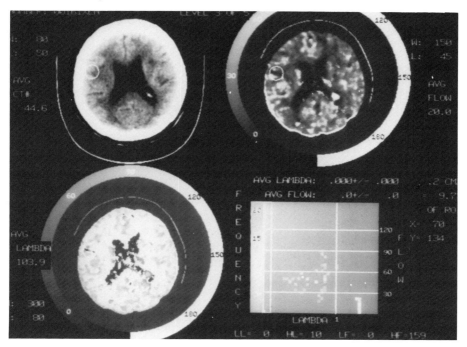

**FIG. 4.** Flow/λ display shows a region of interest drawn around an infarcted region. Here, the λ boundaries are set to select the region of zero xenon absorption.

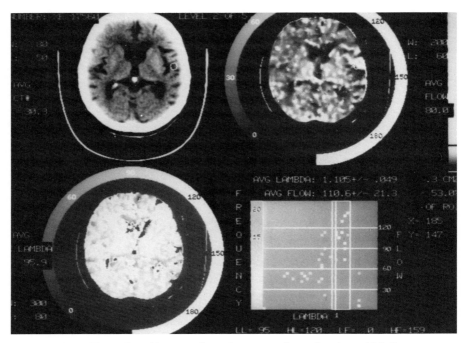

**FIG. 5.** The region of interest, drawn in an area of atrophy, shows high flow.

## CONCLUSIONS

These results illustrate that a mixture of tissue types and health can co-exist within any given ROI. The multiple-ROI display along with the histogram improves gray/white discrimination and enables more efficient data analysis. For example, intra- and inter-subject gray-matter flow averages can be better compared when the varying amounts of white matter can be excluded from the calculation. Gray-matter flow values averaged over a ROI can appear artificially low when the ROI includes white matter. For the ROI in Figs. 2 and 3, the average flow of 38.4 ml/100 g/min with an average λ of 1.06 indicated a mixture of tissue types. The selection of λ boundaries to average flow and λ over homogeneous tissue types yielded the expected higher gray-matter flows (50.6 ± 19.1 ml/100 g/min) and lower white-matter flows (26 ± 12.6 ml/100 g/min).

The ability to measure zero flow is an important advantage of the Xe/CT CBF method. By clearly segregating tissue with zero flow and zero xenon absorption, the histogram can quantify the size of this region within any ROI. Flow averages for other areas with abnormal λ values can also be determined.

Additionally, including λ in CBF analysis allows for more accurate analysis of the flow map, as shown dramatically in Fig. 5, where the ROI on the flow map indicated high flow in the atrophied region. In this instance, the λ values are centered around 1, the λ value of blood not brain tissue. The high flows indicated vessel flow rather than tissue perfusion.

Lastly, the simultaneous display of an ROI on the CT image, flow map, and λ map together with the histogram enables integration of brain anatomy with flow and λ. This display can minimize the limitation presented by extrapolating to xenon saturation in tissue (λ) from a 5-minute xenon-inhalation period; indeed, this feature can be used to identify a problem area. Low-flow gray matter can be mistakenly assigned as white matter (high λ) when extrapolation is made after only 3 or 5 minutes of xenon inhalation. With the CT image as part of the display, however, an ROI drawn in gray matter but indicating high λ and low flow on the histogram would indicate a low-flow problem area.

The clinical potential of Xe/CT CBF monitoring has just begun to be explored. In the United States, only a few hospitals routinely incorporate Xe/CT CBF studies into their clinical evaluation of patients with cerebrovascular diseases and neurological disorders. A step toward more widespread use of the technology may lie in better methods of data analysis and full coverage of the brain as well as in faster flow and λ calculation. The flow/λ histogram display on the Picker 1200, as described here, is a significant advance in analyzing the large amount of data obtained with a Xe/CT CBF study. An interactive histogram display of flow and λ values, along with the simultaneous display of the CT image, and flow map, and λ map, allows full integration of all data. When these features are combined with full brain coverage in up to seven levels and fast calculation time, the Xe/CT CBF method has the potential to become a powerful diagnostic tool.

## ACKNOWLEDGMENTS

The authors would like to express their appreciation to those listed below for their assistance and for the images in this chapter:

Rancho Los Amigos Medical Center, Downey, California
    Department of Medical Imaging
        Angela Wang, M.D., Director of CT and MRI
        Lawrence Greenfield, M.D., Chairman
        Freida Diaz, CRT/AART, CT/MR Technical Supervisor
    Department of Neurological Science
        Helena Chui, M.D., Chairman
Guang An Men Hospital, Beijing, China
    Zhang Zong-mu, M.D., Professor of Radiology

## REFERENCES

1. Yonas H. Xenon-enhanced CT: evaluating cerebral blood flow. *Diagnostic Imaging* 1988;May: 88–94.
2. Meyer JS, Hata T, Imal A, Sakai F. Xenon CT helps reveal blood flow disorders. *Diagnostic Imaging* 1986;May:92–96.
3. Tarr RW, Johnson DW, Rutigliano M, et al. Use of acetazolamide-challenge xenon CT in the assessment of cerebral blood flow dynamics in patients with arteriovenous malformations. *AJNR* 1990;11:441–448.

*Cerebral Blood Flow Measurement with Stable Xenon-Enhanced Computed Tomography,* edited by Howard Yonas. Raven Press, Ltd., New York © 1992.

# Determination of Cerebral Blood Volume by Simultaneous Xenon-Enhanced Computed Tomographic Cerebral Blood Flow Measurement and Dynamic Computed Tomography Enhanced by Intravenous Contrast

Gerrit J. Bouma, Panos P. Fatouros*, J. Paul Muizelaar, Warren A. Stringer*, Donald W. Marion, and Anthony Marmarou

*Division of Neurosurgery and *Department of Radiology, Medical College of Virginia, Virginia Commonwealth University, Box 631, MCV Station, Richmond, Virginia 23298*

It is generally assumed that hyperemia of the brain following severe head injury is a major cause of increased intracranial pressure (ICP), especially in children (1,2). Although the exact cause of this phenomenon is unknown, loss of vasomotor tone is believed to play a role, leading to a decrease in cerebrovascular resistance and a subsequent increase of cerebral blood flow (CBF) above levels necessary to meet the metabolic demands of the brain. This vasodilation also leads to an increase in cerebral blood volume (CBV), which, according to the Monro-Kellie doctrine, would contribute to raised ICP. A recent study by Muizelaar et al., however, found no clear relationship between CBF and ICP in 32 children with severe head injury (3). One possible explanation for this finding is that there is no linear relationship between CBF and CBV; CBF measurements alone, therefore, may not be sufficient for understanding the mechanisms leading to high ICP. This problem could be addressed by measuring CBV in the acute stage of head injury.

Measurement of CBV always has been difficult though. Several attempts have been made, and some of these methods such as the emission computed tomographic studies using radioactively labeled erythrocytes described by Kuhl et al. (4), have indeed proven useful but these methods are not widely available and considered too laborious for routine use. To circumvent these problems, we recently devised a new procedure to measure CBV in the acute stage of head injury without interfering with patient management. The method involves the simultaneous measurement of CBF and the transit time of a nondiffusible indicator using rapid sequential scanning after intravenously injecting a bolus of contrast material. Because the contrast material remains intravascular, principles of indicator dilution analysis can be applied to the time course of the changes in contrast concentration (5).

## SUBJECTS AND METHODS

We performed 15 studies in 12 severely head-injured patients. Most studies were done within the first days after injury, when ICP was monitored with an intraventricular catheter, and the data stored every 30 seconds in a VAX computer. CBF was measured by a stable xenon/computed tomography (CT) study using a GE 9800 scanner. Details of this procedure are described in this volume and elsewhere. In some of our earlier studies, we measured CBF with the intravenous $^{133}$Xe technique of Obrist et al. (2).

Transit time was measured by dynamic CT scanning performed immediately after the CBF study, also using the GE 9800 scanner. A 50-cc bolus of iodine contrast was injected intravenously in 5 seconds; rapid serial CT scanning began simultaneously. We obtained ten scans at a level for which CBF was previously determined. Each scan took 2 seconds, and the minimum interscan delay was 2.3 seconds. By segmenting the raw scan data, we obtained a total of 20 images. Each hemisphere was chosen as a region of interest, and the mean Hounsfield unit in each image was calculated. In this way, we constructed a time-density curve that described the passage of the contrast material through the cerebral blood vessels. To facilitate analysis and to correct for recirculation, the data were fitted to an asymmetric gamma variate curve (6). The appearance time $T_0$ was estimated from the raw data. The interval between the first and second inflection of the curve ("mode transit") was taken as an estimate of the mean transit time (MTT) (7). CBV was calculated by multiplying CBF by MTT. Global CBV and CBF were calculated and used for further analysis.

## RESULTS

All data are presented in Table 1. CBV values ranged between 3.7 and 8.6 ml/100 g, averaging 5.4 ml/100 g. No correlation existed between CBV and CBF, especially in the "physiologic" region (CBF 30–45 ml/100 g/min).

All patients with high CBV in whom ICP was monitored showed larger ICP fluctuations than patients with normal CBV. This is demonstrated by hourly mean ICP graphs for a patient with high CBV (Fig. 1A) and a patient with normal CBV (Fig. 1B). Interestingly, both patients had high CBF and would be considered hyperemic according to Obrist's criteria (2).

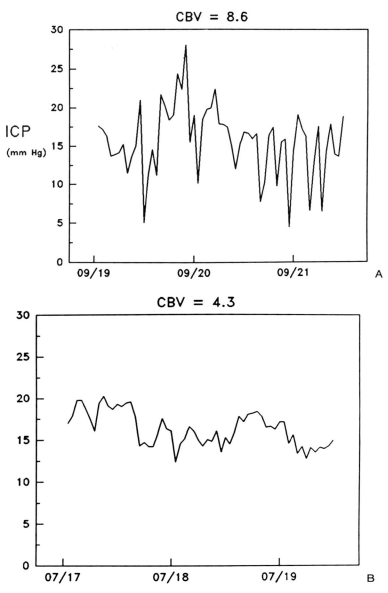

**FIG. 1.** Course of intracranial pressure (ICP; hourly mean values in mm Hg) in two comatose head-injured patients (#9 and #4) during $2\frac{1}{2}$ days in the first week after injury. During this period, cerebral blood volume (CBV) was high (8.6 ml/100 g) in patient 9 (A) and normal (4.3 ml/100 g) in patient 4 (B).

**TABLE 1.** *Results of 15 measurements of mean transit time (MTT), cerebral blod flow (CBF) and volume (CBV), and intracranial pressure (ICP) in 12 comatose head-injured patients*

| Patient | Age (yrs) | MTT (sec) | CBF (ml/100 g/min) | CBV (ml/100 g) | ICP (mm Hg) |
|---|---|---|---|---|---|
| 1 | 24 | 7.2 | 37.6[a] | 4.5 | 16 |
| 2 | 30 | 6.5 | 38.3[a] | 4.1 | 17 |
| 2 | 30 | 9.8 | 38.2[a] | 6.2 | 22 |
| 3 | 64 | 10.9 | 21.0[a] | 3.8 | — |
| 4 | 23 | 5.2 | 50.1[a] | 4.3 | 16 |
| 5 | 31 | 9.4 | 23.8[a] | 3.7 | 15 |
| 6 | 14 | 6.3 | 51.5 | 5.4 | 18 |
| 7 | 28 | 8.3 | 44.2 | 6.1 | 15 |
| 8 | 19 | 6.1 | 52.0 | 5.3 | 19 |
| 9 | 14 | 8.0 | 37.5 | 5.0 | 20 |
| 9 | 14 | 9.1 | 57.0 | 8.6 | 16 |
| 10 | 53 | 9.6 | 37.0 | 5.9 | 20 |
| 11 | 26 | 7.7 | 29.0 | 3.7 | — |
| 12 | 29 | 8.0 | 56.5 | 7.5 | 18 |
| 12 | 29 | 7.3 | 56.5 | 6.9 | 17 |

[a] $^{133}$Xe CBF measurement.

## DISCUSSION

Based on previous studies, normal CBV values in humans appear to be between 4 and 5 ml/100 g (4,8). In the present study, CBV was $\geq 6$ ml/100 g/min on six occasions. In only three of these six studies was CBF also in the "hyperemic" range according to Obrist's criteria (>50 ml/100 g/min). Though CBF above 50 ml/100 g/min was found six times, only in the three cases mentioned above was CBV also elevated; in the other three, we found normal CBV values. This lack of correlation between CBF and CBV indicates that a direct correlation between CBF and ICP should not be expected.

We likewise found no direct correlation between CBV and ICP at the time of CBV measurement. This finding may be at least partially because we almost never allow elevated ICP in severely head-injured patients to run its natural course; instead, we treat it vigorously with ventricular drainage, mannitol, or hyperventilation. When the time course of ICP in patients with normal and elevated CBV is compared, however, fluctuations of ICP appear to be much larger in the latter group. This finding suggests that an increase in CBV reduces the capacity of the intracranial system to compensate for small changes in volume. In other words, CBV is a contributing factor to "stiffness" of the brain. The relationship between CBV and brain stiffness, however, has not yet been examined in depth, and more data are needed before valid conclusions can be drawn.

Measuring CBV by multiplying CBF by MTT was first reported in the early 1970s (9,10). Since then, techniques for CBF measurement have improved and have been further validated. Moreover, CT scanners have become faster, allowing a more accurate estimate of transit time. On the other hand, the potential exists for errors in the measurement of blood volume, both because of the finite duration and subsequent dispersion of the bolus through the cardiopulmonary circulation and because a certain amount of contrast material may begin to leave the region of interest before complete entrance of the bolus ("overlapping effect"). Application of mode transit, as in the present study, is valid only under the assumption that the bolus has entered the system completely before any has left it (7). Nevertheless, this method holds promise for use in both research and clinical practice. It is easy to perform, adds only a few minutes to a regular stable Xe/CT CBF study, and may provide important new information. This contention is supported by our preliminary data that show CBV values that are highly consistent with earlier data and appear to bear a meaningful relationship to ICP dynamics. Even so, the algorithm used to calculate transit time from the data obtained by dynamic CT scanning may need to be modified. Additional studies comparing this technique for deriving CBV to more established methods may provide future guidance.

## REFERENCES

1. Bruce DA, Alavi A, Bilaniuk L, Dolinkas C, Obrist W, Uzzell B. Diffuse cerebral swelling following head injuries in children: the syndrome of "malignant brain edema." *J Neurosurg* 1981;54:170–178.
2. Obrist WD, Langfitt TW, Jaggi JL, Cruz J, Gennarelli T. Cerebral blood flow and metabolism in comatose patients with acute head injury. Relationship to intracranial hypertension. *J Neurosurg* 1984;61:241–253.
3. Muizelaar JP, Marmarou A, DeSalles AA, et al. Cerebral blood flow and metabolism in severely head-injured children. Part 1: relationship with GCS score, outcome, ICP, and PVI. *J Neurosurg* 1989;71:63–71.
4. Kuhl D, Alavi A, Hoffman EJ, et al. Local cerebral blood volume in head injured patients. Determination by emission computed tomography of $^{99m}$Tc-labeled red cells. *J Neurosurg* 1980;52:309–320.
5. Axel L. Cerebral blood flow determination by rapid sequence CT, a theoretical analysis. *Radiology* 1980;137:679–686.
6. Thompson HK, Starmer CF, Whalen RE, et al. Indicator transit time considered as gamma variate. *Circ Res* 1964;14:502–515.
7. Oldendorf WH. Measurement of the mean transit time of cerebral circulation by external detection of an intravenously injected radioisotope. *J Nucl Medicine* 1964;3:382–398.
8. Grubb RL Jr, Raichle ME, Higgins CS, Eichling JO. Measurement of regional cerebral blood volume by emission tomography. *Ann Neurol* 1978;4:322–328.
9. Smith AL, Neufeld GR, Omninsky AJ, Wollman H. Effect of arterial $CO_2$ tension on cerebral blood flow, mean transit time, and vascular volume. *J Appl Physiol* 1971;31:701–707.
10. Mathew NT, Meyer JS, Bell RL, Johnson PC, Neblett CR. Regional cerebral blood flow and blood volume measured with the gamma camera. *Neuroradiology* 1972;4:133–140.

*Cerebral Blood Flow Measurement with Stable Xenon-Enhanced Computed Tomography,* edited by Howard Yonas. Raven Press, Ltd., New York © 1992.

# Discussion

Participants:
Dr. Gerrit Bouma (Richmond, Virginia, USA)
Dr. Walter Obrist (Pittsburgh, Pennsylvania, USA)
Dr. Neils Lassen (Copenhagen, Denmark)

Dr. Bouma's presentation on measuring cerebral blood volume (CBV) using an iodine bolus and sequential computed tomography (CT) images provoked highly critical responses from Dr. Obrist and Dr. Lassen. Dr. Obrist pointed out that, as originally proposed in the 1960s, a gamma-variate function has two unknowns: the time of tracer appearance and the rate of transit through the brain. Dr. Obrist said he did not believe that CT imaging every 4.3 seconds would be able to characterize this curve. He also was concerned that the calculations would require knowing the circulation time from the arm to the carotid artery. Dr. Lassen proposed that the transit time of the iodine bolus from the arm to the brain and then the time for dispersion within the brain must be considered. He maintained height over area should be measured, as reported by Kety, rather than transit time. Both Dr. Obrist and Dr. Lassen suggested the need for extensive cross validation with other CBV-measurement methods.

Dr. Bouma agreed that further validation was needed. Nevertheless, he remained optimistic about the merit of the method he proposed, because even with relatively slow scanning rates, his group was able to produce physiologically reasonable measurements. He was confident that faster scanners would improve their results.

(Editor's note: The availability of anatomic information, local CBF, and local CBV measurements from a single visit to a CT facility would have wide clinical and experimental application. Despite current limitations, efforts to measure CBV with CT and iodinated contrast material should be pursued.)

*Cerebral Blood Flow Measurement with Stable Xenon-Enhanced Computed Tomography,* edited by Howard Yonas. Raven Press, Ltd., New York © 1992.

# Interictal Regional Cerebral Blood Flow in Patients with Refractory Complex Partial Seizures

Karl Broich, *Christian E. Elger, Alexander Hartmann, **Laszlo Solymosi, *Andreas Hufnagel, Stephan Zierz, Christian Dettmers, and ***Willi Kalender

*Departments of Neurology, *Epileptology, and **Neuroradiology, University of Bonn, Sigmund Freud Str. 25, D-5300 Bonn 1, Germany; and ***Siemens Medical Systems, Henkestr. 127, 8520 Erlangen, Germany*

Complex partial seizures, one of the most common forms of epilepsy, are often refractory to standard drug therapy. Recently, temporal lobectomy has been recognized as an effective treatment that results in good clinical outcome in a high proportion of patients (1). This treatment requires preoperative localization of the side of the focus using easily available imaging techniques. In addition to electroencephalographic (EEG) techniques, positron-emission tomography (PET) and single-photon emission tomography (SPECT) have been used to detect lateralizing abnormalities. Interictal measurements with PET have demonstrated a hypometabolic area (2,3) and those with SPECT, a hypoperfused region (4,5) consistent with 75% to 90% of foci indicated by EEG recordings. As another procedure, the inhalation of stable xenon gas and successive recording of its increasing concentration in the brain tissue by computerized tomography (CT) has made it possible to calculate regional cerebral blood flow (rCBF) with high spatial resolution in a variety of clinical applications (6). Theoretically then, stable xenon-enhanced CT (Xe/CT) may be able to identify similar lateralizing abnormalities in patients with complex partial seizures (CPS).

## METHODS

Sixteen patients (9 women and 7 men), 18 to 29 years old (mean age: 22.6 ± 3.3 years) with a unilateral EEG focus completed the protocol. We compared their results to those of seven age-matched, healthy control subjects without central nervous system disease. All patients had undergone multiple EEG recordings, including scalp (10–20 System) and sphenoidal electrodes. The temporal lobe enclosing the EEG focus was defined as the affected side and the contralateral temporal lobe as the unaffected side.

Xe/CT was performed with a commercial inhalation system for xenon delivery and a CT scanner with dynamic imaging capabilities (Siemens DR2; 96 kVp, 0.54 m-As). We selected the levels for rCBF analysis from two baseline scans of the temporal lobe containing the EEG focus. We then obtained six to eight Xe/CT scans during inhalation of 28% stable xenon (mixed with 30% oxygen and room air) over 10 minutes. We defined lateral and medial temporal regions of interest symmetrically for both hemispheres from the anatomical scan. The percentage of the side-to-side difference was estimated as follows: (higher side − lower side)/higher side × 100. For statistical evaluation, we used the paired and unpaired Student's $t$ tests.

## RESULTS

Within the group of patients with CPS, there were no statistically significant differences between rCBF in the affected and unaffected sides, either for the whole temporal lobe or for the lateral or medial parts (Table 1). The partition coefficient, $\lambda$, was significantly lower in the affected side for the whole temporal lobe and its lateral strip, but not in the medial part. The rCBF was lower on the affected side in seven patients but on the unaffected side in four patients; in the other five, we detected only insignificant differences. Lambda was reduced on the affected side in 10 patients, on the unaffected side in only one patient, and was not different in five patients. In the control group, the mean side-to-side difference in rCBF was $18 \pm 8\%$; in $\lambda$, only $10 \pm 5\%$. Thus, $\lambda$ was more sensitive than rCBF to lateralizing abnormalities (Fig. 1).

One patient had a CPS 2 minutes after ending the Xe/CT study. No other major side effects occurred, though some experienced slight agitation, euphoria, light-headedness, and dysesthesia.

TABLE 1. *Comparison of affected and unaffected sides in patients with complex partial seizures*

| | | Mean values ($\pm$ SD) | | |
| | Anatomical region | Affected side | Unaffected side | Significance ($t$ test) |
|---|---|---|---|---|
| Regional blood flow (ml/100 g/min) | temporal | 32.1 (9.5) | 33.2 (8.3) | n.s. |
| | temporolateral | 32.3 (10.9) | 35.7 (10.7) | n.s. |
| | temporomedial | 39.3 (9.1) | 38.8 (7.7) | n.s. |
| Lambda | temporal | 1.07 (0.12) | 1.17 (0.11) | $P \le 0.05$ |
| | temporolateral | 1.10 (0.20) | 1.26 (0.16) | $P \le 0.01$ |
| | temporomedial | 1.03 (0.20) | 1.08 (0.20) | n.s. |

n.s., not significant.

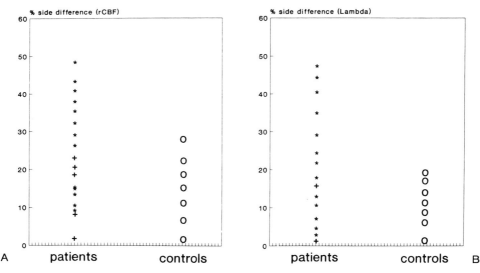

**FIG. 1.** Side-to-side differences in regional cerebral blood flow (A) and λ (B), in both patients with complex partial seizures and healthy control subjects. For the patients, lower values on the affected side are represented by * and on the unaffected side by +. Side-to-side differences in control subjects are indicated by a 0.

## DISCUSSION

The rCBF results of Xe/CT studies in patients with CPS were discouraging. Lambda, however, seemed to be more sensitive to the lateralizing abnormalities found with EEG. In 63% of the patients, λ was significantly lower on the affected side; only one had a reduced value on the opposite side. Fish et al. (7) found Xe/CT-defined rCBF to be more accurate than we did in localizing the focus, but unfortunately, they did not report λ values.

Gur et al. (8) reported that the main disadvantages of Xe/CT were low signal-to-noise ratio and artifacts from patient movement. The special slice position and angle required for temporal scans as used in our study, make them more susceptible to motion artifacts, and the nearby dense petrous bone leads to more beam hardening and consequent streaking artifacts than in other brain regions. Using higher concentrations of xenon would improve the signal-to-noise ratio, but more side effects would result from the anesthetic properties of xenon, and seizures could be triggered due to excitative effects.

In our studies, we detected dysrhythmic and focal EEG abnormalities, particularly of the temporal lobes, in 3 of 11 normal, healthy subjects who inhaled 26% stable xenon. Therefore, one explanation of the low sensitivity of rCBF may be a physiologic activation of the EEG-defined focus with a xenon-induced increase of CBF in the focus itself. The most frequent cause of CPS with an

EEG-defined temporal focus is medial temporal sclerosis (9). This may explain the better ability of λ to detect the side of the focus.

Overall, our study suggests that Xe/CT studies may be useful in patients with CPS and that in two thirds of patients, the side of the epileptogenic focus, as defined by EEG, can be identified correctly by λ values. Regional CBF measured by Xe/CT seems to be of less value.

## REFERENCES

1. Delgado-Escueta AV, Walsh GO. Type 1 complex partial seizures of hippocampal origin: excellent results of anterior temporal lobectomy. *Neurology* 1985;37:143–154.
2. Engel JP Jr, Kuhl DE, Phelps ME, et al. Interictal cerebral glucose metabolism in partial epilepsy and its relation to EEG changes. *Ann Neurol* 1982;12:512–517.
3. Holmes MD, Kelly K, Theodore WH. Complex partial seizures: correlation of clinical and metabolic features. *Arch Neurol* 1988;45:1191–1193.
4. Biersack HJ, Stefan H, Reichmann K, et al. HM-PAO brain SPECT and epilepsy. *Nucl Med Commun* 1987;8:513–518.
5. Ryding E, Rosen I, Elmqvist D, Ingvar DH. SPECT measurements with $^{99m}$Tc-HM-PAO in focal epilepsy. *J Cereb Blood Flow Metab* 1988;8:S95-S100.
6. Yonas H, Gur D, Latchaw RE, Wolfson SK. Xenon computed tomographic blood flow mapping. In: Wood JH, ed. *Cerebral blood flow: physiologic and clinical aspects.* New York: McGraw-Hill, 1987;220–242.
7. Fish DR, Lewis TT, Brooks DJ, et al. Regional cerebral blood flow of patients with focal epilepsy studied using xenon enhanced CT brain scanning. *J Neurol Neurosurg Psychiatry* 1987;50:1584–1588.
8. Gur D, Wolfson SK, Yonas H, et al. Progress in cerebral vascular disease: local cerebral blood flow by xenon enhanced CT. *Stroke* 1982;13:750–758.
9. Engel JP Jr, Brown WJ, Kuhl DE, et al. Pathological findings underlying focal temporal hypometabolism in partial epilepsy. *Ann Neurol* 1982;12:518–528.

*Cerebral Blood Flow Measurement with Stable Xenon-Enhanced Computed Tomography,* edited by Howard Yonas. Raven Press, Ltd., New York © 1992.

# Leuko-araiosis, Cerebral Ischemia, and Cognitive Performance Correlated by Xenon/Computed Tomographic Cerebral Blood Flow Studies

## Jun Kawamura, John S. Meyer, Makoto Ichijo, and Masahiro Kobari

*Cerebral Blood Flow Laboratory, Veterans Affairs Medical Center, 2002 Holcombe Boulevard, Houston, Texas 77211; and Department of Neurology, Baylor College of Medicine, One Baylor Plaza, Houston, Texas 77030*

Hypodense lesions detected by computed tomography (CT) in periventricular white matter have been of interest since Hachinski et al. (1) coined the term "leuko-araiosis" in 1987. Leuko-araiosis has been associated with aging and with risk factors for stroke and dementia, but its exact cause and nature remain unknown. This study was designed to elucidate the clinical correlates and possible contributions of ischemia to the pathogenesis of leuko-araiosis by measuring local cerebral blood flow (CBF) with the stable xenon-enhanced CT CBF method in patients with and without leuko-araiosis.

## SUBJECTS

Our subjects included six neurologically normal volunteers, two patients with chronic cerebral infarction, and 23 patients with dementia. Patients with chronic cerebral infarction had normal cognition. Nine of the patients with dementia had Alzheimer disease, and 14 had multi-infarct dementia (MID). The type of dementia was diagnosed according to the recommendation of *DSM-III-R*, NINCDS-ADRDA Work Group criteria, Hachinski ischemic scores, and the Cognitive Capacity Screening Examination (CCSE). In patients with MID, cerebral infarctions were confirmed by CT and magnetic resonance imaging (MRI).

## METHODS

To measure local CBF, we used the Xe/CT CBF method, details of which have been reported elsewhere (2). After taking two control CT scans, we obtained seven serial scans at 1-minute intervals between the second and eighth minutes of inhalation of 27% xenon gas (Linde XeScan stable xenon in oxygen USP, Union Carbide Rare Gases, Specialty Medical Products, Danbury, CT). We used a specially designed xenon delivery system (Enhancer 3000, Diversified Diagnostic Products) and a high-resolution, rapid CT scanner (Somatom DR version H, Siemens Medical Systems). We also used a polygram to monitor the end-tidal partial pressures of xenon gas and carbon dioxide during the CBF study and a computer program to generate local lambda and local CBF values as color-coded brain images. The two control scans served as baselines, and the seven enhanced scans were used for the xenon saturation curves, computed with Kety's formula.

The MRI was performed with a 0.6-tesla superconductive unit, and spin-echo protocols, 1800–2500/40–120 (TR/TE), were used to evaluate $T_2$-weighted images. We assessed the severity of leuko-araiosis using a baseline CT image. Based on criteria described in an earlier publication (3), we graded the following abnormal findings: periventricular high-intensity signals detected by $T_2$-weighted MRI (MR-PVH); remote high-intensity signals located in subcortical white matter and detected by $T_2$-weighted MRI (MR-SCH); periventricular hypodense areas of leuko-araiosis detected by CT (CT-LEU); and degrees of cerebral atrophy, estimated by enlargement of the third and lateral ventricles and dilatation of sulci measured on both MRI and CT images.

## RESULTS

We found significant correlations between the severity of leuko-araiosis and reductions of pooled local CBF values in the frontal ($r = -0.40$, $P < 0.05$), temporal ($r = -0.40$, $P < 0.05$), and occipital ($r = -0.36$, $P < 0.05$) cortex; the caudate nucleus ($r = -0.43$, $P < 0.05$); the putamen ($r = -0.50$, $P < 0.01$); and the internal capsule ($r = -0.37$, $P < 0.05$). MR-PVH and MR-SCH, however, did not correlate with pooled local CBF values measured within the nine regions.

Table 1 shows the correlation coefficients between MRI-defined lesions, CT findings of leuko-araiosis, cerebral atrophy, age, and CCSE scores. The severity

**TABLE 1.** *Correlation coefficients between magnetic resonance imaging, computed tomography, cerebral atrophy, age, and CCSE scores (n = 31)*

|  | MR-SCH | CT-LEU | Atrophy | Age | CCSE Scores |
|---|---|---|---|---|---|
| MR-PVH | 0.115 | 0.694* | 0.471* | 0.432** | −0.309 |
| MR-SCH | — | 0.046 | −0.004 | 0.097 | 0.052 |
| CT-LEU | — | — | 0.752* | 0.565* | −0.653* |
| Atrophy | — | — | — | 0.659* | −0.641* |
| Age | — | — | — | — | −0.468* |

* $P < 0.01$, ** $P < 0.05$.
CCSE, Cognitive Capacity Screening Examination; MR-PVH, periventricular high-intensity signals detected by $T_2$-weighted magnetic resonance imaging (MR); MR-SCH, remote high-intensity signals in subcortical white matter on MR; CT-LEU, periventricular hypodense lesions on CT.

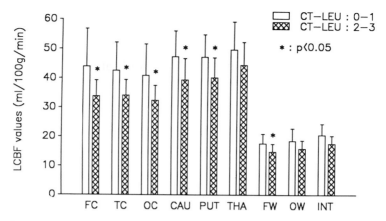

**FIG. 1.** Comparison of the local cerebral blood flow (LCBF) values in nine cerebral regions of the group with no or mild CT findings of leuko-araiosis (CT-LEU: 0–1) to those of the group with moderate to severe periventricular hypodense areas on CT (CT-LEU: 2–3). In the group with moderate to severe periventricular hypodensity, LCBF values for cerebral cortical regions, caudate nucleus (CAU), putamen (PUT), and frontal white matter (FW) were all significantly lower. FC, frontal cortex; OC, occipital cortex; TC, temporal cortex; THA, thalamus; OW, occipital white matter; INT, internal capsule.

of periventricular lesions on MRI correlated significantly with the severity of leuko-araiosis, the degree of cerebral atrophy, and age, but not with CCSE scores. Remote subcortical lesions on MRI did not correlate with periventricular lesions on MRI, leuko-araiosis, cerebral atrophy, age, or CCSE scores. We also found significant correlation between the severity of leuko-araiosis and the severity of periventricular lesions on MRI, the degree of cerebral atrophy, age, and cognitive impairment.

We divided the 31 subjects into two groups according to the severity of leuko-araiosis. Figure 1 compares the local CBF values in nine cerebral regions of the group with no or mild leuko-araiosis to those of the group with moderate to severe leuko-araiosis. In the latter group, local CBF values for cerebral cortical regions, the caudate nucleus, putamen, and frontal white matter were all significantly lower than corresponding values in the first group.

We also divided subjects into two groups according to the severity of periventricular high-intensity lesions on MRI (MR-PVH). Local CBF values for cortical and subcortical gray matter regions tended to be lower in the group with moderate to severe periventricular lesions, but there were no significant differences between the two groups.

## DISCUSSION

As with CT-defined leuko-araiosis, the severity of periventricular white-matter lesions demonstrated by MRI correlated with advancing age and the degree of cerebral atrophy. CT findings of leuko-araiosis also correlated with cognitive impairment, though cognitive impairment was not significantly associated with MR-PVH. This lack of correlation with the MRI findings appears to be because of the extraordinarily high sensitivity of MRI to trivial periventricular white-matter lesions. Periventricular white matter constitutes a watershed territory between cortical pial arteries and the deep penetrating arteries of the white matter, thereby causing a zone of predilection to cerebral ischemia. This accounts for the frequent occurrence of white-matter lesions. Our investigation suggests that diffuse cerebral hypoperfusion combined with the poor collateral circulation in white matter surrounding the lateral ventricle is causally related to leuko-araiosis.

## ACKNOWLEDGMENTS

This work was supported by the Department of Veterans Affairs, Washington D.C., and Siemens, Inc., Iselin, New Jersey.

## REFERENCES

1. Hachinski VC, Potter P, Merskey H. Leuko-araiosis. *Arch Neurol* 1987;44:21–23.
2. Meyer JS, Shinohara T, Imai A, et al. Imaging local cerebral blood flow by xenon-enhanced computed tomography. Technical optimization procedures. *Neuroradiology* 1988;30:283–292.
3. Kobari M, Meyer JS, Ichijo M, Oravez WT. Leuko-araiosis: correlation of MRI and CT findings with blood flow, atrophy, and cognition. *AJNR* 1990;11:273–281.

*Cerebral Blood Flow Measurement with Stable Xenon-Enhanced Computed Tomography,* edited by Howard Yonas. Raven Press, Ltd., New York © 1992.

# Cerebral Blood Flow Determination Within the First Few Hours of Acute Embolic Infarction

Hiroo Sato, Yoshiharu Sakurai, Hiroshi Niizuma, Takamasa Kayama, and *Akira Ogawa

*Department of Neurosurgery, Stroke Center, Sendai National Hospital 2-8-8 Miyagino, Miyagino ku, Sendai, Miyagi 983, Japan; and *Division of Neurosurgery, Institute of Brain Diseases, Tohoku University School of Medicine, 1-1 Seiryo-cho, Aobu ku, Sendai, Miyagi 980, Japan*

In clinical trials of treatments for stroke, determining the size, severity, and location of an ischemic injury during the first few hours after onset is crucial to making treatment decisions. We therefore compared the clinical, conventional computed tomography (CT), and Xe/CT cerebral blood flow (CBF) findings in five patients with acute embolic infarction to provide additional information concerning patient selection, prognostic factors, surgical results, and complications of embolectomy.

## PATIENTS AND METHODS

The five patients were admitted to our clinic within 4 hours of stroke onset. At that time, conventional CT findings were normal in all patients. Four patients had middle cerebral artery (MCA) occlusion, which was located at the MCA trunk in three patients and the bifurcation of M1 and M2 in the other. In the fifth patient, the internal carotid artery (ICA) was occluded at the neck. All patients were given brain protective agents (20% mannitol, 500 ml; vitamin E, 500 mg; phenytoin, 500 mg) as soon as possible after admission.

We conducted Xe/CT studies within the first 7 hours after onset using a standardized Xe/CT system integrated in a TCT 20A head scanner (Toshiba Corp., Tokyo) and a Xetron II AZ-701 stable xenon gas rebreathing system (Anzai Sogyo Corp., Tokyo). To keep patients immobile, we performed endotracheal intubation after sedating them with thiopental sodium. Patients inhaled a 35% xenon/65% oxygen mixture for 5 minutes, followed by 10 minutes of desaturation. The end-tidal chamber scan method was used to measure the xenon concentration in arterial blood. We placed 2.5-cm regions of interest (ROIs) bilaterally in the cortical mantle, putamen, and thalamus and one 1.2-cm ROI in each posterior internal capsule.

Emergency embolectomy through a pterional craniotomy was done within 13.5 hours in three patients with MCA occlusion; spontaneous recanalization occurred in the fourth patient within 4 hours of onset. Revascularization was not done in the patient with ICA occlusion. CBF studies were performed both before and after recanalization.

## RESULTS

Table 1 summarizes the five cases, and Table 2 correlates regional CBF and follow-up CT findings. The functional outcome of surgery was good in one patient and fair in three. Details of individual patients follow.

Case 1: A preoperative Xe/CT scan demonstrated diffusely low CBF (<9 ml/ 100 g/min) in the distribution of the right MCA. After emergency embolectomy, CBF in this area improved markedly, but cerebral edema became exacerbated, and external cranial decompression was performed the next day.

Case 2: CBF values were low in the distribution of the right MCA, the lowest values (7 ml/100 g/min) being in the posterior internal capsule and frontoparietal cortex. Xe/CT on postoperative day 11 showed very low flow in the right posterior

**TABLE 1.** *Summary of five cases of acute embolic infarction studied by Xe/CT*

| Patient | Age (yrs)/ sex | Site of occlusion[a] | Hours to Xe/CT | Hours to recanalization | Outcome |
|---------|------|--------|-------|--------|---------|
| 1 | 50/M | MCA trunk | 2.6 | 7.2 | fair |
| 2 | 66/F | MCA trunk | 4.0 | 8.7 | fair |
| 3 | 44/M | MCA trunk | 6.5 | 13.5 | fair |
| 4 | 44/M | MCA branch | 1.5 | 2–4[b] | good |
| 5 | 53/M | ICA | 7.0 | none | fair |

[a] All occluded arteries were on the right side.
[b] Spontaneous recanalization.
MCA, middle cerebral artery; ICA, internal carotid artery.

**TABLE 2.** *Correlation between regional cerebral blood flow and follow-up CT findings*

| Case | Regional CBF (ml/100 g/min) | | | | | | | |
|------|----|-----|-----|-----|----|------|-----|----|
| | F | aT | mT | pT | P | pIC | Put | Th |
| 1[a] | 23 | <5[b] | 9 | 7 | 43 | 7[b] | 14[b] | 42 |
| 2 | 30 | 7[b] | 7[b] | 12 | 28 | 7[b] | 7[b] | 38 |
| 3 | 36 | 17 | 29 | 11[b] | 32 | <5[b] | 13[b] | 38 |
| 4 | 40 | 5[b] | 18 | 5[b] | 18 | 41 | 45 | 63 |
| 5 | 21 | 11 | 14 | 6[b] | 25 | 5[b] | 8[b] | 32 |

[a] External decompression case.
[b] CT-defined infarction.
F, frontal cortex; aT, anterior temporal cortex; mT, middle temporal cortex; pT, posterior temporal cortex; P, posterior cortex; pIC, posterior internal capsule; Put, putamen; Th, thalamus.

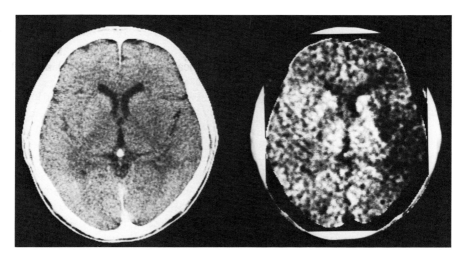

**FIG. 1.** Preoperative conventional CT (*left*) and Xe/CT (*right*) in case 3. LCBF values were diffusely decreased in the distribution of the right MCA, with the greatest reduction occurring in the posterior internal capsule, putamen, and posterotemporal cortex.

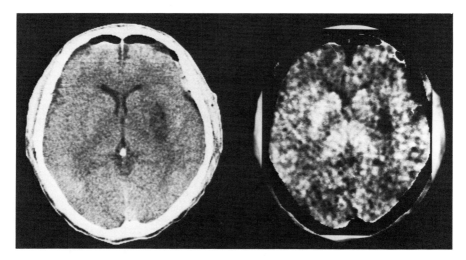

**FIG. 2.** Postoperative conventional CT (*left*) and Xe/CT (*right*) in case 3. Except in the posterior internal capsule and putamen, flow in the right MCA area was remarkably improved after embolectomy.

internal capsule and putamen; a flow increase to 70 ml/100 g/min in the frontoparietal cortex indicated hyperemia. Follow-up CT showed hemorrhagic infarction in the right basal ganglia and low density in the frontoparietal region.

Case 3: Preoperative Xe/CT demonstrated focal flow reduction (<11 ml/100 g/min) in the right posterior internal capsule and posterotemporal cortex and mild reduction (17–32 ml/100 g/min) in the remaining area of the right MCA (Fig. 1). Postoperative Xe/CT showed focal reduction of CBF only in the right posterior internal capsule (Fig. 2). Presumably, fragments of emboli had not been removed from the lenticulostriate artery. Follow-up CT confirmed hemorrhagic infarction in the basal ganglia and posterotemporal cortex (Fig. 3).

Case 4: CBF values were low (5–18 ml/100 g/min) throughout the MCA distribution, whereas flow in the basal ganglia remained in the normal range. Postoperative Xe/CT showed recanalization of only the central branch of the right MCA. Follow-up CT showed that regions that were not recanalized had reduced

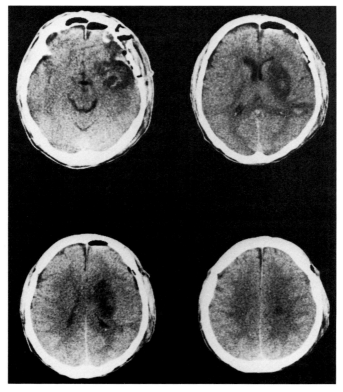

**FIG. 3.** Follow-up conventional CT in case 3, showing hemorrhagic infarction in the right posterior internal capsule, putamen, and posterotemporal cortex.

CT attenuation consistent with infarction. This patient had a left-sided homonymous hemianopsia and no paresis when discharged from our institution.

Case 5: CBF was diffusely low in the distribution of the right ICA. Values were markedly lower (5–8 ml/100 g/min) in the right basal ganglia and posterotemporal cortex. Acute revascularization was not performed in this patient. Follow-up CT confirmed infarction in the areas that had exhibited very low CBF values.

## DISCUSSION

The role of emergency embolectomy for acute occlusion of the MCA remains controversial because the natural course of MCA occlusion has many variations (1,2), and the findings concerning MCA embolectomy have been inconclusive (3–5). For example, severe ischemic edema has been found after fatal embolectomies, whereas in some cases, neurological signs have improved remarkably soon after the procedure.

### Stable Xenon-Enhanced CT CBF Studies

Stable xenon-enhanced CT provides the following advantages. First, examinations can be performed within the first few hours after stroke onset. Second, Xe/CT has produced local CBF measurements with a relatively high degree of spatial resolution. Third, very low local CBF values (<10 ml/100 g/min) can be recorded even in small and centrally located brain regions.

Nevertheless, Xe/CT also has significant disadvantages. For instance, the study demands registration of baseline and xenon-enhanced images. In our method, we immobilized patients using endotracheal intubation following sedation with thiopental. Moreover, even in the total absence of blood flow, Xe/CT does not record a value of 0 ml/100 g/min. Finally, the quantitative value of Xe/CT has been questioned because of the tendency of xenon gas to increase CBF.

### Surgical Results of Acute Embolectomy

Meyer et al. (3) reviewed 20 cases in which emergency embolectomy was used to treat acute MCA occlusion. Two patients had an excellent result, five were left with minimal deficits but were still employable, four did poorly, and two died. The investigators concluded that collateral flow, as judged from preoperative angiograms, was the best predictor of outcome. In our series, cerebral edema was exacerbated and external decompression required after embolectomy in the patient with diffuse and marked reduction of local CBF (<10 ml/100 g/min) in the distribution of the MCA.

Kitami et al. (5) described five emergency embolectomies for MCA occlusion. They found that patients with occlusion beyond the striate vessel origin did not show any hemorrhagic infarction and had a much better recovery than that reported to result from the natural course of embolic MCA occlusions. Patients with occlusion in the area involving perforators, however, all developed hemorrhagic infarction in the basal ganglionic region after revascularization. In our study, the functional outcome for patients with trunk occlusion was worse than for the patient with branch occlusion.

### CBF Study of Acute Cerebral Infarction

Shimada et al. (4) reported that preoperative dynamic CT scans have been done to estimate the degree of ischemia. Patients who had a major stroke with a type 1 pattern on the dynamic CT scan (the peak value of the time-density curve exceeded 50% of the opposite healthy side) had a remarkably good recovery if revascularization was completed within 6 hours after the attack. In patients with a type 3 pattern (the time-density curve was almost flat, or the peak value did not reach even approximately one-third of the opposite side), however, massive cerebral infarction often developed even after acute revascularization. Major stroke cases of the type 2 pattern on dynamic CT scans (the peak value was from one-third to one-half of the normal side) had a poor functional recovery, even if revascularization was performed very early. In our series, the patient who did not undergo recanalization had regions with moderate CBF values ($>13$ ml/100 g/min) that demonstrated normal flow on follow-up CT. In the recanalized patients, however, emergency embolectomy had a salvaging effect in the cortex where CBF values ranged from 7 to 12 ml/100 g/min.

Hughes et al. (6) performed Xe/CT CBF mapping within the first 8 hours after the onset of symptoms in seven patients with cerebral infarction. Three patients with very low blood flow ($<10$ ml/100 g/min) had no clinical improvement after admission, and follow-up CT in these patients confirmed infarction in the area of very low flow. Three patients with moderate flow reductions (15–45 ml/100 g/min) had significant spontaneous clinical improvement with normal follow-up CT findings. One patient had increased blood flow (hyperemia) after stroke and made no clinical recovery.

In our study, in addition to large ROIs in the cortical mantle, we placed small ROIs in the posterior internal capsule to evaluate CBF in the region of the lenticulostriate arteries. We concluded that in the patients with diffuse, severely low local CBF values ($<10$ ml/100 g/min), acute reperfusion of ischemic tissues increased the likelihood of massive hemorrhagic transformation and exacerbation of cerebral edema. The patients with profound loss of flow ($<10$ ml/100 g/min) to the lenticulostriate arteries made no clinical recovery, as defined by follow-up CT studies showing infarction in those regions. Emergency embolectomy had a salvaging effect in the cortex when CBF values there ranged from 7 to 12 ml/100 g/min.

## REFERENCES

1. Yoshimoto T, Ogawa A, Seki H, Kogure T, Suzuki J. Clinical course of acute middle cerebral artery occlusion. *J Neurosurg* 1986;65:326–330.
2. Houkin K, Ueno K, Tada M, Ibahara H. Spontaneous arterial recanalization in the acute stage of cerebral infarction. *Neurol Med Chir (Toyko)* 1988;28:1163–1169.
3. Meyer FB, Piepgras DG, Sundt TM, Yanagihara T. Emergency embolectomy for acute occlusion of the middle cerebral artery. *J Neurosurg* 1985;62:639–647.
4. Shimada T, Kaneko M, Tanaka K, Sugiura M. A clinical study of major stroke cases of a low-perfusion pattern on a dynamic CT scan. *Progress in CT (Tokyo)* 1986;8:529–535.
5. Kitami K, Tsuchida H, Sohma T, Hamajima I, Sakamaki Y, Takeda T. Emergency embolectomy for embolic occlusion of the middle cerebral artery. *Neurol Surg (Tokyo)* 1988;16:977–982.
6. Hughes RL, Yonas H, Gur D, Latchaw R. Cerebral blood flow determination within the first 8 hours of cerebral infarction using stable xenon-enhanced computed tomography. *Stroke* 1989;20: 754–760.

*Cerebral Blood Flow Measurement with Stable Xenon-Enhanced Computed Tomography,* edited by Howard Yonas. Raven Press, Ltd., New York © 1992.

# Cerebral Blood Flow Determination Within the First Eight Hours of Cerebral Infarction

Richard L. Hughes, *Howard Yonas, **David Gur, and **Richard Latchaw

*Department of Neurology, Ochsner Clinic, 1514 Jefferson Highway, New Orleans, Louisiana 70121; and Departments of *Neurological Surgery and **Radiology, University of Pittsburgh School of Medicine, 3459 Fifth Avenue, Pittsburgh, Pennsylvania 15213*

The lack of a practical method to determine the size, cause, and prognosis of an acute neurologic deficit during the first few hours after onset has been a major problem in clinical trials of treatments for stroke. Even after extensive evaluation during a patient's clinical course, the mechanism, size, and location of an ischemic injury often remain uncertain (1).

We reviewed xenon-enhanced computed tomography (Xe/CT) scans obtained within the first 8 hours after a hemispheric cerebral infarction in six patients and a progressive brainstem infarction in one patient. A standardized Xe/CT system integrated in a GE 9800 CT scanner (General Electric Corp., Medical Systems Division, Milwaukee, WI) was used for all seven patients. Xe/CT scanning added approximately 15 minutes to the time required to complete a conventional CT scan, and cerebral blood flow (CBF) maps were available within 15 minutes after the study was completed. By altering the window and level (equal to local [L] CBF in ml/100 g/min) settings on the CT terminal, areas of normal and abnormal CBF were identified in minutes.

The 2-cm regions of interest (ROIs), selected when the Xe/CT studies were obtained, were reviewed retrospectively and have representative and reproducible CBF values. Regions of physiologically low CBF due to excessive amounts of cerebrospinal fluid were appropriately identified using the corresponding CT image. These regions were excluded from analysis.

## CASE REPORTS

Table 1 gives a clinical summary of the seven cases. The following are reports on two of them.

Case 1: A 66-year-old right-handed woman had undergone bilateral carotid endarterectomies 11 years earlier and had a right superficial temporal artery-to-

**TABLE 1.** *Clinical summary of seven cases of cerebral infarction studied by Xe/CT*

| Case | Age (yrs)/sex | Deficit | Hours to CT and Xe/CT | LCBF (ml/100 g/min) | Follow-up CT Results | Day | Improvement at discharge |
|------|---------------|---------|-----------------------|---------------------|----------------------|-----|--------------------------|
| 1 | 66/F | R hemiplegia, R hemianopsia, aphasia | 4 | <10 | + | 3 | No |
| 2 | 67/M | Quadriparesis | 2 | <10 | + | 14 | No |
| 3 | 60/F | L hemiplegia, dysconjugate gaze | 1 | <5 | + | 7 | No |
| 4 | 71/M | L hemiplegia | 2 | 14–44 | NA | | Yes |
| 5 | 65/F | L hemiplegia, L hemianopsia | 1 | 17–27 | – | 7 | Yes |
| 6 | 62/M | R hemiparesis, aphasia | 3 | 32–61 | – | 11 | Yes |
| 7 | 70/F | R hemiparesis | 8 | 67–113 | NA | | No |

R, right; L, left; +, positive; −, negative; NA, not available.

middle cerebral artery bypass 4 years after that. She was admitted to our hospital for two left-hemisphere transient ischemic attacks (TIAs). An angiogram demonstrated bilateral carotid stenosis. Preoperative CT and Xe/CT scans showed evidence of an old right-hemispheric infarction.

Immediately after a left-sided carotid endarterectomy, she had hemiplegia and homonymous hemianopsia on the right side. A Xe/CT scan was obtained in conjunction with the CT study within 4 hours of her admission to the recovery room. It demonstrated LCBF values of 3 to 6 ml/100 g/min in ROIs within the territories of the left middle and anterior cerebral arteries (Fig. 1A, B). The posterior temporal and parietal cortex overlying these areas had higher LCBF values (>20 ml/100 g/min).

Initially alert, she worsened over the next few days and had signs of herniation on postoperative day 3. Regions that had CBF values of <10 ml/100 g/min had reduced CT attenuation consistent with infarction (Fig. 1C, D). Although the signs of herniation resolved, she remained hemiplegic and aphasic. She was discharged to a nursing home.

Case 7: A 70-year-old right-handed woman had three brief hemispheric TIAs and underwent a left-sided carotid endarterectomy with electroencephalographic monitoring. In the recovery room, she had weakness on her right side and therefore underwent reoperation. A fresh thrombus was removed from the area of the original surgical procedure. A CT image obtained within 8 hours after the first endarterectomy demonstrated only an old left frontoparietal infarction. Xe/CT, however, demonstrated abnormally high CBF of 113 ml/100 g/min in cortical regions of the left middle cerebral artery; CBF values in similar areas of the right

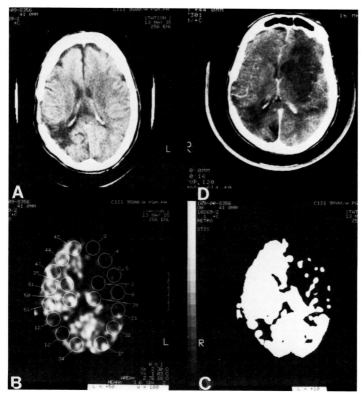

**FIG. 1.** Case 1. **(A)** Conventional CT demonstrating vague decrease in density within left hemispheric white matter. **(B)** Xe/CT 4 hours after infarction showing blood flow in 2-cm regions of interest in ml/100 g/min. **(C)** Xe/CT gray scale adjusted to the level of 10 ml/100 g/min; areas of very low blood flow (<10 ml/100 g/min) appear black. **(D)** Follow-up CT scan on postoperative day 3.

hemisphere were 41 to 76 ml/100 g/min. When discharged, she was able to work but could not move her right arm.

## DISCUSSION

The patterns and absolute LCBF values in these seven patients fall into three categories (Table 2). Case 1 represents the first category (cases 1–3): patients whose Xe/CT CBF study showed cortical regions with CBF values of <10 ml/100 g/min, whose follow-up CT studies showed infarction in those regions, and who had clinically severe and irreversible deficits corresponding to those regions. Similar correlations between LCBF values of <10 to 15 ml/100 g/min and irreversible infarction were found in a study using positron-emission tomography

**TABLE 2.** *Cases of cerebral infarction studied by Xe/CT, categorized by local CBF*

| Category | LCBF (ml/100 g/min) | Follow-up CT Results | n | Clinical improvement |
|---|---|---|---|---|
| I (n = 3) | <10 | + | 1 | No |
| II (n = 3) | 14–61 | − | 2 | Yes |
| III (n = 1) | 67–113 | NA | | No |

LCBF, local cerebral blood flow in appropriate anatomic area; +, positive; −, negative; NA, not available.

(PET) (2) and in experimental measurements of CBF and metabolism that repeatedly found a CBF threshold ≤8 ml/100 g/min for the viability of brain tissue (3,4).

Cases 4 to 6 constitute the second category: patients who had normal or low LCBF values, no evidence of low-density areas on follow-up CT scans, and a better clinical outcome. These patients probably had an ischemic insult that was less severe and/or of shorter duration. It is possible that CT scanning later would have demonstrated their infarctions. Nevertheless, although very few PET studies have been obtained during the initial hours after infarction, PET scans obtained within 48 hours after stroke onset also indicate that these patients generally have a more favorable course (5).

Case 7 was our only example of a third category: patients whose CBF values are significantly higher than normal, suggesting that reperfusion occurred after a significant ischemic challenge (6). Higher-than-normal CBF values indicate an absolute "luxury perfusion," wherein blood flow probably far exceeds metabolic need. Acute hyperemia was associated with severe neurologic deficits when accompanied by reperfusion in animals that died with "large infarcts and considerable swelling of the brain" (7). In one clinical series, however, the delayed appearance of low-density areas on CT images did not consistently follow cortical hyperemia (6). The prognostic significance of identifying a cortical region with such high CBF values remains unclear.

Two important observations can be made from our initial series. One is that CBF examinations can be performed within the first few hours after stroke onset. Because the Xe/CT method uses a CT scanner, this study can be done immediately after the emergency CT scan excludes a mass lesion or intracranial hemorrhage as the cause of a neurologic deficit. The other observation is that Xe/CT can record very low LCBF values (<10 ml/100 g/min), even in small and centrally located brain regions. Experience with animal models (8) and with clinical cases of focal cerebral ischemia (9–11) and brain death (12) suggests that this technology can record the very low LCBF values that consistently are accompanied by irreversible infarction.

Without a well-defined therapy for stroke, it is difficult to state the clinical implications of being able to identify regions that progress within several hours from ischemia to having essentially no, low-normal, or high blood flow. Many current strategies for stroke therapy involve efforts to increase CBF. Those most likely to benefit from such CBF augmentation probably include the group with low-normal CBF and perhaps persons who have infarctions with a surrounding ischemic penumbra (i.e., a significant area of low CBF). On the other hand, the late reintroduction of CBF to infarcted tissues with essentially no viability cannot be clinically beneficial and carries the risk of hemorrhagic transformation or exacerbation of cerebral edema. Efforts to augment CBF in an already hyperemic region obviously can be of no value. Thus, as treatments for stroke are being examined clinically, the inclusion of CBF determinations in the study protocol could clarify which patients are likely to benefit.

## REFERENCES

1. Kunitz SC, Gross CR, Heyman A, et al. The Pilot Stroke Data Bank: definition, design, data. *Stroke* 1984;15:740–746.
2. Powers WJ, Grubb RL, Raichle ME. Physiological response to focal cerebral ischemia in humans. *Ann Neurol* 1984;16:546-552.
3. Bell BA, Symon L, Branston NM. CBF and time thresholds for the formation of ischemic cerebral edema, and effect of reperfusion in baboons. *J Neurosurg* 1985;62:31–41.
4. Jones TH, Moraiwetz RB, Crowell RM, et al. Threshold of focal cerebral ischemia in awake monkeys. *J Neurosurg* 1981;54:773–782.
5. Hakim AM, Pokrupa RP, Villanueva J, et al. The effect of spontaneous reperfusion on metabolic function in early human cerebral infarcts. *Ann Neurol* 1987;21:279–289.
6. Olson TS, Lassen NA. A dynamic concept of middle cerebral artery occlusion and cerebral infarction in the acute state based on interpreting severe hyperemia as a sign of embolic migration. *Stroke* 1984;15:458–468.
7. Heiss WD, Hayakawa T, Waltz AG. Patterns of changes of blood flow and relationships to infarction in experimental cerebral ischemia. *Stroke* 1976;7:454–459.
8. Yonas H, Gur D, Claassen D, Wolfson SK Jr, Moossy J. Stable xenon enhanced computed tomography in the study of clinical and pathologic correlates of focal ischemia in baboons. *Stroke* 1988;19:228–238.
9. Yonas H, Wolfson SK Jr, Gur D, et al. Clinical experience with the use of xenon-enhanced CT blood flow mapping in cerebral vascular disease. *Stroke* 1984;15:443–450.
10. Yonas H, Good WF, Gur D, et al. Mapping cerebral blood flow by xenon-enhanced tomography: clinical experience. *Radiology* 1984;152:435–442.
11. Meyer JS, Okayasu H, Tachibana H, Okabe T. Stable xenon CT CBF measurements in prevalent cerebrovascular disease (stroke). *Stroke* 1984;15:80–90.
12. Darby JM, Yonas H, Gur D, Latchaw RE. Xenon-enhanced computed tomography in brain death. *Arch Neurol* 1987;44:551–554.

*Cerebral Blood Flow Measurement with Stable Xenon-Enhanced Computed Tomography,* edited by Howard Yonas. Raven Press, Ltd., New York © 1992.

# Cerebral Hemodynamics of Occlusive Cerebrovascular Disease

Kimito Tanaka, Yasuhiro Yonekawa, Akira Kobayashi, Yasunobu Gotoh, and Kousuke Yamashita

*Department of Neurosurgery, National Cardiovascular Center, 5-7-1 Fujishiro dai, Suita, Osaka 565, Japan*

Because hemodynamic dysfunction can have a significant influence on the natural course of occlusive cerebrovascular disease, investigations of cerebral hemodynamics can yield important clinical information. Several types of studies have been developed to analyze hemodynamic status, including positron-emission tomography (PET) (1–5). This chapter explains why we find the xenon-enhanced computed tomographic cerebral blood flow (Xe/CT CBF) method coupled with dynamic CT more clinically useful for such analyses than single-photon emission computed tomography using N-isopropyl-(p)-[$^{123}$I]-iodoamphetamine (IMP-SPECT).

## SUBJECTS AND METHODS

We conducted a study of 19 patients with chronic occlusive cerebrovascular disease who had not had an ischemic attack for more than 3 months (Table 1). We used Xe/CT to calculate their CBF. To obtain mean transit time (MTT), we used dynamic CT. Cerebral blood volume (CBV) was calculated by multiplying CBF by MTT. We also evaluated vascular reactivity by measuring CBF after giving patients an intravenous injection of acetazolamide (10 mg/kg up to 1 g). We then classified patients according to cerebral hemodynamic status as estimated by Xe/CT and dynamic CT (Table 2). Finally, we performed IMP-

TABLE 1. *Cerebrovascular disease in the 19 study subjects*

|  | Number of patients |
|---|---|
| Internal carotid artery occlusion | 4 |
| Internal carotid artery stenosis | 4 |
| Middle cerebral artery occlusion | 3 |
| Middle cerebral artery stenosis | 1 |
| Moya Moya disease | 7 |

**TABLE 2.** *Classification of hemodynamic status in relation to delayed IMP-SPECT findings*

| Hemodynamic status | Xenon and dynamic CT findings | | | | Re-uptake image on IMP-SPECT |
| --- | --- | --- | --- | --- | --- |
| | Regional CBF | Reactivity to acetazolamide | MTT | CBV | |
| Group 1 | Normal or slightly reduced | Impaired | Prolonged | Slightly increased | Complete |
| Group 2 | Slightly or moderately reduced | Impaired | Prolonged | Normal or slightly reduced | Incomplete |
| Group 3 | Moderately or severely reduced | Impaired | Prolonged | Reduced | Incomplete |

MTT, mean transit time; CBV, cerebral blood volume.

SPECT to obtain both early and delayed images for evaluating the degree of tracer redistribution in the hemodynamically compromised region. The early and delayed scans were taken 30 minutes and 4 hours, respectively, after IMP administration.

## ILLUSTRATIVE CASES

Case 1 (hemodynamic status, group 1): A 46-year-old man was suffering from left-sided hemiparesis. CT demonstrated small low-density areas in the right

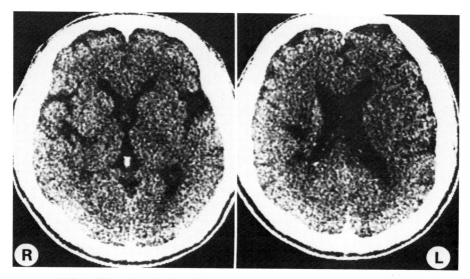

**FIG. 1.** This patient had small low-density areas in the right hemisphere (**R**).

R                                                                    L

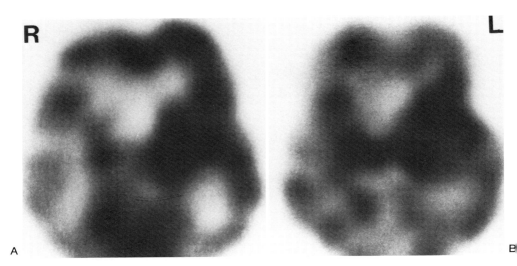

A                                                                    B

**FIG. 2.** Early (**A**) and delayed (**B**) IMP-SPECT images revealed a complete re-uptake in the right hemisphere (**R**).

hemisphere (Fig. 1), and cerebral angiography showed an occlusion of the right middle cerebral artery (MCA). Both early and delayed SPECT images revealed a complete re-uptake of IMP in the right hemisphere (Fig. 2). The Xe/CT study found CBF to be normal in the right MCA territory; the flow decreased after the patient received acetazolamide (Fig. 3). In the corresponding MCA territory, MTT was prolonged and CBV slightly increased.

Case 2 (hemodynamic status, group 2): A 50-year-old man had left-sided hemiparesis and left-sided homonymous hemianopsia. Upon admission to the hospital, CT demonstrated multiple low-density areas in the right hemisphere (Fig. 4). Cerebral angiography revealed occlusion of the right internal carotid artery, with its distal territory being supplied by the external carotid artery via the ophthalmic artery. Re-uptake of IMP was incomplete in the right hemisphere (Fig. 5). Xe/CT showed slightly decreased CBF and a steal phenomenon in the MCA territory after the administration of acetazolamide (Fig. 6A, B). The MTT was prolonged and CBV reduced in the right MCA territory (Fig. 6C, D).

Case 3 (hemodynamic status, group 3): A 67-year-old man had right-sided hemiparesis associated with dysarthria. CT showed low densities in the left hemisphere (Fig. 7). Occlusion of the left internal carotid artery and multiple stenotic lesions in the major arteries were evident on angiograms. IMP-SPECT revealed an incomplete re-uptake in the left frontotemporal region (Fig. 8). Xe/CT indicated severely decreased CBF (Fig. 9A) and a steal phenomenon in the frontotemporo-parietal region after the administration of acetazolamide (Fig. 9B). The MTT was prolonged (Fig. 9C) and CBV accordingly decreased in that region (Fig. 9D).

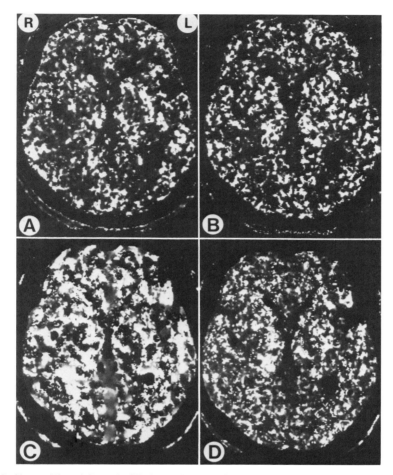

**FIG. 3.** Xenon (**A**) and dynamic CT showed normal CBF values with impaired CBF reactivity to acetazolamide (**B**), prolonged mean transit time (**C**), and slightly increased cerebral blood volume (**D**) in the right MCA territory. R, right hemisphere; L, left hemisphere.

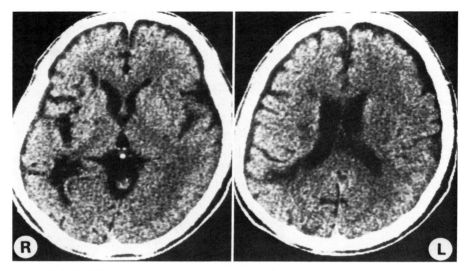

**FIG. 4.** This patient had multiple low-density areas in the right hemisphere (**R**).

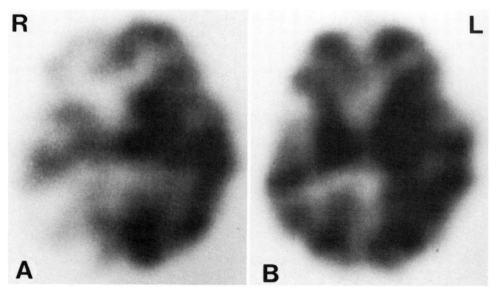

**FIG. 5.** Early (**A**) and delayed (**B**) IMP-SPECT images revealed an incomplete re-uptake of IMP in the right hemisphere (**R**).

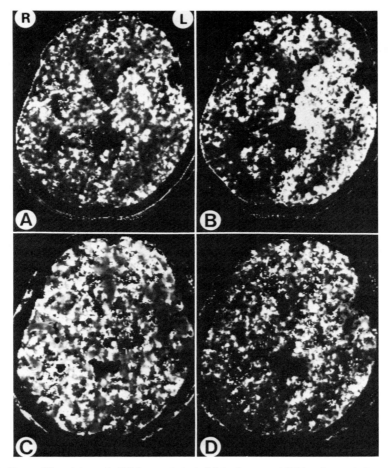

**FIG. 6.** Xenon (**A**) and dynamic CT demonstrated slightly decreased CBF and a steal phenomenon after the administration of acetazolamide (**B**), prolonged mean transit time (**C**), and reduced cerebral blood volume (**D**) in the right MCA territory. R, right hemisphere; L, left hemisphere.

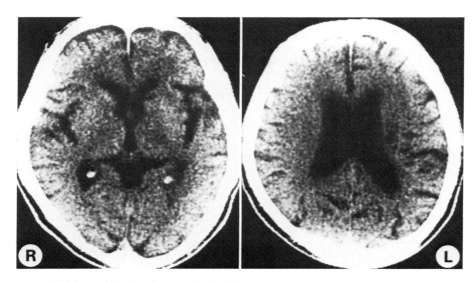

**FIG. 7.** CT showed low-density spots in the left hemisphere in this patient. R, right hemisphere; L, left hemisphere.

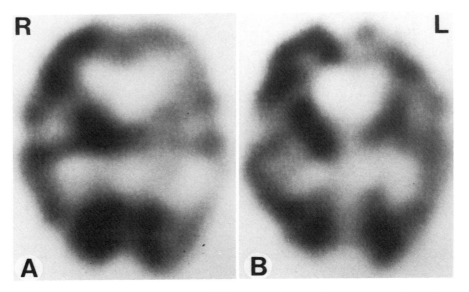

**FIG. 8.** Early (**A**) and delayed (**B**) IMP-SPECT showed an incomplete re-uptake in the left frontotemporal region. R, right; L, left.

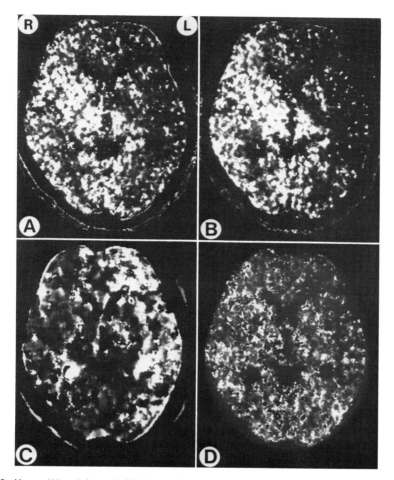

**FIG. 9.** Xenon (**A**) and dynamic CT showed remarkably decreased CBF and a steal phenomenon after the administration of acetazolamide (**B**). Mean transit time was prolonged (**C**), and cerebral blood volume decreased (**D**) in the frontotemporo-parietal region. R, right hemisphere; L, left hemisphere.

## DISCUSSION

It is generally believed that re-uptake of the contrast material on delayed IMP-SPECT images qualitatively indicates the viability of the ischemic tissue, which can be an important criterion in selecting candidates for surgical treatment (5). But because both groups 2 and 3 were characterized by incomplete IMP re-uptake, IMP-SPECT alone could not distinguish the degree of hemodynamic compromise. By providing a quantitative assessment of physiological parameters, expressed by the CBF, CBV, MTT, and CBF response to acetazolamide, Xe/CT

CBF and dynamic CT studies enable analysis of the hemodynamic compromise in the region in question. We thus conclude that Xe/CT and dynamic CT scanning produce enough information to assess hemodynamic dysfunction and that the results are more accurate and detailed than obtainable with IMP-SPECT alone.

## REFERENCES

1. Powers WJ, Grubb RL, Raichle ME. Physiological responses to focal cerebral ischemia in humans. *Ann Neurol* 1984;16:546–552.
2. Gibbs JM, Wise RJS, Leenders KL, Jones T. Evaluation of cerebral perfusion reserve in patients with carotid artery occlusion. *Lancet* 1984;11:310–314.
3. Gibbs JM, Wise RJS, Leenders KL, Herold S, Frackowiak RSJ, Jones T. Cerebral hemodynamics in occlusive carotid artery disease. *Lancet* 1985;20:933–934.
4. Powers WJ, Press GA, Grubb RL, Gado M, Raichle ME. The effect of hemodynamically significant carotid artery disease on the hemodynamic status of the cerebral circulation. *Ann Intern Med* 1987;106:27–35.
5. Kanno I, Uemura K, Higano S, et al. Oxygen extraction fraction at maximally vasodilated tissue in the ischemic brain estimated from the regional $CO_2$ responsiveness measured by positron emission tomography. *J Cereb Blood Flow Metab* 1988;8:227–235.

*Cerebral Blood Flow Measurement with Stable Xenon-Enhanced Computed Tomography,* edited by Howard Yonas. Raven Press, Ltd., New York © 1992.

# Comparison of Color-Coded Xenon-Enhanced Computed Tomography and Angiography in Cerebrovascular Disease

Hartmut Becker, Thomas Berger, Bernd Haubitz, *Michael R. Gaab, *Kurt Holl, *Mohammad-Nabi Nemati, and *Hermann Dietz

*Departments of Neuroradiology and *Neurosurgery, Hannover School of Medicine, Konstanty-Gutschow-Straße 8, D-3000 Hannover 61, Germany*

Thromboembolic cerebrovascular disease has been difficult to distinguish from cerebrovascular insufficiency. Nevertheless, the distinction is important because of the consequences of treatment. In patients with hemodynamic insufficiency, the use of an intraluminal shunt is warranted during carotid thromboendarterectomy. Evidence of hemodynamic deficiency also may indicate extra-intracranial bypass surgery (1). Before the introduction of the stable xenon/computed tomography cerebral blood flow (Xe/CT CBF) method, cerebral angiography was considered the most useful procedure to determine whether cerebrovascular disease was of thromboembolic or hemodynamic origin. Our study was designed to compare the accuracy of cerebral angiography and stable Xe/CT CBF monitoring in the diagnosis of these two disorders.

We performed Xe/CT CBF studies on a GE 9800 scanner using the commercially available xenon hardware and software system. At the beginning of our investigations, the flow maps were displayed on a monitor in 16 gray tones from black to white and documented on multiformat film with a fixed level of 50 Hounsfield units (HU) and a fixed window of 100 HU. Later we used a color-coded flow map created by transforming the gray tones into a color scale corresponding to the natural color spectrum from violet to white. Colors correlated with CBF in ml/100 g/minute: violet = 0 ml, blue = 25 ml, green = 50 ml, red = 75 ml, and white = 100 ml and above. The color-coded flow maps were displayed on a color monitor and printed with a color plotter (Delta Scan CH-5301) (2).

Such color images offer a diagnostic advantage over the black-and-white ones used previously. For instance, the color method enables better differentiation of flow levels, especially in regions of extremely low CBF. Areas of extremely high CBF are also more identifiable. With the increased color gradations, small differences in CBF are simply recognized more easily. In addition, the degree of

**TABLE 1.** *Angiographic findings in the two study groups*

|  | Thromboembolic patients (n = 40) Number (%) | Hemodynamic patients (n = 28) Number (%) |
|---|---|---|
| Occlusion & stenosis | 8 (20) | 23 (82) |
| Multiple-vessel stenoses | 19 (48) | 19 (68) |
| One-vessel stenosis | 9 (23) | 1 (4) |
| Collaterals[a] | 1 (3) | 13 (46) |
| Ulceration | 8 (20) | 11 (39) |

[a] Ophthalmic artery, anterior and posterior communicating arteries, parenchymal and leptomeningeal collaterals.

CBF alteration can be readily determined, especially in follow-up studies before and after the administration of acetazolamide (Diamox).

To differentiate between thromboembolic and hemodynamic causes, we established an angiographic rating of diagnostic criteria in 68 patients (recognizing, of course, that CBF alterations can have a combination of these two causes). We assigned 40 patients to the thromboembolic group and 28 to the hemodynamic group (Table 1). In the thromboembolic group, 23% of the patients had single-vessel stenosis, far more than in the hemodynamic group. On the other hand, patients in the hemodynamic group had more multiple stenoses, and a combination of occlusion with stenosis was found in 82%, four times the incidence in the thromboembolic group.

We compared the results of cerebral angiography with those of stable Xe/CT CBF studies for all 68 patients. After determining resting CBF with a control study, we gave patients 1 g of acetazolamide intravenously and then performed another Xe/CT CBF study. Because acetazolamide normally stimulates CBF increases (3–6), it enabled us to determine the cerebral reserve capacity. A reduced cerebral reserve capacity indicates a hemodynamic insufficiency.

Unilateral carotid stenosis usually did not significantly decrease the CBF or the cerebrovascular reserve capacity. The presence of clinical symptoms in such patients thus suggests a thromboembolic cause. Nevertheless, some patients with stenosis of only the internal carotid artery were assigned to the thromboembolic group based on angiography but were later found to have a hemodynamic insufficiency with Xe/CT CBF studies (Fig. 1). In patients with multiple stenotic and/or occlusive vascular lesions, we often saw a reduction of the cerebrovascular reserve capacity as a sign of hemodynamic insufficiency. Some of these patients had normal resting CBF. In contrast, some patients with an occlusion on one side of the internal carotid artery and stenosis on the other had both normal CBF values at rest and a normal reserve capacity after stimulation (Fig. 2).

In comparing the angiographic and Xe/CT CBF results, we found more hemodynamic insufficiencies with Xe/CT CBF (Fig. 3). Thirteen patients who had been assigned to the thromboembolic group based on angiographic findings were transferred to the hemodynamic group after we examined their Xe/CT CBF

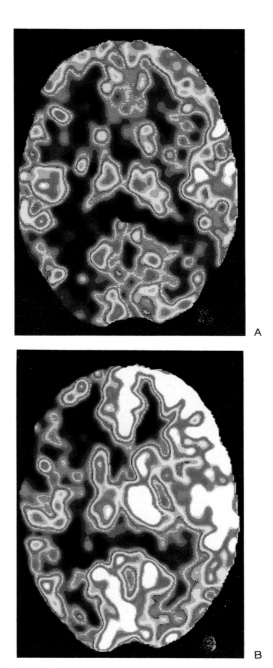

**FIG. 1.** Xe/CT in a patient with unilateral high-grade stenosis of the right internal carotid artery shows reduced cerebral blood flow at rest (**A**) and reduced cerebral reserve capacity of the right hemisphere after stimulation with acetazolamide (**B**).

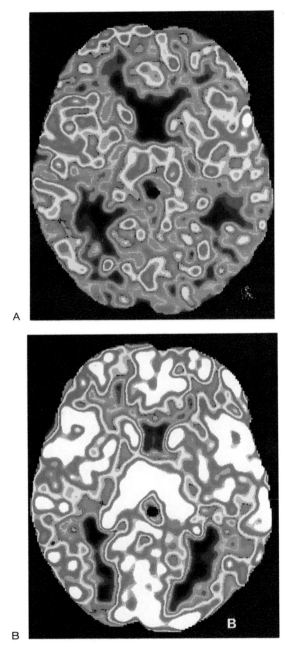

**FIG. 2.** This patient had occlusion of the left internal carotid artery and stenosis of the right internal carotid artery. Xe/CT shows normal resting cerebral blood flow (**A**) and normal cerebrovascular reserve capacity (**B**).

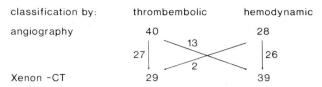

**FIG. 3.** Angiographically defined symptoms in patients classified as hemodynamic or thromboembolic on the basis of Xe/CT cerebral blood flow studies.

results. Only two patients in the hemodynamic group were classified as thromboembolic after the Xe/CT study. These findings confirm that a single stenotic vessel usually correlates with a thromboembolic cause of the cerebrovascular disease, whereas patients with vascular occlusion tend to have more hemodynamic disturbances. We found that angiography was not as successful as the Xe/CT CBF method in differentiating between these two groups.

We conclude that cerebral angiography alone cannot differentiate between a thromboembolic and hemodynamic cause of cerebrovascular disease. Nevertheless, a definite distinction between these causes is possible with Xe/CT CBF studies. The Xe/CT CBF method provides important information that angiography does not. This information is especially useful in surgical planning.

## REFERENCES

1. Gaab MR, Holl K, Nemati MN, Rzesacz E, Becker H, Dietz H. Mapping of rCBF and cerebrovascular reserve capacity by stable xenon CT in cerebrovascular disease: pathophysiological aspects and effects of operative therapy. *Psychiatry Res* 1989;29:309-312.
2. Becker H, Haubitz B, Gaab M, Holl K, Nemati MN, Dietz H. Optimized demonstration of cerebral blood flow with colour coded xenon CT. In: Nadjmi M, ed. *XVth Congress of the European Society of Neuroradiology.* Würzburg, September 13–17, 1988. Berlin: Springer-Verlag, 1989: 509–512.
3. Kreisig T, Schmiedek P, Leinsinger G, Einhäupl K, Moser E. [133]Xe-DSPECT: normal values of resting cerebral blood flow and reserve capacity. *Nuklearmedizin* 1987;26:192-197.
4. Majewski A, Holl K, Nemati MN, Gaab MR, Dietz H, Becker H. The cerebral circulation in xenon-CT. *Rontgenpraxis* 1988;41:311–318.
5. Rogg J, Rutigliano M, Yonas H, Johnson DW, Pentheny S, Latchaw RE. The acetazolamide challenge: imaging techniques designed to evaluate cerebral blood flow reserve. *AJNR* 1989;10: 803–810.
6. Sullivan HG, Kingsbury TB, Morgan ME, et al. The rCBF response to Diamox in normal subjects and cerebrovascular disease patients. *J Neurosurg* 1987;67:525–534.

*Cerebral Blood Flow Measurement with Stable Xenon-Enhanced Computed Tomography,* edited by Howard Yonas. Raven Press, Ltd., New York © 1992.

# Stable Xenon-Enhanced Computed Tomography in Moya Moya Disease: A Case Study Using the Calcium Channel Blocker Nifedipine

Kathleen Hurwitz, Stephen Ashwal, Lawrence Tomasi, Sanford Schneider, and *Joseph Thompson

*Departments of Pediatrics and *Radiation Sciences, Loma Linda University School of Medicine, Loma Linda, California 92350*

Moya Moya disease is a cerebrovascular disorder characterized by progressive occlusion of the distal internal carotid and proximal cerebral arteries. The classic angiographic findings are these occlusions and anastomotic networks of vessels (1). Clinical findings include seizures, hemiparesis, loss of vision, and progressive intellectual deterioration. Although surgical and medical treatment modalities have offered some improvement, the prognosis is poor, especially in children under 2 years of age (2).

Direct and indirect extracranial-to-intracranial anastomoses via various neurosurgical procedures have led to the best outcome in these patients (3). The progressive nature of the disease, however, limits the long-term success of surgical correction. Medical treatment with a calcium channel blocker (verapamil) has also been described; the drug-induced vasodilation resulted in clinical improvement in one 7-year-old patient (4).

We examined cerebral perfusion using the stable xenon-enhanced computed tomography cerebral blood flow (Xe/CT CBF) method in a 10-month-old girl with Moya Moya disease. We also studied the changes in CBF during hyperventilation to determine if flow would reach ischemic thresholds in different brain regions. In addition, we measured CBF before and after the administration of the calcium channel blocker nifedipine to determine whether this drug would help to increase CBF.

## CASE HISTORY

J.N. was first seen at 4 months of age for failure to thrive. At 7 months of age, she had acute left-sided hemiplegia, though it improved over the next month.

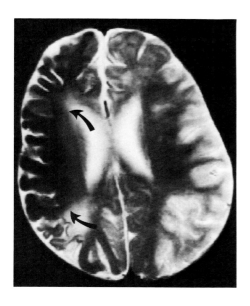

**FIG. 1.** Axial T$_2$-weighted spin echo magnetic resonance image at upper lateral ventricular level. Overall signal is inhomogeneous with the low signal (*dark areas*) caused by the paramagnetic effects of hemorrhagic infarctions from a combination of old and recent ischemic insults. Right frontal and parietal regions (*arrows*) have low signal due largely to deoxyhemoglobin. Computed tomography showed petechial hemorrhagic densities in the same area.

When 9 months old, she had left-sided and then right-sided seizures, followed several days later by a dense hemiplegia on the right side. When examined, she was found to be lethargic with right-sided hemiplegia and hemianopsia. Her CT scan demonstrated a subacute right frontotemporal infarction with acute petechial changes and an acute left hemispheric infarction. Magnetic resonance images (MRI) were somewhat unusual in appearance, thought to be related to the petechial hemorrhage and confirmed the acute ischemic injury on the left (Fig. 1).

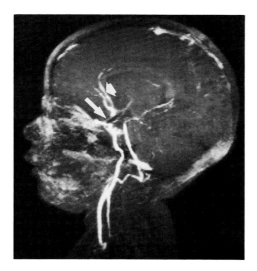

**FIG. 2.** Sagittal magnetic resonance angiographic findings, later confirmed with conventional angiography. Compare the small distal supraclinoid internal carotid artery segment (*arrow*) to the pericallosal artery (*arrow head*). This marked distal internal carotid artery tapering was present bilaterally.

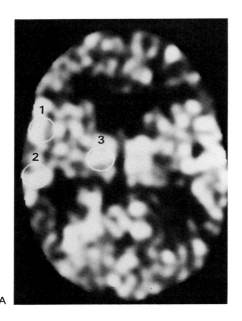

A

**FIG. 3A.** Xenon/CT cerebral blood flow map from baseline study, performed 7 days after magnetic resonance angiogram, at the level of the frontal horns in the same plane. Regions of interest labeled *1*, *2*, and *3* show increased flows of 63, 70, and 62 ml/100 g/min, respectively, at a $pCO_2$ of 39 torr. Note some peripheral areas of flow inhomogeneity and poor correlation with areas of insult seen on magnetic resonance image 7 days earlier (Fig. 1).

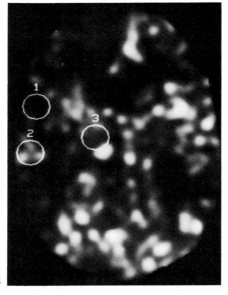

B

**FIG. 3B.** Xenon/CT cerebral blood flow map at a location identical to that in Fig. 3A after adequate xenon wash-out and at a $pCO_2$ of 25 torr. Identical regions of interest *1*, *2*, and *3* now have flows measuring 8, 28, and 21 ml/100 g/min, respectively. In addition to this dramatic response to hyperventilation, note the relatively greater flow reduction ($CO_2$ response) in the right frontal lobe (anterior to region of interest *1*) and the right temporal lobe (dorsal to region of interest *2*). Also see Tables 1 and 3.

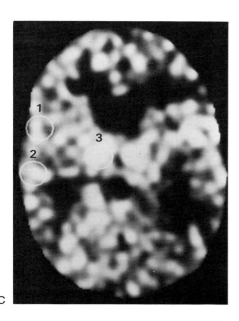

C

**FIG. 3C.** Xenon/CT cerebral blood flow map at a location identical to that in Figs. 3A, B after adequate xenon wash-out and at a $pCO_2$ of 41 torr. Now flow in the same regions of interest *1*, *2*, and *3* post-nifedipine measures 54, 60, and 76 ml/100 g/min, respectively. Overall hemispheric flows show some improvement. See Tables 2 and 3.

Magnetic resonance angiography (Fig. 2) and cerebral angiography confirmed a diagnosis of Moya Moya disease.

## METHODS

We performed Xe/CT CBF studies using the General Electric 9800 xenon blood flow system with the patient breathing a 33% nonradioactive xenon/oxygen mixture (Linde XeScan stable xenon in oxygen USP, Union Carbide Rare Gases, Specialty Medical Products, Danbury, CT) (5). Over a period of 4 minutes, we obtained images in three planes, 1 cm apart, to visualize the upper brainstem, subcortical nuclei, and cortex. Flow values (ml/100 g/min) were determined with the region-of-interest cursor for the subacutely infarcted right hemisphere and the acutely infarcted left hemisphere and the following regions: frontal gray and white matter; temporal, parietal, and occipital gray matter; thalamus; caudate nucleus; midbrain; and cerebellar cortex.

The patient underwent three Xe/CT CBF studies over 2 hours (Fig. 3): one before hyperventilation ($pCO_2$ = 39 torr), one after hyperventilation for 20 minutes ($pCO_2$ = 25 torr), and another 30 minutes later ($pCO_2$ = 41 torr) after 0.16 mg/kg nifedipine was administered sublingually in increments of 0.4 mg/kg. The patient had been intubated electively before the study and sedated with midazolam (Versed) (0.1 mg/kg). We monitored her blood pressure and pulse every 3 minutes throughout the study and began the post-nifedipine Xe/CT CBF study when her systolic blood pressure decreased.

## RESULTS

### Baseline Global and Regional CBF ($pCO_2 = 39$)

Table 1 lists global and regional CBF values. The patient's global CBF was low but still within the normal range for her age. Her regional CBF varied; flow was slightly low in the frontal gray and white matter, temporal gray matter, and caudate nuclei. Despite the early cerebral atrophy and subacute infarction, flow values were only slightly below normal in the right hemisphere (see Table 3).

### CBF/$CO_2$ Reactivity

After hyperventilation, all regions of the brain showed markedly decreased CBF. Global and regional flow in the frontal gray and frontal white matter had fallen below the ischemic threshold. The change in global CBF/$CO_2$ reactivity was 1.7 ml/100 g/min/torr. Local CBF/$CO_2$ responsiveness varied in different regions, with decreases in CBF ranging from 21% to 68%.

After the administration of nifedipine at a $pCO_2$ of 41 torr, CBF was elevated in most regions, the increase averaging 25% with a range of 9% to 37% (Table 2). In the lenticular nucleus, however, we observed an 8% reduction. Mean arterial blood pressure dropped from 138 to 67 torr. Thus the increased flow was not caused by a passive increase in perfusion due to a loss of autoregulation.

**TABLE 1.** *Regional cerebral blood flow (CBF) before and after hyperventilation*

| | CBF (ml/100 g/min) | | | |
| | Before hyperventilation (ET $pCO_2$ = 39 torr) | After hyperventilation (ET $pCO_2$ = 25 torr) | CBF/torr $CO_2$ (ml/100 g/ min/torr) | % Decrease in CBF |
|---|---|---|---|---|
| Global | 40 | 16 | 1.7 | 60 |
| Frontal gray | 36 | 15 | 1.5 | 58 |
| Frontal white | 19 | 6 | 0.9 | 68 |
| Temporal | 37 | 21 | 1.1 | 43 |
| Parietal | 57 | 22 | 2.5 | 61 |
| Occipital | 43 | 31 | 0.9 | 28 |
| Caudate | 33 | 26 | 0.5 | 21 |
| Thalamic | 65 | 24 | 2.9 | 63 |
| Lenticular | 51 | 29 | 1.6 | 43 |
| Midbrain | 63 | 22 | 2.9 | 65 |
| Cerebellar | 40 | 19 | 1.5 | 53 |

ET, end-tidal.

**TABLE 2.** Regional cerebral blood flow before and after nifedipine administration

| | Blood flow (ml/100 g/min) | | |
| | Before nifedipine | After nifedipine | % Change |
|---|---|---|---|
| Global | 36 | 45 | 25 |
| Frontal gray | 36 | 40 | 11 |
| Frontal white | 19 | 22 | 16 |
| Temporal | 37 | 48 | 23 |
| Parietal | 57 | 56 | -2 |
| Occipital | 43 | 47 | 9 |
| Caudate | 33 | 46 | 21 |
| Thalamic | 65 | 74 | 14 |
| Lenticular | 51 | 47 | -8 |
| Midbrain | 63 | 86 | 37 |
| Cerebellar | 40 | 54 | 35 |
| End-tidal $pCO_2$ | 39[a] | 41[a] | 5 |
| Mean arterial blood pressure | 138[a] | 67[a] | -51 |

[a] Blood flow (mm Hg).

## CBF in the Actively Infarcted versus Previously Subacutely Infarcted Brain Regions

Table 3 compares CBF changes in the left hemisphere regions that were acutely infarcted with those in the previously subacutely infarcted right hemisphere. The CBF control values in both the infarcted and uninfarcted regions were similar, and reduced flow was seen in several areas.

The decrease in CBF after hyperventilation in the previously infarcted right hemisphere showed greater $CBF/CO_2$ reactivity, averaging 56% for the five regions

**TABLE 3.** Effects of hyperventilation and nifedipine on cerebral blood flow (CBF) in acutely infarcted versus previously subacutely infarcted brain regions

| | CBF (ml/100 g/min) | % Decrease in CBF after hyperventilation | % Increase in CBF after nifedipine[a] |
|---|---|---|---|
| Anterior frontal | | | |
| Acute infarct | 33 | 31 | 23 |
| Previous infarct | 27 | 38 | 53 |
| Mid frontal | | | |
| Acute infarct | 35 | 62 | 0 |
| Previous infarct | 39 | 71 | 30 |
| Opercular cortex | | | |
| Acute infarct | 52 | 45 | 0 |
| Previous infarct | 50 | 79 | -5 |
| Subcortical | | | |
| Acute infarct | 49 | 54 | 8 |
| Previous infarct | 49 | 33 | 14 |
| Posterior temporal | | | |
| Acute infarct | 44 | 59 | 3 |
| Previous infarct | 33 | 58 | -2 |

[a] Compared to control CBF.

compared to only 50% in the acutely infarcted left hemisphere. Similarly, after nifedipine administration, the increase in CBF in the previously infarcted areas averaged 18% in the five regions, whereas in the acutely infarcted areas, the increase averaged 7%.

## DISCUSSION

The principal finding of this study was that nifedipine increased CBF an average of 25%. This finding suggests that nifedipine, or other calcium entry blockers more selective for the cerebral circulation, may be clinically useful in the medical treatment of children with Moya Moya disease, either in combination with surgical anastomosis or as primary treatment (4,6). Nevertheless, further controlled studies are needed to determine the efficacy of such agents in treating this disease.

The response to nifedipine varied in different brain regions. The effects were greater in the subcortical regions and posterior circulation than in the more superficial or peripheral cortical regions supplied by the anterior and middle cerebral arteries. This difference may have occurred because these peripheral regions, where flow was already low because of the proximal vascular occlusive disease, were near maximal vasodilation (7). This suggests that calcium entry blockers may have limited pharmacologic benefit in the treatment of Moya Moya disease and that their use in combination with surgical treatment would be more effective.

Most patients with Moya Moya disease suffer bilateral cerebral infarctions during the course of their illness. A patient is thus likely to have infarctions at different stages of insult and/or recovery. Our results showed that nifedipine increased CBF in both the acutely infarcted (7%) and subacutely infarcted (18%) regions, although in some areas, it had no effect or caused a slight reduction in flow ($-2\%$ to $-5\%$). The difference in the effect of nifedipine on the acute and subacute infarctions was not related to the average CBF (43 versus 40 ml/100 g/min). It may have been associated with other phenomena, such as nifedipine's effect on local brain metabolic activity or, perhaps, the presence of more vascular spasm in the acutely infarcted areas of brain resulting from the release of parenchymal vasoconstrictor substances that are less sensitive to the effects of calcium channel blockers. In addition, no correlation was apparent between the response to hyperventilation and the response to nifedipine in the acute versus previously infarcted brain regions. This finding was to be expected, because the mechanisms of vasodilation and constriction for carbon dioxide and the calcium channel blockers are, for the most part, independent.

Another major finding in this study was that hyperventilation reduced global CBF below the presumed ischemic threshold. Some previous studies have shown that CBF may be lower in children with Moya Moya disease (3,7–11), although other investigators have reported abnormally high values (12). CBF has been much lower in patients with cerebral infarction than in those whose symptoms suggest transient ischemic attacks (3,9).

In previous studies, the response to hyperventilation also has been dramatic. Nishimoto et al. (9) demonstrated a 5–36% decrease in global CBF, whereas in this study, we observed a 21–68% decrease in local CBF. Nishimoto's group did not report the $pCO_2$ changes accompanying the reductions in flow. They did, however, make the interesting observation that, in young children, crying was sufficient to induce hypocapnia and precipitate irreversible ischemic symptoms.

Tagawa et al. (12) found the $CBF/CO_2$ response to be 1.3 ml/100 g/min/torr without evidence of regional differences in this response. In contrast, we noted marked variations. The difference in our findings may be related to the technique of CBF measurement. With the Xe/CT method, local measurements of flow are made with good reliability. The fact that the patients in Tagawa's series had high CBF values may explain why hyperventilation did not induce ischemia. These authors also suggested that younger children with Moya Moya disease have more ischemic episodes because they have greater $CBF/CO_2$ reactivity. Nevertheless, this theory was not supported by data in their 20 patients nor in our patient.

In one patient, Takeuchi et al. (7) found a $CBF/CO_2$ response of 2.58 ml/100 g/min/torr (right hemisphere) and 3.13 ml/100 g/min/torr (left hemisphere). Although their data suggest results similar to ours, where hyperventilation decreased peripheral cortical flow of the anterior circulation more than it decreased subcortical flow, they reported that no regional differences were present.

In a recent study of intraoperative continuous measurement of $CBF/CO_2$ reactivity, researchers noted three different responses to hyperventilation, which correlated with angiographic findings: transient reduction in prolonged reduction, and transient increase in CBF (13). Based on that study, it is likely that our patient would manifest a prolonged reduction in CBF in response to hyperventilation. Considering the degree of flow reduction that we observed after hyperventilation in the patient, whose baseline flow was already low, our findings suggest that certain patients with Moya Moya disease may be much more susceptible to ischemic injury with hyperventilation. This effect would result from a combination of low baseline CBF, preservation of $CBF/CO_2$ reactivity even in severely affected patients, and a prolonged response to hyperventilation. Thus, Xe/CT CBF studies may be of value in predicting which patients are at greater risk for further cerebral infarction. Our study also suggests that the Xe/CT CBF method may be beneficial in assessing the effectiveness of specific cerebrovascular vasodilators, such as calcium entry blockers, in the treatment of Moya Moya disease.

## REFERENCES

1. Fukuyama Y, Umezu R. Clinical and cerebral angiographic evolutions of idiopathic occlusive disease of the circle of Willis ("moyamoya" disease) in children. *Brain Dev* 1985;7:21–37.
2. Gordon N, Isler W. Childhood moyamoya disease. *Dev Med Child Neurol* 1989;31:103–107.

 3. Suzuki J, Takaku A, Kodama N, Sato S. An attempt to treat cerebrovascular "moyamoya" disease in children. *Childs Brain* 1975;l:193–206.
 4. McLean MJ, Gebarski SS, van der Spek AF, Goldstein GW. Response of moyamoya disease to verapamil [letter]. *Lancet* 1985;1:163–164.
 5. Ashwal S, Schneider S, Thompson J. Xenon computed tomography measuring cerebral blood flow in the determination of brain death in children. *Ann Neurol* 1989;25:539–546.
 6. Conen D, Ruttimann S, Noll G, Schneider K, Muller J. Short- and long-term cerebrovascular effects of nitrendipine in hypertensive patients. *J Cardiovasc Pharmacol* 1988;12(Suppl 4):S64–68.
 7. Takeuchi S, Tanaka R, Ishii R, Tsuchida T, Kobayashi K, Arai H. Cerebral hemodynamics in patients with moyamoya disease. A study of regional cerebral blood flow by the [133]Xe inhalation method. *Surg Neurol* 1985;23:468–474.
 8. Ebihara S, Gotoh F, Kanda T, et al. Cerebral blood flow and metabolism in moyamoya disease (occlusion of the circle of Willis). *Acta Neurol Scand* 1977;56(Suppl 64):404–405.
 9. Nishimoto A, Onbe H, Ueta K. Clinical and cerebral blood flow study in moyamoya disease with TIA. *Acta Neurol Scand* 1979;60(Suppl 72):434–435.
10. Ishii R, Takeuchi S, Ibayashi K, Tanaka R. Intelligence in children with moyamoya disease: evaluation after surgical treatments with special reference to changes in cerebral blood flow. *Stroke* 1984;15:873–877.
11. Suzuki R, Matsushima Y, Takada Y, Nariai T, Wakabayashi S, Tone O. Changes in cerebral hemodynamics following encephalo-duro-arterio-synangiosis (EDAS) in young patients with moyamoya disease. *Surg Neurol* 1989;31:343–349.
12. Tagawa T, Naritomi H, Mimaki T, Yabuuchi H, Sawada T. Regional cerebral blood flow, clinical manifestations, and age in children with moyamoya disease. *Stroke* 1987;18:906-910.
13. Nakao K, Yamada K, Hayakawa T, et al. Intraoperative measurement of cortical blood flow and its $CO_2$ response in childhood moyamoya disease. *Neurosurgery* 1987;21:509–514.

*Cerebral Blood Flow Measurement with Stable Xenon-Enhanced Computed Tomography,* edited by Howard Yonas. Raven Press, Ltd., New York © 1992.

# Cerebral Blood Flow and $CO_2$ Reactivity in Children with Bacterial Meningitis

Stephen Ashwal, *Warren A. Stringer, Lawrence Tomasi, Sanford Schneider, *Joseph Thompson, and Ron Perkin

*Departments of Pediatrics and *Radiation Sciences, Loma Linda University School of Medicine, Loma Linda, California 92350*

Bacterial meningitis in children can cause a variety of cerebral insults, including infarction, dural sinus thrombosis, cerebritis, subarachnoid hemorrhage, and subdural effusion (1). Many of these insults are due to vasculitis of cerebral arteries or veins. Cerebral edema with raised intracranial pressure (ICP) also contributes to the morbidity by reducing cerebral perfusion (2,3).

We examined cerebral perfusion using the stable xenon computed tomographic cerebral blood flow (Xe/CT CBF) method in children with bacterial meningitis. We were interested in determining whether CBF is reduced during the acute phase of the infection and whether perfusion varies in different brain regions. Because hyperventilation is used to treat increased ICP, we also wanted to learn the extent to which CBF is affected by reducing the carbon dioxide tension.

## PATIENTS AND METHODS

We performed Xe/CT CBF determinations in 20 children, aged 7 days to 8 years, with bacterial meningitis. As previously reported (4), the scans were obtained within 48 hours after admission using the General Electric 9800 xenon blood flow system while patients breathed a 33% nonradioactive xenon-oxygen mixture (Linde XeScan stable xenon in oxygen USP, Union Carbide Rare Gases, Specialty Medical Products, Danbury, CT). Over a 4-minute interval, CT images were obtained in three planes, with slices 1 to 2 cm apart, to allow visualization of the upper brain stem, subcortical nuclei, and peripheral cortex (5). Flow values were determined with the region-of-interest cursor on the CT scanner.

Of the 20 patients, 13 had a single Xe/CT CBF study; two of these patients

---

Dr. Stringer's present address is Department of Radiology, Medical College of Virginia, Virginia Commonwealth University, Box 615, MCV Station, Richmond, Virginia 23298.

were brain dead within the first 24 hours. The other seven patients had double Xe/CT CBF studies at two $pCO_2$ levels averaging $40 \pm 3$ and $29 \pm 3$ torr. Data were analyzed using a Student's $t$ test and were reported as the mean $\pm$ standard deviation (SD) at a significance level of $P < 0.05$.

## RESULTS

Symptoms and signs observed within the first 24 hours included coma (12 patients), seizures (15 patients), paralysis (7 patients), cranial nerve dysfunction (8 patients), respiratory impairment (10 patients), herniation (4 patients), hearing or visual loss (6 patients), and brain death (2 patients). The bacterial organisms that caused the meningitis were *Haemophilus influenzae* (8 patients), *Streptococcus pneumoniae* (4 patients), *Neisseria meningitidis* (5 patients), and Group B *Streptococcus* (3 patients). During Xe/CT scanning, mean values (±SD) for relevant physiologic variables were the following: arterial blood pressure, 79 (13) torr; heart rate, 145 (29) beats per minute; temperature, 97.5° F (2.1°) (36.4° ± 1.4° C); arterial pH, 7.42 (0.14); $pCO_2$, 35 (14) torr; $pO_2$, 95 (51) torr; and end-tidal $pCO_2$, 33 (7) torr. CT findings were normal in 5 of the 18 patients who were not brain dead at the time of Xe/CT CBF. Four scans demonstrated diffuse low-attenuation changes; seven showed mild to moderate edema; four patients had small extracerebral fluid collections; one had intrafalcial herniation; and one, scattered infarcts.

**TABLE 1.** *Global and regional cerebral blood flow values in 18 children with bacterial meningitis*[a]

| | Flow values (ml/100 g/min) | |
| --- | --- | --- |
| | Normal-flow group (n = 13) Mean (±SD) | Reduced-flow group (n = 5) Mean (±SD) |
| Global | 62 (20) | 26 (10)[b] |
| Frontal gray | 61 (29) | 30 (15) |
| Frontal white | 41 (17) | 11 (05) |
| Temporal | 67 (27) | 36 (18) |
| Parietal | 66 (27) | 22 (18) |
| Occipital | 70 (27) | 36 (22) |
| Caudate | 63 (20) | 25 (18)[b] |
| Thalamic | 63 (21) | 27 (13) |
| Lenticular | 72 (25) | 32 (16)[b] |
| Midbrain | 79 (30) | 49 (08)[b] |
| Cerebellar | 60 (23) | 40 (11)[b] |

[a] Two of the twenty children originally in this study were brain dead at the time of the Xe/CT cerebral blood flow study; their flows averaged 3 ml/100 g/min.
[b] Significantly different from normal group ($P < 0.05$).

### Global and Regional CBF

Table 1 presents global and regional CBF determinations. In 13 children, global CBF ($62 \pm 20$ ml/100 g/min) was within the normal range for age based on our previous studies and those reported in the literature (4,6). There was some regional variability. Cortical, subcortical, and posterior fossa flows were similar. In many patients, local areas had reduced flow.

In five children, global and most regional flows were reduced significantly. Global flow averaged $26 \pm 10$ ml/100 g/min; average flows were $30 \pm 15$ ml/100 g/min in frontal gray matter and $11 \pm 5$ ml/100 g/min in white matter. None of these patients were hypotensive or hypoxic, and only one had an end-tidal pCO$_2$ below 30 torr. In some patients, regional flow reductions were considerable (below 5–10 ml/100 g/min).

### CBF/CO$_2$ Reactivity

In six of the seven patients who had double studies (at pCO$_2$ levels of $40 \pm 3$ torr and $29 \pm 3$ torr), hyperventilation significantly reduced (by 33%) global CBF and the majority of regional flows (Fig. 1). In one patient, however, global CBF paradoxically increased 25% after hyperventilation, rising from 56 ml/100 g/min (at pCO$_2$ = 45 torr) to 75 ml/100 g/min (at pCO$_2$ = 35 torr). In two patients, hyperventilation reduced blood flow to levels considered to be below

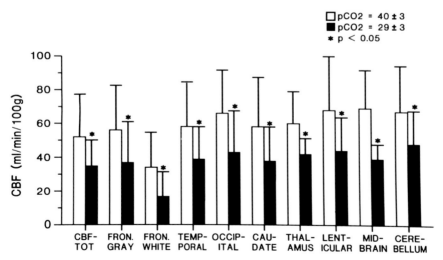

**FIG. 1.** Global (CBF TOT) and regional CBF/CO$_2$ reactivity in six children with bacterial meningitis. Values represent the mean ($\pm 1$ SD) CBF, demonstrating reduction of global and regional CBF with hyperventilation. FRON., frontal.

the ischemic threshold. In one patient, the $pCO_2$ level decreased from 37 to 25 torr with hyperventilation; global CBF decreased from 22 to 14 ml/100 g/min; and perfusion decreased from 27 to 2 ml/100 g/min in the frontal gray matter and from 13 to 1 ml/100 g/min in the frontal white matter. This patient was brain dead 2 days later.

## DISCUSSION

Increased ICP resulting from severe cerebral edema and decreased cerebrospinal fluid reabsorption is a common and early complication of bacterial meningitis in children. It is also associated with other serious neurologic complications (7–9). In three recent studies in which ICP was monitored continually, morbidity and mortality, due primarily to decreased cerebral perfusion pressure, were found to be greater in children with elevated ICP (2,3,10).

One of the principal findings of our study, that CBF was reduced in 5 of 18 (28%) children with meningitis, confirms the concerns raised by previous investigators. Even in the children with normal global CBF values, we frequently observed regions where flow was significantly reduced, presumably because of isolated cerebral vascular involvement. Four of these infants with reduced CBF had serious neurologic sequelae.

Another important observation in our study was that hyperventilation significantly reduced CBF. In two of six children, flow fell below ischemic thresholds in several brain regions. After hyperventilation, two other patients had local flows in the range of 15–20 ml/100 g/min when their end-tidal $pCO_2$ was 31 torr. Had they been hyperventilated to a $pCO_2$ of 20–25 torr, their CBF presumably would have been further reduced to a level of potential ischemia.

Hyperventilation often is used to decrease ICP in many acute neurologic disorders by causing cerebral vasoconstriction and decreasing cerebral blood volume (11). However, such treatment potentially can lead to severe cerebral ischemia (12). Because baseline CBF values were already significantly reduced in 28% of the children in this study, this potential ischemic effect is of even greater concern. Assuming that these children maintain $CBF/CO_2$ reactivity, it is possible that hyperventilation in patients with meningitis could further reduce CBF below ischemic thresholds. Ischemic thresholds for infants and children, however, have not yet been determined. In infants under 1 month of age, these thresholds are lower than the 15–18 ml/100 g/min cited for adults. This determination is based on studies by Griesen (13) and by Altman et al. (14) and on the observation in our study of a 1-week-old patient who survived intact despite a global CBF of 13 ml/100 g/min. Additional studies are needed, however, to establish the ischemic threshold for infants and children and to determine how it changes with maturation.

Our findings raise concerns about the routine use of hyperventilation in the management of increased ICP. In patients with meningitis whose CT or magnetic resonance imaging scans suggest ischemic insults not associated with increased ICP, hyperventilation should be used with caution. Further studies examining the optimal management of elevated ICP in children with meningitis should be conducted to correlate the changes in ICP with CBF, oxygen delivery, and the long-term neurologic outcome.

## ACKNOWLEDGMENT

The authors wish to thank Ann Elliott for secretarial assistance in preparing this manuscript.

## REFERENCES

1. Cabral DA, Floodmark O, Farrell K, Speert DP. Prospective study of computed tomography in acute bacterial meningitis. *J Pediatr* 1987;111:201–205.
2. Goiten KJ, Tamir I. Cerebral perfusion pressure in central nervous system infections of infancy and childhood. *J Pediatr* 1983;103:40–43.
3. McMenamin JB, Volpe JJ. Bacterial meningitis in infancy: effects on intracranial pressure and cerebral blood flow velocity. *Neurology* 1984;34:500–504.
4. Ashwal S, Schneider S, Thompson J. Xenon computed tomography measuring cerebral blood flow in the determination of brain death in children. *Ann Neurol* 1989;25:539–546.
5. Gur D, Yonas H, Good WF. Local cerebral blood flow by xenon-enhanced CT: current status, potential improvements, and future directions. *Cerebrovascular and Brain Metabolism Reviews* 1989;1:68–86.
6. Tachibana H, Meyer JS, Okayasu H, Kandula P. Changing topographic patterns of human cerebral blood flow with age measured by xenon CT. *AJR* 1984;142:1027–1034.
7. Horwitz SJ, Boxerbaum B, O'Bell J. Cerebral herniation in bacterial meningitis in childhood. *Ann Neurol* 1980;7:524–528.
8. Kaplan SL, Fishman MA. Supportive therapy for bacterial meningitis. *Pediatr Infect Dis J* 1987;6: 670–677.
9. Hahn SM. Current concepts in bacterial meningitis. *West J Med* 1989;151:180–186.
10. Rebaud P, Berthier JC, Hartemann E, Floret D. Intracranial pressure in childhood central nervous system infections. *Intensive Care Med* 1988;14:522–525.
11. Bruce DA. Treatment of intracranial hypertension. In: McLaurin RL, Schut L, Venes JL, Epstein F, eds. *Pediatric neurosurgery*. New York: Saunders, 1989:245–254.
12. Cold GE. Does acute hyperventilation provoke cerebral oligaemia in comatose patients after acute head injury? *Acta Neurochir (Wein)* 1989;96:100–106.
13. Griesen G. Cerebral blood flow in preterm infants during the first week of life. *Acta Paediatr Scand* 1986;75:43–51.
14. Altman DI, Powers WJ, Perlman JM, et al. Cerebral blood flow requirements for brain viability in newborn infants is lower than in adults. *Ann Neurol* 1988;24:218–226.

*Cerebral Blood Flow Measurement with Stable Xenon-Enhanced Computed Tomography,* edited by Howard Yonas. Raven Press, Ltd., New York © 1992.

# Discussion

Participants:
Dr. Karl Broich (Erlangen, Germany)
Dr. John Meyer (Houston, Texas, USA)
Dr. Steven Ashwal (Loma Linda, California, USA)
Dr. Walter Obrist (Pittsburgh, Pennsylvania, USA)
Dr. Alexander Hartmann (Bonn, Germany)
Dr. David Gur (Pittsburgh, Pennsylvania, USA)

In response to Dr. Broich's paper concerning the study of patients with epilepsy, Dr. Meyer related his experience using excitatory techniques to identify epileptogenic foci. He and his colleagues found that the withdrawal of anticonvulsants combined with sleep deprivation better enabled them to identify ictal and interictal flow abnormalities. He maintained that, compared to a routine CBF study, such provocative methods produce a far greater yield of focal high and low flow values that correlate with ictal and interictal seizure foci.

Dr. Ashwal's report of a study in children with meningitis provoked two areas of discussion. Dr. Obrist was concerned by Dr. Ashwal's assumption that normal flow values in children were known, because CBF data in 1- to 5-year-olds is currently lacking. Even so, he acknowledged that some studies suggest CBF may be twice as high in children as in adults. Dr. Ashwal said that he was also aware of a report indicating that normal flow values in children range between 60 and 80 ml/100 g/min. He added that, in his experience, Xe/CT CBF measurements of 50 to 80 ml/100 g/min were common in children under 3 years of age.

Dr. Hartmann was concerned about the reliability of Xe/CT-derived CBF measurements, especially at very low levels. Dr. Ashwal agreed that very low flow values can be difficult to interpret, but said that he had found global flow values in brain-dead infants to be <5 ml/100 g/min (Ashwal S, *Ann Neurol* 1989;25:539–546). Values in near-drowning victims who remained comatose were about 30 ml/100 g/min, a typical range for coma. (Editor's note: Two published articles [Darby et al., *Arch Neurol* 1987;44:551–554; Pistoia et al., *AJNR* 1991;12:97–103] have indicated that Xe/CT CBF studies are sensitive to very low [<5 ml/100 g/min] flow values throughout the entire brain and that these measurements are consistent with clinical criteria for brain death.)

Dr. Gur believed that the issue was not whether $\frac{1}{2}$ or 1 Hounsfield unit of enhancement could be detected reliably in a given voxel under conditions of near-zero flow. Rather, the question was whether flow values recorded as low as 1 to 2 ml/100 g/min in a relatively large brain region accurately reflect the actual flow. The consistent observation of very low CBF values with a very small standard deviation within thousands of adjacent voxels does, in fact, correlate with the near absence of perfusion, Gur said. A flow value of $2 \pm 1$ ml/100 g/min obtained in 5,000 adjacent voxels would be 14 standard deviations from the threshold for reversible ischemia (15 ml/100 g/min). Therefore, he concluded, there is an extremely low probability that flow values in this region are actually consistent with viability.

*Cerebral Blood Flow Measurement with Stable Xenon-Enhanced Computed Tomography,* edited by Howard Yonas. Raven Press, Ltd., New York © 1992.

# Acetazolamide and Stable Xenon-Enhanced Computed Tomography: Benefits and Adverse Reactions

Bruce L. Dean, *John A. Hodak, *Burton P. Drayer, Charles Lee, **Thomas W. Grahm, and Gary R. Conrad

*Department of Radiology, Albert B. Chandler Medical Center, University of Kentucky, Lexington, Kentucky 40536; and Departments of *Neuroradiology and **Neurosurgery, Barrow Neurological Institute, St. Joseph Hospital and Medical Center, 350 W. Thomas St., Phoenix, Arizona 85013*

Acetazolamide (Diamox; Lederle, Pearl River, NY) is a potent dilator of the cerebral vasculature. When stable xenon-enhanced computed tomographic (Xe/CT) scanning is performed before and after the intravenous (IV) administration of acetazolamide (1), the functional reserve of cerebral blood flow (CBF) can be assessed. This cerebrovascular "stress test" highlights underperfused areas of normal-appearing brain (2). Even so, safety is an important consideration in repeating an entire sequence of Xe/CT scans following the infusion of a potent cerebral vasodilator. The technique prolongs scanning and exposes the patient to a second course of xenon inhalation. Acetazolamide also places additional demands on brain tissue that may have a marginal reserve of CBF and can elevate intracranial pressure (ICP) by increasing cerebral blood flow and volume. This chapter reports our experience in 119 patients in whom we performed Xe/CT scanning before and after the infusion of acetazolamide. We also discuss the safety of this technique.

## SUBJECTS AND METHODS

### Patient Selection

We reviewed 119 Xe/CT scans performed in adult patients before and after they received acetazolamide. The indications for obtaining the Xe/CT CBF studies are listed in Table 1. Patients with closed head injuries or an otherwise high likelihood of elevated ICP were excluded from this study. Patients with an allergy to sulfa or a history of liver or renal failure were not given acetazolamide and also were excluded from the study.

**TABLE 1.** *Patient history or reason for scan*

| History | Number of patients | Percent of total |
|---|---|---|
| Stroke, TIA, carotid stenosis, post-endarterectomy | 42 | 35.3 |
| Subarachnoid hemorrhage, suspected vasospasm | 33 | 27.7 |
| Intracranial tumor | 24 | 20.2 |
| Motor vehicle accident, gunshot wound, other trauma | 7 | 5.9 |
| EC-IC bypass evaluation, giant aneurysm, middle cerebral artery stenosis | 4 | 3.3 |
| Arteriovenous malformation | 3 | 2.5 |
| Seizures (temporal lobectomy planning) | 3 | 2.5 |
| Moya Moya disease | 2 | 1.7 |
| Post-arrest | 1 | 0.8 |

## Scanning Technique

Total scanning time during xenon inhalation was limited to 4.5 minutes to lessen adverse reactions and improve patient compliance. If needed, some patients received sedatives, generally IV midazolam (Versed; Roche Labs, Nutley, NJ) or fentanyl (Sublimaze; Elkins-Sinn, Cherry Hill, NJ). We usually acquired six CT scans at each of three preselected brain levels: at each level, two baseline scans were obtained and averaged, and then four scans were taken during xenon inhalation. In uncooperative patients, scans were done at only one or two levels. CT scanning was performed on a GE 9800 scanner (General Electric, Milwaukee, WI) using the standard GE xenon blood flow analysis package. For each patient, we recorded the hematocrit measured within a few days of the CBF study.

Most patients inhaled the 33% xenon/67% oxygen mixture (Linde XeScan stable xenon in oxygen USP, Union Carbide Rare Gases, Specialty Medical Products, Danbury, CT) through a mask. For claustrophobic patients, we used a mouthpiece with a nose clamp. A technologist "coached" the patients throughout the procedure to lessen anxiety and decrease patient motion. The end-tidal xenon concentration was measured continually using a thermoconductivity analyzer.

Following the initial multi-level Xe/CT CBF study, we administered 1 g of IV acetazolamide. After a 20-minute delay to assure maximal cerebral vasodilation (3), we began a second set of scans at the same brain levels.

## Patient Monitoring

During all studies, a physician or nurse monitored the patient. Vital signs were taken routinely throughout the scanning process, and arterial saturations were monitored continually by a pulse oximeter. In patients with ICP monitors, ICP levels were checked intermittently during scanning. After scanning, we evaluated all patients for changes in clinical condition. We asked those able to respond verbally about their level of discomfort and symptoms during the procedure.

We classified any adverse reactions as the result of either xenon inhalation or acetazolamide. The physiologic changes we attributed to xenon inhalation included respiratory delay, diaphoresis, light-headedness, tingling in extremities, headaches, and anxiety (4–6). Reactions ascribed to acetazolamide included drowsiness, allergic reactions (acetazolamide cross reacts with other sulfa compounds), ICP elevation, and headaches (7–9).

## Scan Evaluation

Neuroradiologists evaluated the scans retrospectively to identify abnormalities on images obtained before or after acetazolamide and to determine if scans taken after acetazolamide offered any additional information than those obtained prior to acetazolamide administration.

## RESULTS

### Adverse Reactions

Expressed symptoms and objective findings attributable to xenon inhalation are presented in Table 2. Other than drowsiness and headaches, which could have been caused by either the xenon or acetazolamide, there were no adverse reactions that could be ascribed solely to acetazolamide. No new cerebral infarctions or extension of existing infarctions were evident, and no changes in neurologic status were found in post-scan examinations. In patients with ICP monitors, we observed no unusual ICP elevations during scanning that could be attributed to acetazolamide.

### Scan Results

Regions of abnormal blood flow not seen on images taken before acetazolamide were identified on images taken after giving this agent in 31.1% (37/119) of the

**TABLE 2.** *Adverse reactions due to xenon inhalation*

| Adverse reactions | Number of patients[a] | Percent of total |
|---|---|---|
| Respiratory delay > 10 seconds | 10 | 8.4 |
| Drowsiness or somnolence[b] | 8 | 6.7 |
| Emotional lability | 7 | 5.9 |
| "Out of control" | 5 | 4.2 |
| Headache[b] | 5 | 4.2 |
| Hallucinations | 2 | 1.7 |
| Seizure | 1 | 0.8 |

[a] Some patients experienced more than one adverse reaction.
[b] May have been related to either acetazolamide or xenon inhalation.

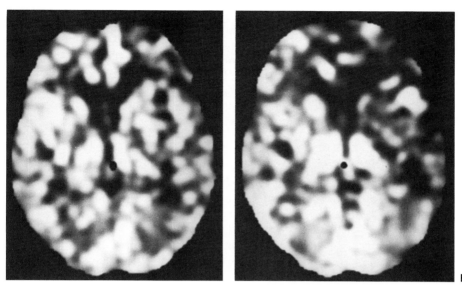

A
B

**FIG. 1.** An angiogram revealed bilateral carotid and left vertebral artery occlusions in this patient with TIAs. The pre-acetazolamide Xe/CT scan (**A**) was nondiagnostic and revealed minimal hemispheric asymmetry. The post-acetazolamide Xe/CT study (**B**) showed relative hyperperfusion in the thalamus and occipital lobes not evident in the pre-acetazolamide scan. Of the four main vessels supplying these regions via thalamoperforator and posterior cerebral artery branches, the right vertebral artery was the only vessel remaining patent. Hypoperfusion is highlighted in the left cerebral hemisphere in the distribution of the left anterior and middle cerebral arteries.

patients (Fig. 1). A hypoperfused area was seen in 54.6% of subjects in either pre- or post-acetazolamide images. The improved detection of hypoperfusion after infusion of acetazolamide was most evident in patients with subarachnoid hemorrhage who were being evaluated for vasospasm. The post-acetazolamide scans were least beneficial in patients with intracranial tumors.

## DISCUSSION

Xe/CT scanning after the administration of acetazolamide allows assessment of the functional reserve of brain tissue. Acetazolamide's vasodilating properties generally highlight areas of fixed hypoperfusion by increasing flow to the surrounding normal brain tissues. In nearly one third of our patients, this effect revealed a perfusion abnormality not apparent on conventional Xe/CT images.

In fact, acetazolamide can increase surrounding normal brain perfusion to the point that a patient with marginal flow may have preferential "steal" of flow from areas of marginal reactivity, resulting in increased flow to acetazolamide-responsive areas. This phenomenon actually can decrease flow to poorly responsive areas. Vorstrup et al. (10) reported that this steal phenomenon enabled the prediction of patients who would benefit from an extracranial-intracranial bypass.

The vasodilation associated with acetazolamide frequently enhances the interhemispheric asymmetry in low-flow states caused by either significant carotid stenosis or intrahemispheric regional differences in flow secondary to arterial spasm (2,11). In particular, the regional perfusion abnormalities were better delineated on post-acetazolamide scans in the patients evaluated for vasospasm.

Several physiological symptoms are expected with xenon inhalation. The most common include light-headedness and tingling in the extremities (5). The most alarming side effect is respiratory delay (12); Latchaw et al. (4) reported an incidence of 3.6% in a series of 1,830 patients. In our study, 8.4% of patients experienced respiratory delays longer than 10 seconds, slightly greater than twice the rate previously reported. This higher rate may be related to longer total scanning times, each patient having undergone the Xe/CT scanning sequence both before and after receiving acetazolamide. The incidence also may be related to our patient sample, which generally consisted of inpatients with acute and significant neurological findings. However, all patients were easily stimulated and reminded to breathe. One patient, who was being evaluated for frequent seizures, had a seizure after the post-acetazolamide Xe/CT scan.

Acetazolamide (1 g, IV) has been found to cause a 31% to 75% increase in CBF (3,7,13–15). The rise in CBF peaks at about 25 minutes, then decreases with a half-life of about 95 minutes (3). This increase is also coupled to an increase in cerebral blood volume (16). Wilkinson (8) described a canine model with elevated ICP in which the vasodilator response from acetazolamide stimulated a dangerous rise in ICP. None of our patients with ICP monitors experienced unusual elevations in ICP after receiving acetazolamide. We checked pressure monitors frequently during the study and drained cerebrospinal fluid to lower ICP when appropriate.

Given the tenuous blood supply to infarcted areas and, more importantly, to surrounding ischemic areas, altering vascular dynamics with acetazolamide can be deleterious. Vorstrup et al. (17) demonstrated that infarcted tissue had a reduced but detectable response to vasoreactive medications. The loss of the Bohr effect in red blood cells after acetazolamide administration (caused by inhibition of carbonic anhydrase that shifts the oxygen dissociation curve) creates the potential for a small drop in tissue oxygenation. This may be balanced, though, by the slight increase in CBF.

The potential for reduction of flow to the ischemic area also exists if acetazolamide elicits the steal phenomenon or elevates ICP significantly. Nevertheless, we found no clinical evidence of change in neurological status following the use of acetazolamide in our series.

## CONCLUSIONS

In 31.1% of our patients, Xe/CT CBF studies with acetazolamide showed a perfusion abnormality not present on the conventional Xe/CT CBF examination.

There were no significant complications in any of our 119 patients. We recommend avoiding the use of acetazolamide in patients with clinical evidence of increased ICP. In other patients, the use of acetazolamide should be accompanied by proper monitoring to eliminate prolonged respiratory delays and dangerous elevations of ICP. Used according to these guidelines, the pre- and post-acetazolamide Xe/CT technique is a relatively safe and useful method to evaluate regional CBF in a variety of clinical settings.

## REFERENCES

1. Rogg J, Rutigliano M, Yonas H, Johnson D, Pentheny S, Latchaw R. The acetazolamide challenge: imaging techniques designed to evaluate cerebral blood flow reserve. *AJNR* 1989;10:803–810.
2. Vorstrup S. Tomographic cerebral blood flow measurements in patients with ischemic cerebrovascular disease and evaluation of the vasodilatory capacity by the acetazolamide test. *Acta Neurol Scand* 1988;114(Suppl):1–48.
3. Hauge A, Nicolaysen G, Thorensen M. Acute effects of acetazolamide on cerebral blood flow in man. *Acta Physiol Scand* 1983;117:233–239.
4. Latchaw R, Yonas H, Pentheny S, Gur D. Adverse reactions to xenon-enhanced CT cerebral blood flow determination. *Radiology* 1987;163:251–254.
5. Yonas H, Grundy B, Gur D, Shabason L, Wolfson S, Cook E. Side effects of xenon inhalation. *J Comput Assist Tomogr* 1981;5:591–592.
6. Winkler S, Turski P. Potential hazards of xenon inhalation. *AJNR* 1985;6:974–975.
7. Sullivan H, Kingsbury T, Morgan M, et al. The RCBF response to Diamox in normal subjects and cerebrovascular disease patients. *J Neurosurg* 1987;67:525–534.
8. Wilkinson H. Cerebral blood flow response to acetazolamide. *J Neurosurg* 1989;70:156.
9. Schroede T. Cerebrovascular reactivity to acetazolamide in carotid artery disease. *Neurol Res* 1986;8:231–236.
10. Vorstrup S, Brun B, Lassen N. Evaluation of the cerebral vasodilatory capacity by the acetazolamide test before EC-IC bypass surgery in patients with occlusion of the internal carotid artery. *Stroke* 1986;17:1291–1298.
11. Yonas H, Sekhar L, Johnson D, Gur D. Determination of irreversible ischemia by xenon-enhanced computed tomographic monitoring of cerebral blood flow in patients with symptomatic vasospasm. *Neurosurgery* 1989;24:368–372.
12. Holl K, Nemati N, Kohmura E, Gaab M, Samii M. Stable-xenon-CT: effects of xenon inhalation on EEG and cardio-respiratory parameters in the human. *Acta Neurochir (Wien)* 1987;87:129–133.
13. Vorstrup S, Boysen G, Brun B, Engell H. Evaluation of the regional cerebral vasodilatory capacity before carotid endarterectomy by the acetazolamide test. *Neurol Res* 1987;9:10–18.
14. Bickler P, Litt L, Banville D, Severinghaus J. Effects of acetazolamide on cerebral acid-base balance. *J Appl Physiol* 1988;65:422–427.
15. Severinghaus J, Cotev S. Carbonic acidosis and cerebral vasodilation after Diamox. *Scand J Clin Lab Invest* 1968;22:(Suppl 102):I;E.
16. Bickler P, Litt L, Severinghaus J. Effects of acetazolamide on cerebrocortical NADH and blood volume. *J Appl Physiol* 1988;65:428–433.
17. Vorstrup S, Paulson O, Lassen N. Cerebral blood flow in acute and chronic ischemic stroke using xenon-133 inhalation tomography. *Acta Neurol Scand* 1986;74:439–451.

*Cerebral Blood Flow Measurement with Stable Xenon-Enhanced Computed Tomography,* edited by Howard Yonas. Raven Press, Ltd., New York © 1992.

# Selecting Patients for Extracranial-Intracranial Bypass Using Xe/CT Blood Flow Studies and the Diamox Test

Tetsuo Yamashita, Shiro Kashiwagi, Shigeki Nakano, Teiichi Takasago, Seisho Abiko, Yujiro Shiroyama, Masaaki Hayashi, and Haruhide Ito

*Department of Neurosurgery, Yamaguchi University School of Medicine, 1144 Kogushi Ube, Yamaguchi 755, Japan*

The report of the Extracranial-Intracranial (EC-IC) Arterial Bypass Study Group (1) concluded that the procedure has no value in preventing stroke. However, this study has been criticized for failing to identify and separately analyze patients with reduced regional cerebral perfusion pressure distal to the symptomatic arterial lesion, patients who might be most likely to benefit from the surgery (2,3). Vorstrup et al. (4) reported that resting cerebral blood flow (CBF) usually was not changed after bypass surgery. Other variables, such as the oxygen extraction fraction (OEF), cerebral blood volume (CBV), $CO_2$ response, and acetazolamide (Diamox) response, as well as resting CBF, must be examined to evaluate the effect of bypass. Patients with "misery perfusion," decreased $CO_2$ response, increased CBV/CBF, or acetazolamide-induced "steal effect" would seem to be among those that the surgery could help (5–10).

We used stable xenon-enhanced computerized tomography (Xe/CT) and a Diamox test to identify patients with reduced CBF and/or cerebrovascular reserve capacity (CRC) due to preoperatively compromised collateral circulation. We also evaluated postoperative changes in resting CBF and CRC and consequently propose criteria for selecting proper candidates for EC-IC bypass.

## SUBJECTS AND METHODS

This study included 15 consecutive patients (13 men and 2 women) who had cerebral ischemic symptoms (Table 1). Their ages ranged from 46 to 71 years (mean: 60 years). Ten patients had suffered minor strokes; four, transient ischemic attacks (TIAs); and one, a reversible ischemic neurological deficit (RIND). Selection for surgery was based on clinical symptoms and the findings on angiograms, CT scans, and CBF studies. All patients had stenosis or occlusion in the

TABLE 1. *Summary of patients*

| Patient | Age (yrs)/sex | Clinical diagnosis | Angiographic findings | Size of infarct on CT | Operative procedure[a] | Outcome |
|---|---|---|---|---|---|---|
| 1 | 57/M | TIA | ICA oc | none | proximal | NRA |
| 2 | 51/M | TIA | ICA oc | none | proximal | NRA |
| 3 | 71/M | TIA | ICA oc | none | single | NRA |
| 4 | 66/M | minor stroke | ICA oc | small | double | improved |
| 5 | 60/M | minor stroke | ICA oc | small | double | improved |
| 6 | 59/M | minor stroke | ICA st | none | single | NRA |
| 7 | 60/M | minor stroke | ICA st | none | double | NRA |
| 8 | 64/M | minor stroke | ICA oc + ICA oc | moderate | proximal | NRA |
| 9 | 61/M | minor stroke | ICA oc + ICA oc | none | single | improved |
| 10 | 59/M | minor stroke | ICA oc + ICA st | none | double | NRA |
| 11 | 46/M | minor stroke | MCA oc | moderate | single | NRA |
| 12 | 61/F | minor stroke | MCA oc | small | proximal | NRA |
| 13 | 57/F | TIA | MCA st | none | proximal | NRA |
| 14 | 64/M | RIND | MCA st | small | proximal | NRA |
| 15 | 66/M | minor stroke | MCA st | small | double | NRA |

[a] Superficial temporal artery to middle cerebral artery (MCA) anastomosis.

TIA, transient ischemic attack; RIND, reversible ischemic neurological deficit; ICA, internal carotid artery; oc, occlusion; st, stenosis; NRA, no recurrent attack.

internal carotid or middle cerebral artery (MCA). Patients with CT-defined large infarcts ($\geq 20$ cm$^2$) were excluded from this study. Fifteen EC-IC bypass operations were performed: four single superficial temporal artery (STA) to MCA anastomoses, five double STA-MCA anastomoses, and six STA to proximal MCA anastomoses. Postoperative angiograms showed a patent bypass in all cases.

## Study Protocol

We performed CBF studies (preoperatively) at least 1 month after the cerebrovascular accident and postoperatively. Resting CBF was studied with the subject's eyes closed. End-tidal $CO_2$, respiratory and pulse rates, and blood pressure were monitored. After the resting CBF measurement, we drew an arterial blood sample to evaluate hematocrit, pH, and $PaCO_2$, and then administered 1 g of Diamox intravenously. Twenty minutes later, we again measured CBF and drew another arterial blood sample.

The CBF studies were conducted with a DR3 CT scanner (Siemens Medical Systems), a Xetron III closed rebreathing xenon inhalator (Anzai Sogyo), an AZ-723-XS end-tidal xenon monitor (Anzai Sogyo), and Evax CBF imaging software (Siemens Medical Systems). The theoretical background, validity, and clinical applications of the Xe/CT CBF method are discussed elsewhere (11).

## Data Analysis

We evaluated the resting mean regional (r) CBF, mean Diamox-induced rCBF, and rCRC of the MCA distribution at the level of the basal ganglia both pre-

## Correlation Between Preoperative Grouping and
## Postoperative Increase in rCBF or rCRC

We compared the results of bypass surgery with postoperative increases in the resting rCBF or rCRC (Fig. 3). An increase in rCBF of 5 ml or more was considered significant. No patient in group I ($n = 4$) had an increase in resting rCBF and rCRC values. In group II ($n = 3$), rCRC was postoperatively higher in the three patients; none had a significant increase in rCBF though. In group III ($n = 2$), rCRC was higher in only one patient. Three patients in group IV ($n = 6$) had postoperative increases in resting rCBF; four had higher rCRC values.

## Representative Case

A 66-year-old man had sudden left-sided hemiparesis 6 months before admission to our hospital. Neurologic examination at the time of admission found mild hemiparesis and dysarthria. CT showed a small infarct in the right putamen, and an angiogram of the right common carotid artery revealed proximal occlusion of the internal carotid artery. He underwent right-sided double STA-MCA anastomoses, and postoperative angiography showed excellent flow through the MCA branches. Preoperative Xe/CT CBF images had detected a low perfusion state and absent rCRC in the right hemisphere (Fig. 4). The postoperative CBF images indicated that his resting rCBF was 5 ml/100 g/min higher than preoperative rCBF values and that the hemispheric asymmetry had decreased. Diamox caused CBF to increase in both hemispheres. In this case, bypass surgery not only in-

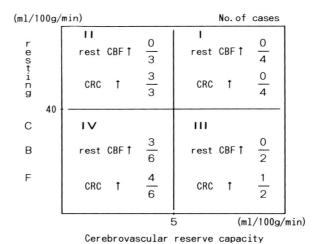

**FIG. 3.** Postoperative hemodynamic changes in each group. Numerators show number of patients who had a postoperative increase in resting CBF or cerebrovascular reserve capacity (CRC). Denominators show total number of patients in the groups.

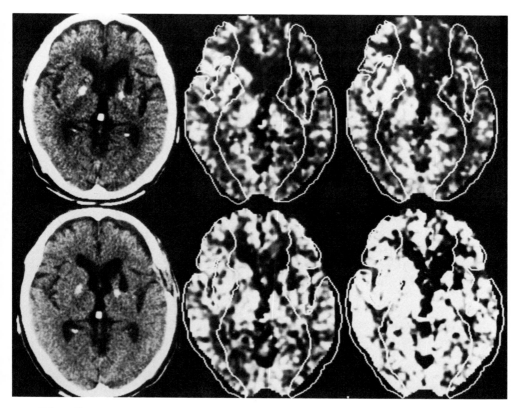

**FIG. 4.** Top, preoperative images; bottom, postoperative images. Left, plain CT; center, resting CBF; right, Diamox-induced CBF. Preoperative Xe/CT CBF images showed a low perfusion state and absent regional cerebrovascular reserve capacity (rCRC) in the right hemisphere. Postoperative CBF images indicated that both the resting CBF and CRC had increased.

creased the resting CBF, but also restored CRC. His hemiparesis improved after the surgery.

## DISCUSSION

Critics have faulted the EC-IC Bypass Study Group for failing to identify and separately analyze patients with "chronic hemodynamic insufficiency," those most likely to gain by having the surgery (2,3). To identify such patients preoperatively, some investigators have measured CBF using $CO_2$ inhalation, acetazolamide injections, or hypotension; others have measured the OEF or CBV (5–10). Based on these examinations, the patient with reduced $CO_2$ response, misery perfusion, or an acetazolamide-induced steal effect appears to belong to a subgroup that could benefit from the operation (5–10).These investigations used positron-emission tomography, single-photon emission CT, or dynamic CT. Unlike these techniques, the Xe/CT method we used has the advantages of being easily repeated, cost effective, and providing both high resolution and quantitative blood flow values.

Symptomatic arterial trunk occlusion produces reduced regional cerebral perfusion pressure following dilation of the cerebral vessel distal to the occlusive site. Under this condition, a vasodilating agent causes a smaller-than-expected increase in CBF, and rCBF decreases with hypotension, indicating the presence of reduced rCRC. Although CRC can be evaluated with $CO_2$ inhalation or hypotension, the former makes many patients uncomfortable, and the latter risks inducing an irreversible ischemic attack. Diamox, a carbonic anhydrase inhibitor, causes tissue acidosis, which leads to vasodilation and an increase in CBF (12). Vorstrup et al. (10) reported that the Diamox test was more convenient than other methods for evaluating CRC in the ischemic brain. In our institution, more than 100 Diamox tests have been conducted without complications.

In normal control subjects (mean age: 63 years), Vorstrup's group found a mean CBF value of 55 ml/100 g/min; this increased by 31% (range: 13–46%) 20 minutes after the intravenous injection of 1 g of Diamox (10). Our data were consistent with theirs. In our normal adult subjects (mean age: 28 years), resting rCBF in the MCA territory was 60.4 (3.1) ml/100 g/min, and the rCRC was 19.0 (3.3) ml/100 g/min.

In another report, Vorstrup et al. (4) noted that resting CBF did not change in most patients after bypass surgery because both blood flow and metabolism were reduced preoperatively. Likewise, we found that in the global analysis of all cases, EC-IC bypass did not increase the resting CBF but did increase the rCRC. These results suggest that bypass is more effective in improving rCRC than in increasing resting CBF.

Theoretically, patients in group II with normal rCBF and decreased rCRC and those in group IV with decreased rCBF and rCRC would be expected to have postoperative increases in rCBF or CRC. This theory was supported by our findings that bypass surgery improved the rCRC in group II and improved both the rCRC and resting rCBF in group IV. EC-IC bypass certainly increases perfusion pressure in the area distal to arterial occlusion and decreases vasodilation, resulting in an increase in the rCRC. In the area of severely reduced perfusion pressure, which is likely in a state of misery perfusion, bypass increases the resting rCBF.

## CONCLUSION

We concluded that Xe/CT with the Diamox test is a useful and simple way to evaluate cerebral hemodynamics. The preoperative grouping according to resting rCBF and rCRC was helpful in evaluating the effect of EC-IC bypass surgery. We also propose that maximal vasodilation (as seen in group II) and severe perfusion pressure reduction (as seen in group IV) are proper indications for EC-IC bypass surgery.

## REFERENCES

1. The EC-IC Bypass Study Group. Failure of extracranial-intracranial arterial bypass to reduce the ischemic stroke. *N Engl J Med* 1985;313:1191–1200.
2. Ausmann JI, Diaz FG. Critique of the extracranial-intracranial bypass study. *Surg Neurol* 1986;26: 218–221.
3. Day AL, Rhoton AL, Little JR. The extracranial-intracranial bypass study. *Surg Neurol* 1986;26: 222–226.
4. Vorstrup S, Lassen NA, Henriksen L, et al. CBF before and after extracranial-intracranial bypass surgery in patients with ischemic cerebrovascular disease studied with xenon-133 inhalation tomography. *Stroke* 1985;16:616–626.
5. Baron JC, Bousser MG, Rey A, Guillard A, Comar D, Castaigne P. Reversal of focal "misery-perfusion syndrome" by extra-intracranial arterial bypass in hemodynamic cerebral ischemia: a case study with $^{15}$O positron emission tomography. *Stroke* 1981;12:454–459.
6. Gibbs JM, Wise JR, Leenders KL, Jones T. Evaluation of cerebral perfusion reserve in patients with carotid-artery occlusion. *Lancet* 1984;1:310–314.
7. Herold S, Brown MM, Frackowiak RSJ, Mansfield AO, Thomas DJ, Marshall J. Assessment of cerebral hemodynamic reserve—correlation between PET parameters and $CO_2$ reactivity measured by intravenous $^{133}$Xe injection technique. *J Neurol Neurosurg Psychiatry* 1988;51:1045–1050.
8. Norrving B, Nilsson B, Risberg J. rCBF in patients with carotid occlusion--resting and hypercapnic flow related to collateral pattern. *Stroke* 1982;13:155–162.
9. Sullivan HG, Kingsbury TB 4th, Morgan ME, et al. The rCBF response to Diamox in normal subjects and cerebrovascular disease patients. *J Neurosurg* 1987;67:525–534.
10. Vorstrup S, Brun B, Lassen NA. Evaluation of the cerebral vasodilatory capacity by the acetazolamide test before EC-IC bypass surgery in patients with occlusion of the internal carotid artery. *Stroke* 1986;17:1291–1298.
11. Kashiwagi S, Yamashita T, Abiko S, et al. Measurement and imaging of cerebral blood flow with stable xenon and computed tomography (Xe-CT). *Electromedica* 1986;54:136–144.
12. Vorstrup S, Henriksen L, Paulson OB. Effect of acetazolamide on cerebral blood flow and cerebral metabolic rate for oxygen. *J Clin Invest* 1984;74:1634–1639.

*Cerebral Blood Flow Measurement with Stable Xenon-Enhanced Computed Tomography,* edited by Howard Yonas. Raven Press, Ltd., New York © 1992.

# Irreversible Ischemia Determined by Xenon-Enhanced Computed Tomographic Cerebral Blood Flow Studies

Howard Yonas and *David Johnson

*Departments of Neurological Surgery and *Radiology, University of Pittsburgh School of Medicine, 3459 Fifth Avenue, Pittsburgh, Pennsylvania 15213*

Although exactly how subarachnoid hemorrhage (SAH) results in vascular constriction remains unclear, ischemia is generally believed to be the final pathway by which SAH produces the delayed neurological deficits that are often accompanied by infarction (1). Studies involving experimental models of cerebral ischemia have established low cerebral blood flow (CBF) thresholds for brain function and viability (2,3), but only one clinical study has been able to correlate CBF values, neurological symptoms, and imaging-defined infarction (4). Most attempts to relate these factors have relied on [133]Xe external scintillation counting, a method known to have limitations in measuring and identifying regions with low blood flow (5,6). However, in a recent study using positron-emission tomography, investigators found a CBF threshold for infarction in the range predicted by laboratory methods. In four patients with vasospasm, they observed a correlation between regional low flow values (below 15 ml/100 g/min) and local infarction (4).

The relatively new xenon-enhanced computed tomography (Xe/CT) method overcomes many of the limitations of other technologies in determining CBF. It provides direct anatomical correlation, direct calculation of the partition coefficient, and relatively high-resolution quantitative CBF information (7,8). In experimental studies of focal cerebral ischemia, the Xe/CT method has recorded flow values near zero that have consistently predicted infarction (9). To clarify this technique's sensitivity to ischemia and, particularly, to define the significance of specific low flow values that it records, we reviewed the clinical CT and CBF information in a series of patients with SAH. We focused on patients in whom clinical vasospasm developed.

## PATIENTS AND METHODS

Between May 1984 and April 1987, 51 patients with SAH due to an angiographically diagnosed aneurysm underwent a total of 124 Xe/CT CBF studies;

each patient had one to six studies. The first 24 patients were either examined before surgery, after the onset of delayed neurological deterioration, or in both instances. The other 27 patients underwent these studies as part of the treatment protocol, which included sequential Xe/CT studies and transcranial Doppler (TCD) examinations. In this protocol, a Xe/CT CBF study was performed after hemorrhage on days 0 to 1, 4 to 6, and 8 to 10 if the patient's neurological course was stable. If neurological deterioration had occurred, then we obtained an emergency CT scan. If this scan revealed no structural cause for the deterioration, we performed a Xe/CT study immediately, with two or three follow-up Xe/CT studies at 2- to 4-day intervals to evaluate the effectiveness of therapy for vasospasm. TCD examinations were performed at least every other day according to a protocol in which the intracranial internal carotid, middle cerebral, anterior cerebral, and posterior cerebral arteries were examined as feasible and maximal mean velocities greater than 155 cm/s were labeled as "high" (see Table 1).

The CBF studies were performed using the Xe/CT CBF system integrated within the GE 9800 CT scanner (General Electric Medical Systems Division, Milwaukee, WI) and the medical-grade gas XeScan, obtained from Union Carbide Rare Gases (Danbury, CT). Obtaining a combined CT and CBF study required 45 to 90 minutes (average: 60 minutes). Details of our Xe/CT method of mapping CBF have been described previously. In brief, it involves indirectly characterizing the arterial build-up curve by recording the end-tidal build-up curve. The tissue build-up curve is obtained by analyzing sequential CT images taken while the patient inhales the xenon mixture for 4.5 minutes. Then, a blood flow measurement for each CT voxel ($1 \times 1 \times 5$ or $1 \times 1 \times 10$ mm$^3$) is calculated (there are 20,000–30,000 voxels per CT image), and a map of blood flow is compiled. The flow data are displayed on the CT console on a gray scale (the usual window-level setting, 0–100 ml/100 g/min, determines the breadth of the scale). To calculate the flow values and display the CBF map currently requires 14 minutes after data acquisition.

We derived cortical blood flow values by placing 18 to 22 regions of interest (ROIs), each 2 cm in diameter, about the cortical mantle. Differences in flow values in two adjacent cortical ROIs were considered significant, assuming good-quality studies with little motion artifact. In most cases, regions with significant flow alterations include four or more adjacent ROIs. Flow values were used without normalization for $pCO_2$, which varied less than 3 to 4 mm Hg between sequential studies in each patient.

## RESULTS

Neurological deficits developed 3 to 10 days after SAH (average: 5.8 days) in 14 patients, with no anatomic or medical cause for the deficits apparent on the CT study or from serum electrolyte levels. Table 1 displays the relevant clinical information for these patients. The CT studies of all 14 at admission had shown

**TABLE 1.** Clinical findings in patients with symptomatic vasospasm

| Patient | Aneurysm location[a] | Cisternal blood | Transcranial Doppler velocity | Site of lowest cerebral blood flow[a] | Lowest value of cerebral blood flow (ml/100 g/min) | Follow-up CT finding[b] | Deficit severity[c] |
|---|---|---|---|---|---|---|---|
| 1 | A-Com | Thick | NA | Right and left ACA, MCA, PCA | 2 | + | 0 |
| 2 | Right MCA | Thick | NA | Right MCA | 18 | − | 2 |
| 3 | Right MCA | Thick | NA | Right MCA | 20 | − | 2 |
| 4 | A-Com | Thick | NA | Right and left ACA | 0 | + | 0 |
| 5 | Basilar tip | Moderate | NA | Right ACA | 10 | + | 5 |
| 6 | Right ICA | Thick | High | Right and left MCA | 28 | − | 3 |
| 7 | Left ICA | Thick | Normal | Left MCA | 15 | + | 0 |
| 8 | A-Com | Thick | High | Right and left ACA, MCA, PCA | 5 | NA | 0 |
| 9 | Right ICA | Thick | High | Right MCA | 15 | + | 0 |
| 10 | Left ICA | Thick | Normal | Right MCA | 10 | + | Coma |
| 11 | Right ICA | Thick | High | Right ACA, MCA, PCA | 20 | − | 2 |
| 12 | Right MCA | Thick | Normal | Right PCA | 15 | + | 0 |
| 13 | Right MCA | Thick | High | Right ACA, MCA, PCA | 20 | NA | 0 |
| 14 | A-Com | Thick | High | Right ACA | 2 | + | 0 |

[a] A-Com, anterior communicating artery; ACA, anterior cerebral artery; MCA, middle cerebral artery; PCA, posterior cerebral artery; ICA, internal carotid artery.
[b] +, late conversion to low density; −, no sign of infarction; NA, not available.
[c] 0, paralysis; 1–2, antigravity; 3–4, paresis; 5, no deficit.

either a focal or a generalized cisternal clot. In 12 of these patients, the neurological focal deficit was consistent with ischemia within a vascular territory distal to the aneurysm site.

The first CBF study after the onset of deficit showed a regional or global compromise of CBF in the 14 patients. In nine of these, the pattern and measurement of local CBF were dramatically different from what has been observed in one or more prior studies; no previous study was available for comparison with the other five. In none of the remaining 37 patients did a similarly abrupt reduction of CBF occur, although several patients with a Hunt and Hess grade of 4 or 5 consistently maintained cortical flow values between 20 and 30 ml/100 g/min throughout their clinical course.

Cortical CBF values of 18 to 30 ml/100 g/min were identified in four of the 14 patients who had moderately altered levels of consciousness and hemiparesis. Follow-up CT scans did not demonstrate infarction in this group. CT scans did reveal infarction in the other 10 patients. Flow values fell to or below 15 ml/100 g/min in all cortical ROIs within one or more vascular territories that progressed to infarction (Fig. 1). Of the ten patients in this group, eight had paralysis

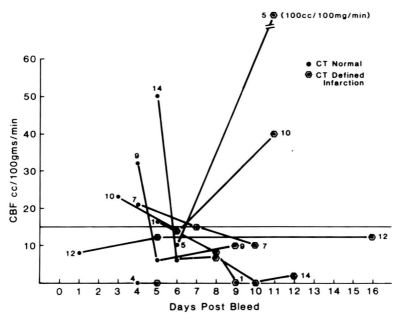

**FIG. 1.** Lowest flow values in two or more adjacent regions of interest in patients with symptomatic vasospasm who developed CT-defined infarctions. Patient numbers on the graph correspond with Table 1. Note that although the CT image retained the appearance of an infarction in patients 5 and 10, flow either normalized or reached elevated levels. This suggested a resolution of vasospasm. Patient 5, however, suffered a catastrophic hemorrhage.

and a severe sensory deficit. One patient whose flow values in both frontal lobes were focally low had only a flat affect.

## DISCUSSION

Sequential TCD studies are simple to perform at the bedside and can provide an early clinical awareness of narrowing of the larger vessels. Therefore, we have used TCD in combination with Xe/CT-derived CBF information to validate the diagnosis of symptomatic vasospasm. Studies have demonstrated a correlation among TCD-detected elevations in velocities, the neurological course, and the presence of subarachnoid blood (10,11). Cognizance of a trend toward higher flow velocities on sequential daily studies thus has proven especially useful in identifying a vascular territory at high risk for developing ischemia. Information from TCD alone, however, cannot disclose significant narrowing of second- or third-order vessels.

Unlike TCD velocity measurements, CBF values correlate closely with clinical symptoms. Like Symon (12), we have observed CBF values between 18 and 30 ml/100 g/min in patients with an altered level of consciousness and a mild to moderate motor or sensory deficit. In our series, cortical regions where flow remained at or above 18 ml/100 g/min did not progress to CT-defined infarction and usually were associated with clinical resolution of the deficit. Furthermore, we found—as did Powers et al. (4)—large cortical regions with flow at or below 15 ml/100 g/min in patients with more severe neurological deficits, and those regions tended to convert to infarction on follow-up CT studies. Conversion to infarction occurred inconsistently in regions with flow values between 12 and 17 ml/100 g/min, whereas values below 12 ml/100 g/min were invariably accompanied by either concurrent or later infarctions as defined by CT.

Several studies have demonstrated the validity of both normal and very low Xe/CT-derived CBF measurements. Xe/CT measurements of CBF correlate closely with values obtained by the microsphere method (13,14). Clinical norms of CBF obtained with Xe/CT have also been consistent with normative values obtained with $^{133}$Xe. In addition, our experience demonstrates that flow values derived with Xe/CT are sensitive to a threshold for infarction. Even so, we have not yet observed flows of 10 to 20 ml/100 g/min often enough to define an absolutely predictive threshold with greater confidence.

## REFERENCES

1. Heros RC, Zervas NT, Varos V. Cerebral vasospasm after subarachnoid hemorrhage: an update. *Ann Neurol* 1983;14:599–608.
2. Heiss WD, Rosner G. Functional recovery of cortical neurons as related to degree and duration of ischemia. *Ann Neurol* 1983;14:294–301.
3. Jones TH, Morawetz RB, Crowell RM, et al. Thresholds of focal cerebral ischemia in awake monkeys. *J Neurosurg* 1981;54:773–782.
4. Powers WJ, Grubb RL, Baker RP, Mintun MA, Raichle NE. Regional cerebral blood flow and metabolism in reversible ischemia due to vasospasm. *J Neurosurg* 1985;62:539–546.
5. Mallet BN, Veall N. The measurement of regional cerebral clearance rates in man using xenon-133 inhalational and extracranial recording. *Clin Sci* 1985;29:179–191.
6. Mickey B, Vorstrup S, Voldby B, Lindewald H, Harmsen A, Lassen NA. Serial measurement of regional cerebral blood flow in patients with SAH using Xe-133 inhalation and emission computerized tomography. *J Neurosurg* 1984;60:916-922.
7. Gur D, Good WF, Wolfson SK Jr, Yonas H, Shabason L. In vivo mapping of local cerebral blood flow by xenon-enhanced computed tomography. *Science* 1982;5:1267–1268.
8. Kishore PR, Rao GU, Fernandez RE, et al. Regional cerebral blood flow measurements using stable xenon-enhanced computed tomography: a theoretical and experimental evaluation. *J Comput Assist Tomogr* 1984;8:619–630.
9. Yonas H, Gur D, Claussen D, Wolfson SK Jr, Moossy J. Stable xenon enhanced computed tomography in the study of clinical and pathologic correlates of focal ischemia in baboons. *Stroke* 1988;19:228–238.
10. Fisher CM, Kistler JP, Davis JM. Relation of cerebral vasospasm to subarachnoid hemorrhage visualized by computerized tomographic scanning. *Neurosurgery* 1980;6:1–9.
11. Seiler RW, Grolimund P, Aaslid R, Huber P, Nornes H. Cerebral vasospasm evaluated by transcranial ultrasound correlated with clinical grade and CT-visualized subarachnoid hemorrhage. *J Neurosurg* 1986;64:594–600.
12. Symon L. Disordered cerebro-vascular physiology in aneurysmal hemorrhage. *Acta Neurochir (Wien)* 1978;41:7–22.
13. Gur D, Yonas H, Jackson DL, et al. Simultaneous measurements of cerebral blood flow by the xenon/CT method and the microsphere method. A comparison. *Invest Radiol* 1985;20:672–677.
14. Fatouros PP, Marmarou A, Keenan R, Kantos H. Comparison of improved stable xenon/CT method for cerebral blood flow measurements with radiolabelled microspheres technique. *Radiology* 1985;158:334.

*Cerebral Blood Flow Measurement with Stable Xenon-Enhanced Computed Tomography,* edited by Howard Yonas. Raven Press, Ltd., New York © 1992.

# Correlation of Xenon-Enhanced Computed Tomography and Angiography in Patients with Intracerebral Arteriovenous Malformations and Clinical Symptoms of Steal

Michael P. Marks, Barton Lane, *Gary K. Steinberg, and Dieter R. Enzmann

*Departments of Diagnostic Radiology and *Neurosurgery, Stanford University Medical Center, Stanford, California 94305*

Patients with arteriovenous malformations (AVMs) can have a variety of symptoms, including gradually progressive neurologic deficits and intellectual deterioration (1), both symptoms attributed to the steal phenomenon (1,2). We have previously identified size and angiomatous change (prominent transcortical collateral supply to the AVM nidus) as vascular characteristics that predispose to steal (3). Physiologic studies have also shown that cerebral blood flow must fall below 10 to 15 ml/100 g/min to affect electrophysiologic neuronal activity (4). Moreover, in patients without steal, we have found a statistically significant reduction in blood flow in selected cortical regions of the hemisphere ipsilateral to an AVM compared to identical regions in the contralateral hemisphere (5). In this study, we compared regional cerebral blood flow (rCBF) in patients who had AVM with clinical steal to rCBF in patients having AVMs without steal symptoms.

## SUBJECTS AND METHODS

We identified eight patients with intracerebral AVMs who had symptoms of gradually progressive neurologic deficits or intellectual deterioration believed to be due to clinical steal. They were selected from a group of more than 125 patients seen at our institution. Patients were eliminated from this group if they had a prior episode of hemorrhage or ictus that left them with a fixed neurologic deficit. They were also excluded if they had undergone neurosurgical procedures that could affect flow. The patients chosen included five men and three women, aged 20 to 61 years (mean: 45 years). In addition to symptoms of steal, four patients had a history of headache and one had seizures. We compared these patients with 20 others (7 male, 13 female) with AVMs who had no clinical evidence of steal. Their age range was 11 to 59 years (mean: 35.5 years). Of these patients, eight had a seizure history, seven had headaches, and six had a history of hemorrhage. The rCBF in the 20 has been reported elsewhere (5).

All patients underwent biplane angiography to determine AVM volume. Non-contrast axial computed tomography (CT) scans (10-mm slice thickness) were performed on a GE 9800 scanner fitted with a specially designed hardware and software system. We selected two levels for study: one through the basal ganglia and another through the centrum semiovale. Patients inhaled a 33% xenon/67% oxygen mixture (Linde XeScan stable xenon in oxygen USP, Union Carbide Rare Gases, Specialty Medical Products, Danbury, CT). We used a previously described method (6,7) to calculate blood flow and generate blood flow maps.

At each axial level, we drew regions of interest (ROI) corresponding to the cortical regions supplied by the three major cerebral arteries feeding each hemisphere (the anterior, middle, and posterior cerebral arteries). This yielded a set of ROI values ipsilateral and contralateral to the AVM. For each patient, we subtracted the blood flow value of the region (or regions) adjacent to the AVM from that in the same area on the contralateral side to obtain a mean difference.

We used angiograms to predict areas where flow would be expected to be low, by identifying those cortical regions supplied by vessels feeding the AVM more proximally. The rCBF values from cortical regions of "predicted steal" were subtracted from identical ROI values in the contralateral hemisphere to determine the mean difference.

## RESULTS

In the eight patients with symptoms of steal, the AVM locations were random throughout the supratentorial compartment. Three patients had parietal AVMs, two had frontal lesions; two, basal ganglia/thalamic lesions; and one, temporal lesions. Of the 20 patients without steal, five had lesions in a parieto-occipital location, four in the parietal lobe, four in the temporal lobe, three in the basal ganglia/thalamic region, and one each in the frontal and occipital lobes, quadrigeminal cistern, and lateral ventricle.

In the steal group, mean differences in rCBF in adjacent cortical regions ranged from $-9$ to $+30$ ml/100 g/min (average: 14.6 ml/100 g/min). In patients without steal, the range was -20 to $+29$ ml/100 g/min (average: 9.5 ml/100 g/min). Although the mean difference showed a trend toward being greater for patients with steal, this difference was not statistically significant ($P = 0.39$, two-sample $t$ test). The mean differences in rCBF in areas of angiographically predicted steal were $-9$ to $+30$ ml/100 g/min (average: 15.3 ml/100 g/min). We compared these figures to those for the patients without steal, in whom the mean difference ranged from -12 to $+29$ ml/100 g/min (average, 8.9 ml/100 g/min). Again, there

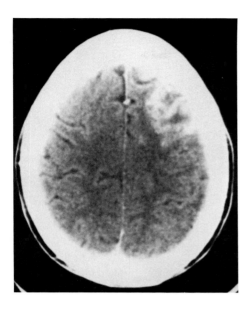

**FIG. 1.** Contrast-enhanced CT demonstrates high left frontal AVM.

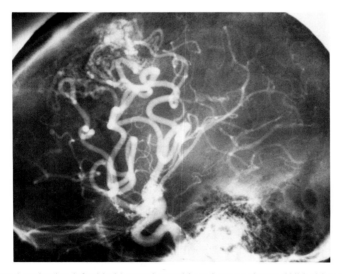

**FIG. 2.** Lateral projection left-sided internal carotid angiogram shows AVM nidus supply from multiple opercular branches. There was additional supply from the right-sided carotid injection with cross filling to the left anterior cerebral artery (not shown). Regions of predicted steal would be the distal territories supplied by the middle cerebral artery in the parietal and parieto-occipital lobes.

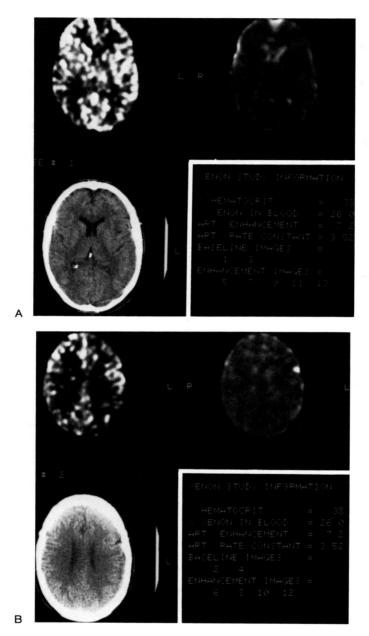

**FIG. 3.** Two levels evaluated with Xe/CT showing the CT levels chosen, the CBF map, and confidence images. Note flow-map areas of lower flow in the left frontal lobe on both slices and in the posterior parietal lobe on the higher slice (**B**).

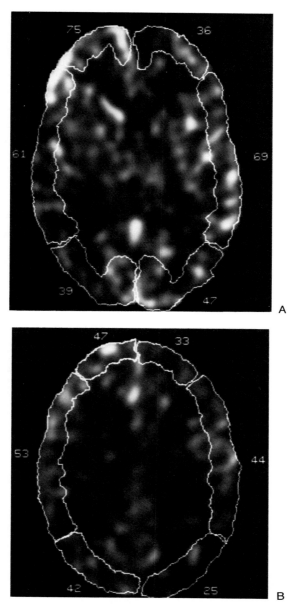

**FIG. 4.** Blood flow maps windowed to show regions of interest (ROI) and their respective flow values in ml/100 g/min. Adjacent cortical areas on the higher slice (**B**) in the frontal and parietal lobes show a mean difference of 14 (47 − 33) and 9 (53 − 44) ml/100 g/min. Areas of predicted steal in the parietal and parieto-occipital lobes on the high slice (**B**) show a mean difference of 9 (53 − 44) and 17 (42 − 25) ml/100 g/min.

was a trend toward higher mean differences in the patients with steal, but the differences were not statistically significant ($P = 0.22$).

AVM size correlated with rCBF results. In the patients without steal, AVM size ranged from 1 to 20 cm$^3$ (mean: 8.7 cm$^3$); in those with steal, the AVMs were 31–125 cm$^3$ (mean: 68 cm$^3$). When we evaluated regions of angiographically predicted steal using linear regression analysis, we found a significant correlation between increasing AVM size and increasing mean difference ($P < 0.027$). However, when we evaluated the cortices adjacent to the AVM, the mean difference was not significant ($P < 0.068$).

We used blood-flow maps to identify those routine ROIs we had drawn in regions where the absolute rCBF value was low (<30 ml/100 g/min). We found areas of low flow in three (15%) of the 20 patients without symptoms of steal and in six (75%) of the eight patients with steal symptoms.

Figures 1–4 show the images, including CBF maps and ROIs, of a 45-year-old woman with a history of seizures. She had progressive memory loss and intermittent aphasia thought to be due to steal.

## DISCUSSION

Comparison of rCBF between cortical regions ipsilateral to the AVM and identical contralateral regions showed a statistically significant decrease in blood flow adjacent to the AVM in patients without clinical steal (5). This study demonstrates that patients with symptoms of clinical steal have a more profound decrease in rCBF than do patients without these symptoms, though the decreases are not statistically significant. We also found that patients with clinical steal are more likely to have cortical regions in which flow is below normal values (<30 ml/100 g/min).

Previous evaluation of angiographic characteristics in patients with AVMs showed that larger size correlates with symptoms of steal (3). Indeed, a larger nidus would be expected to produce a greater shunt. The trend toward lower flow found in this study may thus be explained by the increased shunt present with larger AVMs. Perfusion breakthrough bleeding has also been reported mainly in larger AVMs (2,8–10). This phenomenon occurs because maximally dilated and unresponsive vessels surrounding the AVM are prone to hemorrhage when the AVM is excised. It is likely that the greater declines in blood flow observed near large AVMs are accompanied by maximally dilated vessels—vessels more susceptible to normal perfusion breakthrough bleeding.

The lower blood flow found in this study may have been due to other factors. Cerebral diaschisis has been invoked as a possible reason for the observation of lower flow around the AVM (5,11). Size could contribute to this phenomenon too. The term "diaschisis" has been used to explain blood flow decreases in a region of brain distant from an area of observed neuronal injury. Several studies have proposed that the injury of afferent or efferent fiber tracts results in remote blood flow changes (12,13). The AVM nidus would cause focal loss of neurons seen as areas of gliosis within AVM nidi (14). Presumably, larger nidi would produce more neuronal loss.

Alternatively, the decline in blood flow may be caused by stenosis of vessels proximal to the AVM. Stenosis and occlusions have been implicated in the high flow occurring in AVM feeding vessels (15). Nevertheless, although arterial stenosis was present in one of our patients with steal symptoms, the other patients were not affected in this way. Reduced flow may also be the result of recent or more remote hemorrhage. We attempted to control for this variable by excluding patients with steal who had a prior episode of hemorrhage that contributed to their neurologic deficit. Whereas six (30%) of the 20 patients without steal had a history of intracranial hemorrhage, none in the steal group had any previous clinically significant hemorrhage.

Overall, we have shown that selection of ROIs corresponding to regions of angiographically predicted steal will demonstrate decreases in flow dependent on AVM size. Correlating stable Xe/CT studies with angiography enables the selection of regions that are likely to have relative and absolute decreases in rCBF. Finally, in ROIs adjacent to an AVM, mean differences in rCBF between patients with and without steal were not statistically significant.

## ACKNOWLEDGMENT

The authors wish to thank Paul Chang, M.D., for his invaluable assistance with statistical analysis.

## REFERENCES

1. Luessenhop AJ. Natural history of cerebral arteriovenous malformations. In: Wilson CB, Stein BM, eds. *Intracranial arteriovenous malformations.* 1st ed. Baltimore: Williams & Wilkins, 1984: 12–23.
2. Spetzler RF, Selman WR. Pathophysiology of cerebral ischemia accompanying arteriovenous malformations. In: Wilson CB, Stein BM, eds. *Intracranial arteriovenous malformations.* 1st ed. Baltimore: Williams & Wilkins, 1984:24–31.
3. Marks MP, Lane B, Steinberg G, et al. Angiomatous change: characteristic of vascular architecture associated with steal in intracerebral arteriovenous malformations. *Radiology* 1989;173P:220 (abst).
4. Meyer FB, Sundt TM Jr, Yanagihara T, Anderson RE. Focal cerebral ischemia: pathophysiologic mechanisms and rationale for future avenues of treatment. *Mayo Clin Proc* 1987;62:35–55.
5. Marks MP, O'Donahue J, Fabrikant JI, et al. Cerebral blood flow evaluation of arteriovenous malformations with stable xenon CT. *AJNR* 1988;9:1169–1175.
6. Gur D, Wolfson SK Jr, Yonas H, et al. Progress in cerebrovascular disease: local cerebral blood flow by xenon enhanced CT. *Stroke* 1982;13:750–758.
7. Yonas H, Good WF, Gur D, et al. Mapping cerebral blood flow by xenon-enhanced computed tomography: clinical experience. *Radiology* 1984;152:435–442.
8. Spetzler RF, Wilson CB, Weinstein P, Mehdorn M, Townsend J, Telles D. Normal perfusion pressure breakthrough theory. *Clin Neurosurg* 1978;25:651–672.

9. Day AL, Freidman WA, Sypert GW, Mickle JP. Successful treatment of the normal perfusion pressure breakthrough syndrome. *Neurosurgery* 1982;11:625–630.
10. Batjer HH, Devous MD Sr, Meyer YJ, Purdy PD, Samson DS. Cerebrovascular hemodynamics in arteriovenous malformation complicated by normal perfusion pressure breakthrough. *Neurosurgery* 1988;22:503–509.
11. Tarr RW, Johnson DW, Rutigliano M, et al. Use of acetazolamide-challenge xenon CT in the assessment of cerebral blood flow dynamics in patients with arteriovenous malformations. *AJNR* 1990;11:441–448.
12. Meyer JS, Naritomi H, Sakai F, Ishihara N, Grant P. Regional cerebral blood flow, diaschisis, and steal after stroke. *Neurol Res* 1979;1:101–109.
13. Takano T, Kimura K, Nakamura M, et al. Effects of small deep hemispheric infarction on the ipsilateral cortical blood flow in man. *Stroke* 1985;16:64–69.
14. Stein B, Wolpert SM. Arteriovenous malformations of the brain: current concepts and treatment. *Arch Neurol* 1980;37:1–5.
15. Mawad ME, Hilal SK, Michelsen WJ, Stein B, Ganti SR. Occlusive vascular disease associated with cerebral arteriovenous malformations. *Radiology* 1984;153:401–408.

*Cerebral Blood Flow Measurement with Stable Xenon-Enhanced Computed Tomography,* edited by Howard Yonas. Raven Press, Ltd., New York © 1992.

# Flow Studies Before and During Operative Treatment of Arteriovenous Malformations

## Takahito Yazaki, Takeshi Kawase, and Shigeo Toya

*Department of Neurosurgery, School of Medicine, Keio University, 35 Shinanomachi, Shinjuku-ku, Tokyo 160, Japan*

Understanding the hemodynamics in cerebrovascular malformations and its influence on the surrounding normal cerebral tissue is important in assessing the clinical symptoms of the malformation and the propriety of surgical treatment. Various findings have been reported regarding the cerebral hemodynamics in the area surrounding an intracranial arteriovenous malformation (AVM) (1). Of particular interest was a report that a low-perfusion area located around the AVM and induced by the steal phenomenon contributes to the onset of normal perfusion pressure breakthrough (NPPB) (2,3).

We determined the cerebral blood flow (CBF) at the AVM periphery by performing xenon-enhanced/computed tomography (Xe/CT) studies before and during AVM excision. We also measured CBF in some patients who demonstrated low flow in the surrounding area by using a laser Doppler measuring apparatus before and after excision. We examined the prognostic influences of both CBF kinetics at the AVM periphery before and after excision and the blood flow variations.

## SUBJECTS AND METHODS

Our subjects were 16 patients with AVMs, 17 to 49 years old (mean age: 31.7 years). The subjects were grouped according to the size of the nidus on cerebral angiograms: 4 to 6 cm was considered large; 2 to 4 cm, moderate; and <2 cm, small.

We performed Xe/CT CBF studies as follows. First, with the patient lying on the CT table, the head and limbs were stabilized. The patient wore a mask fitted tightly to his or her face. The mask was connected to a recirculating xenon-inhalation apparatus equipped with a xenon sensor. After denitrogenation for 10 minutes through the inhalation of 100% oxygen, we chose three scanning levels. Scanning was done continually for 25 minutes during slow respiration while 600 to 1,000 ml/min of 100% xenon gas was delivered to the inhalation circuit. The final concentration of inspired xenon was 35% to 60%. We also analyzed the end-tidal concentration of xenon in the blood. Finally, a functional image (CBF map, λ map, and $k$ map) of each slice was produced.

In four patients, we used a laser Doppler tissue blood flow-measuring apparatus to determine intraoperative CBF (4,5). The sites of CBF determination during craniotomy were the normal cerebral surface (control), the cerebral surface around the feeding artery (at the upper part of the nidus, proximal region), and the cerebral surface around the draining vein (at the lower part of nidus, distal region). Direct cortical CBF measurements were obtained before and after resection of the AVM at all of these sites.

## RESULTS

Preoperative Xe/CT CBF studies demonstrated low flow in all four patients with large AVMs and in six patients with moderate AVMs (Table 1). Before excision, four of these patients also had low flow values in the proximal region on the intraoperative CBF study.

Patient 13 was a 37-year-old man who had been experiencing syncope. Right-sided carotid arteriography (CAG) demonstrated an extremely expanded angular artery as the main feeder (Fig. 1). Right-sided vertebral arteriography (VAG)

**TABLE 1.** Clinical and xenon/CT blood flow data in patients with cerebral arteriovenous malformations

| Patient | Age (yrs)/sex | Signs and symptoms | AVM location | Low flow on Xe/CT | MABP (mm Hg) | PaCO$_2$ |
|---------|---------------|--------------------|--------------|-------------------|--------------|----------|
| Small AVM | | | | | | |
| 1 | 32/M | Seizures | R frontal | − | 95 | 48 |
| 2 | 16/M | Seizures | L frontal | − | 90 | 49 |
| 3 | 57/M | Seizures | R parietal | − | 97 | 41 |
| 4 | 29/F | Seizures | L frontal | − | 93 | 45 |
| Moderate AVM | | | | | | |
| 5 | 25/M | Headache | R frontal | + | 91 | 49 |
| 6 | 35/M | R hemiparesis | L pareital | + | 88 | 40 |
| 7 | 17/M | Headache | R frontal | − | 98 | 46 |
| 8 | 29/F | Seizures | L parietal | + | 70 | 50 |
| 9 | 22/M | Headache Visual disturbance | R occipital | − | 93 | 48 |
| 10 | 45/M | Seizures | L temporal | + | 77 | 43 |
| 11 | 49/M | Headache | R temporal | + | 91 | 42 |
| 12 | 22/M | Seizures | L occipital | + | 90 | 46 |
| Large AVM | | | | | | |
| 13 | 37/M | Seizures | R temporo-occipital | + | 92 | 46 |
| 14 | 38/M | Seizures | L frontoparietal | + | 90 | 42 |
| 15 | 34/M | Seizures | L parietal | + | 98 | 46 |
| 16 | 20/M | Seizures | R frontoparietal | + | 95 | 46 |

Xe/CT, xenon-enhanced computed tomography; MABP, mean arterial blood pressure; R, right; L, left.

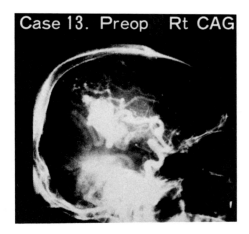

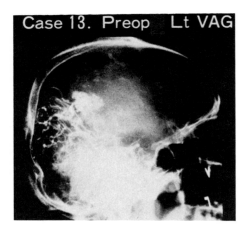

FIG. 1. Patient 13. Preoperative angiograms. Top, right carotid artery; bottom, left vertebral artery.

confirmed other feeders from the parieto-occipital artery and the lateral posterior choroidal artery. Preoperative Xe/CT revealed low flow in the area surrounding the AVM (Fig. 2). A parietotemporal craniotomy was performed, and perioperative CBF was determined at four sites, as shown in Fig. 3: a control site (#1), proximal areas around the feeding artery (#2 and #3), and the distal area around the draining vein (#4). At the control site, CBF was 47 ml/100 g/min before resection and 30 ml/100 g/min after (63.8% decrease). In the proximal regions, CBF values were markedly low before resection (18 ml/100 g/min at each), but rose to 92 ml/100 g/min after (511% increase). The flow value in the distal area decreased slightly before resection to 31 ml/100 g/min. Although uncontrollable hemorrhage and cerebral swelling did not occur during the operation, postoperative CT showed a slight hemorrhage at the periphery of the excision site.

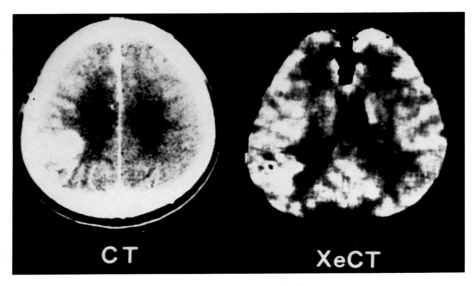

**FIG. 2.** Patient 13. Preoperative images.

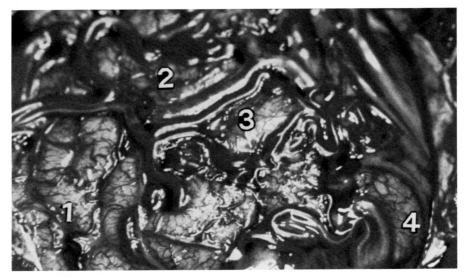

**FIG. 3.** Patient 13. Cerebral blood flow measurement sites.

**TABLE 2.** *Intraoperative cerebral blood flow (CBF) measurements in patient 14*

| Location | CBF (ml/100 g/min) | | % Change |
|---|---|---|---|
| | Before resection | After resection | |
| 1. Control | 68 | 73 | 107 |
| 2. Proximal | 50 | 140 | 280 |
| 3. Proximal | 57 | 175 | 307 |
| 4. Proximal | 18 | 130 | 722 |
| 5. Distal | 80 | 41 | 51.3 |
| 6. Distal | 80 | 76 | 95 |

Patient 14 was a 38-year-old man with symptoms of convulsion and depression. Left-sided CAG revealed distal middle cerebral and lenticulostriate arterial feeders to an AVM in the motor area. Preoperative Xe/CT confirmed low flow at the periphery of the AVM. Direct cortical CBF measurements were obtained at six sites (Table 2). The flow values at the control site (#1) were 68 and 73 ml/100 g/min, respectively, before and after AVM excision; no marked changes were seen. In the proximal areas #2 and #3 and especially in area #4, CBF values were considerably lower before AVM resection. After resection, CBF values approximately tripled. In the distal regions (#5 and #6), CBF was not reduced before excision, but it did decrease postoperatively in area 5. Although this patient also had no intractable hemorrhage during the operation, evidence of slight hemorrhage was seen via CT. Postoperative hemorrhage such as this was seen in three patients with moderate AVMs and three with large AVMs.

## DISCUSSION

Most of the patients with low flow around the AVM on their preoperative study were in the groups with a moderate or large nidus. Low flow can be caused by the steal phenomenon (3). This phenomenon is believed to occur when arteriovenous shunting increases along with the size of an AVM, and the inner pressure of the feeding vessel flowing into the surrounding normal cerebral tissue decreases below the threshold of autoregulation. In short, the size of the AVM, itself seems to have some influence on CBF.

Intraoperative CBF studies confirmed the presence of low flow proximal to the AVM, as had been demonstrated in preoperative Xe/CT images. In addition, we saw markedly increased CBF after resection in patients with low CBF values before resection. Slight hemorrhages also were evident on postoperative CT images in these hyperemic patients. It is very likely that these hemorrhages were caused by hyperperfusion occurring at the previous sites of steal-induced ischemia. The feeder with low pressure and high flow preoperatively may also have suffered vascular overload as a result of higher pressures after resection (6), leading to the so-called NPPB.

## CONCLUSIONS

Based on our study, we conclude that the degree of preoperative hypoperfusion correlates with the size of an AVM. We also believe that Xe/CT CBF studies may be useful for predicting NPPB before surgery.

## REFERENCES

1. Nornes H, Grip A, Winkeby P. Intraoperative evaluation of cerebral hemodynamics using directional Doppler technique. *J Neurosurg* 1979;50:145–151.
2. Spetzler RF. Normal perfusion pressure breakthrough theory in large AVMs. *Neurosurgeons* 1988;7: 27–33.
3. Spetzler RF, Wilson CB, Weinstein P, Mehdorn M, Townsend J, Telles D. Normal perfusion pressure breakthrough theory. *Clin Neurosurg* 1978;25:651–672.
4. Barnett GH, Little JR, Ebrahim ZY, et al. Cerebral circulation during arteriovenous malformation operation. *Neurosurgery* 1987;20:836–842.
5. Rosenblum BR, Bonner RF, Oldfield EH. Intraoperative measurement of cortical blood flow adjacent to cerebral AVM using laser Doppler velocimetry. *J Neurosurg* 1987;66:396-399.
6. Nornes H. Hemodynamic aspect of cerebral arteriovenous malformations. *J Neurosurg* 1980;53: 456–464.

*Cerebral Blood Flow Measurement with Stable Xenon-Enhanced Computed Tomography,* edited by Howard Yonas. Raven Press, Ltd., New York © 1992.

# Hemodynamics in Patients with Brain Tumors

Mitsuharu Tsuura, Tomoaki Terada, Hideyoshi Yokote, Genhachi Hyotani, Kazuki Miyamoto, Yoshinari Nakamura, Takashi Nishiguchi, Toru Itakura, Seiji Hayashi, and Norihiko Komai

*Department of Neurological Surgery, Wakayama Medical College, 7 bancho 27, Wakayama City 640, Japan*

We developed stereotactic local hyperthermia therapy for malignant brain tumors and have achieved successful results (1). However, this therapy has two problems. One is that high blood flow in and about the tumor causes the local temperature to fall, producing the so-called cooling effect. The other is the risk of bleeding that can occur in a hypervascular lesion treated by the stereotactic approach. To assess the feasibility of this therapy, then, we measured the pattern of blood flow in brain tumors.

## PATIENTS AND METHODS

We used xenon-enhanced computed tomography (Xe/CT) to measure the local blood flow in brain tumors in 30 patients. Fifteen patients had gliomas, five had metastatic brain tumors, three had malignant lymphomas, and seven had meningiomas. All patients underwent Xe/CT, iodinated contrast-enhanced CT, magnetic resonance imaging, and histological examination of the tumor.

We used a Toshiba TCT 60-A CT scanner and a special head frame to prevent patient motion. Patients were given 35% stable xenon gas to breathe for 6 minutes, followed by 100% oxygen for 9 minutes. We obtained images at two levels in each patient. The end-tidal xenon gas concentration was monitored continually to obtain input data for analysis. The blood flow and λ values were calculated with the Kety-Schmidt equation, and cerebral blood flow and λ maps were also produced (2).

We compared the tumor blood flow (TBF) with blood flow values in normal tissue without edema or tumor invasion. We then classified TBF into six groups: group 1, TBF from zero to one-half of normal white-matter flow values; group

2, TBF below, but greater than one-half of, normal white-matter flow values; group 3, TBF equal to white-matter flow; group 4, TBF above normal white-matter flow values but less than normal gray-matter flow; group 5, TBF equal to normal gray-matter flow; and group 6, TBF above normal gray-matter values. In each patient, we measured the TBF in three regions: the nonenhanced low-density central area surrounded by the contrast-enhanced region, in the contrast-enhanced region, and in the low-density area around the contrast-enhanced region.

## RESULTS

### Glioma Group

Figure 1 shows an anaplastic astrocytoma. The low-density area on the CT image indicates a blood flow value near that of normal white-matter, and tumor invasion in this area was confirmed histologically. The tissue invaded by tumor had a higher blood flow value than tissue that was edematous but uninvaded, as shown in a patient with a glioblastoma multiforme (Fig. 2). The low-density area around the contrast-enhanced region, where the flow value was less than half of normal white-matter flow, was regarded as having edema without tumor invasion. There was thus a difference between flow values in the low-density

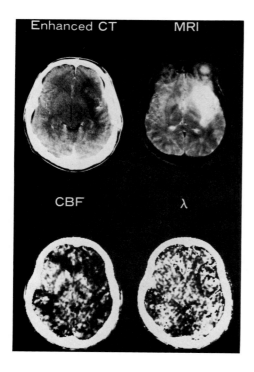

**FIG. 1.** An anaplastic astrocytoma from our study.

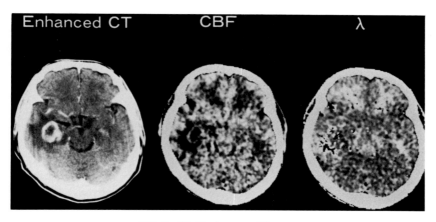

**FIG. 2.** Glioblastoma multiforme.

area without tumor invasion and that with tumor invasion. In another glioblastoma multiforme, flow values in the contrast-enhanced region were near those of normal white matter. Histological examination found no necrosis or cyst but did find a viable tumor. In contrast, flow in the low-density area within the tumor tended to be less than half of normal white-matter flow, and most of this tissue was necrotic.

Figure 3 summarizes the blood flow data for gliomas. In five of the gliomas, flow in the outer low-density area was greater than half of normal white-matter

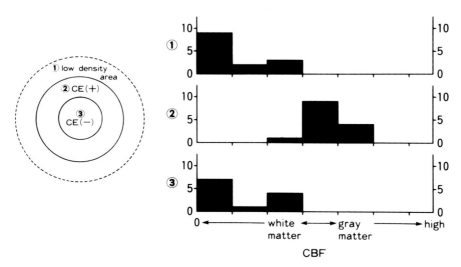

**FIG. 3.** Summary of blood flow data for gliomas. Vertical axes of bar graphs show number of cases.

flow. This tissue was thought to be invaded by tumor. In the area with positive contrast enhancement, the blood flow values ranged from normal white-matter to normal gray-matter values. The inner low-density area with markedly low blood flow (near zero) was regarded as necrotic or cystic tissue. In some cases, however, blood flow in this inner area was nearly that of white matter, suggesting the presence of viable tumor.

### Metastatic Brain Tumor Group

An example of a metastatic brain tumor in the right temporo-occipital region is shown in Fig. 4. The degree of the enhancement was quite uniform in the contrast-enhanced area. However, blood flow in the medial part of the tumor was lower than in the lateral part. Histological examination found hypervascular and hypercellular tumor tissue in the lateral part and hypovascular tumor tissue with necrotic components in the medial. This case showed that contrast enhancement does not always reflect the vascularity of the tumor tissue.

Flow data for the metastatic brain tumors is summarized in Fig. 5. The low-density area around the contrast enhancement had remarkably low flow, almost zero. Flow values within the contrast-enhanced area ranged from those of normal white matter to those of gray matter.

### Malignant Lymphoma and Meningioma Groups

Figure 6 shows a malignant lymphoma. The flow values within the contrast enhancement were between those of white-matter and those of gray-matter. The meningiomas had higher blood flow than that found in normal gray matter (Fig. 7).

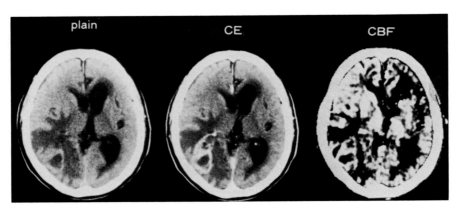

**FIG. 4.** Metastatic brain tumor.

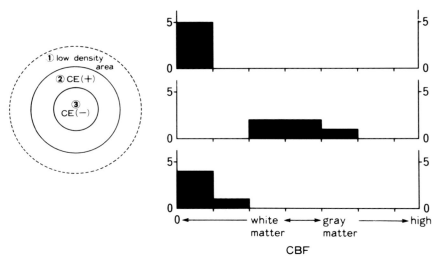

**FIG. 5.** Summary of blood flow data for metastatic brain tumors. Vertical axes of bar graphs show number of cases.

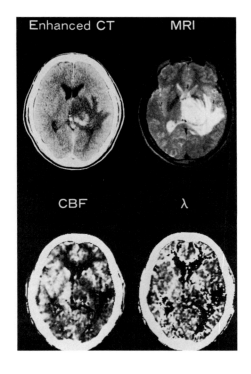

**FIG. 6.** Malignant lymphoma.

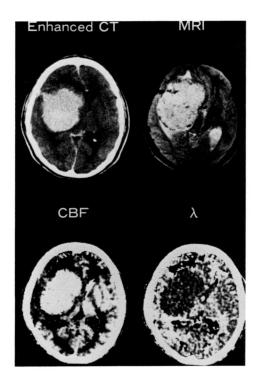

**FIG. 7.** Meningioma.

## DISCUSSION

The difference between contrast-enhanced CT and Xe/CT is that contrast-enhanced CT is influenced by the blood volume of the tissue and the vascular permeability (3), whereas Xe/CT reflects the tissue flow (4,5). Therefore, Xe/CT is a useful method for investigating the blood flow in tissue that is thought to reflect tissue vascularity. It is also useful in estimating the cooling effect and tissue viability. In the gliomas, flow in the low-density area around the contrast enhancement was higher than flow typically found in peritumoral edema seen in meningiomas and metastatic brain tumors. Tumor invasion was suspected in these areas.

Three factors—heat conductance, the cooling effect, and tissue vulnerability—must be considered in estimating the effect of the local hyperthermia therapy. The TBF, which influences the cooling effect, was examined with the data of 30 patients who had various brain tumors. We expected successful results from local hyperthermia therapy for malignant brain tumors in which flow values were equal to or less than gray-matter flow, because thalamotomy for tremor is performed successfully in normal tissue with stereotactic heat coagulation technique. Nevertheless, hyperthermia therapy must be tailored to the individual patient, because we found that blood flow values in and around tumors were not the same for all lesions.

## CONCLUSION

In patients with gliomas and metastatic tumors, blood flow in the tumor tissue was the same as or less than that of gray matter in the normal brain. Therefore, these tumors would be good candidates for stereotactic hyperthermia therapy.

## REFERENCES

1. Yokote H, Komai N, Nakai E, Itakura T, Hayashi S. Stereotactic hyperthermia for brain tumors. Tenth Meeting of the World Society for Stereotactic and Functional Neurosurgery, 1989 (Abstract).
2. Nakamura Y, Hyotani G, Terada T, et al. Regional cerebral blood flow measurement by stable xenon-enhanced CT: methodology and problems. *J Wakayama Med Soc* 1990;41 [*in press*].
3. Sage MR. Kinetics of water-soluble contrast media in the central nervous system. *AJR* 1983;141: 815–824.
4. Drayer BP, Wolfson SK Jr, Reinmuth OM, Dujovney M, Boehnke M, Cook EE. Xenon enhanced CT for analysis of cerebral integrity, perfusion, and blood flow. *Stroke* 1978;9:123-130.
5. Gur D, Yonas H, Wolfson SK Jr, et al. Xenon and iodine enhanced cerebral CT: a closer look. *Stroke* 1981;12:573-578.

*Cerebral Blood Flow Measurement with Stable Xenon-Enhanced Computed Tomography,* edited by Howard Yonas. Raven Press, Ltd., New York © 1992.

# Local Blood Flow in Malignant Brain Tumors: The Effect of Induced Hypertension

Tomoaki Terada, Kazuki Miyamoto, Genhachi Hyotani, Mitsuharu Tsuura, Yoshinari Nakamura, Takashi Nishiguchi, Toru Itakura, Seiji Hayashi, and Norihiko Komai

*Department of Neurological Surgery, Wakayama Medical College, 7 bancho 27, Wakayama City 640, Japan*

Conventional chemotherapy is not always effective for malignant brain tumors. Successful treatment requires that a large amount of the chemotherapeutic agent be preferentially delivered only to the tumor tissue (1–3). We studied the changes in blood flow that occur in tumors under a hypertensive state to determine whether induced hypertensive chemotherapy is an effective treatment for malignant brain tumors.

## PATIENTS AND METHODS

We measured the blood flow in tumors under both a resting state and an induced hypertensive state in 12 patients. Six patients had gliomas, including three with glioblastoma multiformes, two with anaplastic astrocytomas, and one with an ependymoma. The other six patients had metastatic brain tumors with histological findings of adenocarcinoma (see Table 1). Patients with ischemic heart disease or other heart problems were excluded from this study.

Stable xenon-enhanced computed tomography (Xe/CT) was used to measure blood flow in the tumors. The CT scanner was a Toshiba TCT 60-A. The inhaled xenon gas concentration was 35%, and the method was the 6-minute "wash-in"/9-minute "wash-out" protocol. We studied two 10-mm-thick CT slices. The end-tidal xenon concentration was monitored continually, and the resulting data were used as the input function for computing flow values with the Kety–Schmidt equation.

We first measured cerebral blood flow (CBF) under a "resting" state. Then we measured CBF under a hypertensive state that was 40% above the systemic

**TABLE 1.** *Summary of cases*

| Patient | Age (yrs)/ sex | Tumor type | BP (mm Hg) rest/HT | PaCO$_2$ (mm Hg) rest/HT | Blood flow (ml/100 g/min) Tumor rest/HT | Blood flow (ml/100 g/min) Contralateral rest/HT | % Change |
|---|---|---|---|---|---|---|---|
| 1 | 38/M | AA | 80/120 | 44.0/43.1 | 20.1/29.4 | 31.8/28.9 | 60 |
| 2 | 68/M | AA | 115/140 | 41.2/37.5 | 18.8/15.6 | 19.2/11.2 | 42 |
| 3 | 48/M | GM | 90/140 | 34.9/31.7 | 18.7/20.1 | 31.4/29.5 | 14 |
| 4 | 70/F | GM | 103/140 | 40.9/32.4 | 20.8/26.1 | 38.2/38.3 | 48 |
| 5 | 27/F | Ep | 88/110 | 31.7/32.5 | 32.2/34.9 | 59.3/58.8 | 9 |
| 6 | 75/M | GM | 105/140 | 48.5/48.0 | 25.9/30.8 | 23.5/21.1 | 32 |
| 7 | 63/F | Met | 90/140 | 32.5/36.0 | 10.3/13.1 | 21.7/27.1 | 2 |
| 8 | 74/M | Met | 85/140 | 42.6/42.0 | 20.5/19.6 | 28.6/24.1 | 14 |
| 9 | 56/F | Met | 85/120 | 35.1/36.1 | 14.1/14.7 | 36.3/35.2 | 11 |
| 10 | 67/M | Met | 95/134 | 31.8/31.4 | 23.8/25.5 | 50.1/42.5 | 28 |
| 11 | 76/M | Met | 93/140 | 34.4/32.1 | 19.8/44.9 | 29.1/30.2 | 119 |
| 12 | 57/M | Met | 93/140 | 37.4/36.1 | 18.8/15.0 | 29.4/30.5 | 17 |
| Mean | | | 94/134 | 37.9/36.6 | 20.3/24.1 | | 30 |

BP, blood pressure; AA, anaplastic astrocytoma; GM, glioblastoma multiforme; Ep, ependymoma; Met, metastatic; rest, resting; HT. hypertension.

blood pressure, which we induced with angiotensin II. We sampled blood gases during each examination. The change in the tumor blood flow (TBF) was defined as the percentage of TBF change over the change in normal brain-tissue blood flow in the contralateral hemisphere. This was evaluated as follows:

$$\% \text{ TBF changes} = \text{TBF}_{HT}/\text{TBF}_{cont}/\text{CBF}_{HT}/\text{CBF}_{cont} \times 100 - 100\%$$

where $\text{TBF}_{HT}$ is tumor blood flow during hypertension, $\text{TBF}_{cont}$ is tumor blood flow during the resting state, $\text{CBF}_{HT}$ is CBF in the normal tissue during hypertension, and $\text{CBF}_{cont}$ is CBF in the normal tissue during the resting state.

## RESULTS

In the glioma group, TBF increased to varying degrees, depending on changes in blood pressure. Although the increase in TBF did not always correlate with the degree of malignancy of the tumor, the least activation was observed in the least malignant tumor (i.e., ependymoma) (Table 1). In the metastatic tumor group, TBF increased in all but one patient. This increase was marked in patients with highly vascular tumors.

Table 1 also shows the changes in physiological study parameters. The average increase in blood pressure for all patients was from 93 to 134 mm Hg. The PaCO$_2$ did not change significantly. The increase in TBF was from 20.3 to 24.1 ml/100 g/min. The TBF values were lower than the gray-matter flow values within individual patients. A 30% increase in TBF was a statistically significant change when compared with the change contralaterally ($P < 0.05$). Following are reports of two representative cases.

Patient 4 had a glioblastoma multiforme. After administering angiotensin II, we saw an increase in the TBF in the peripheral tumor tissue (Fig. 1). Under this induced hypertension, the appearance of the tumor typified glioblastoma, although the center of the tumor was mainly necrotic tissue.

Patient 11 had a metastatic brain tumor in the right temporo-occipital region. Our flow study demonstrated a 119% increase in the TBF after blood pressure elevation (Fig. 2). Histological examination of the tumor found it to be a hypervascular metastatic adenocarcinoma without necrotic components.

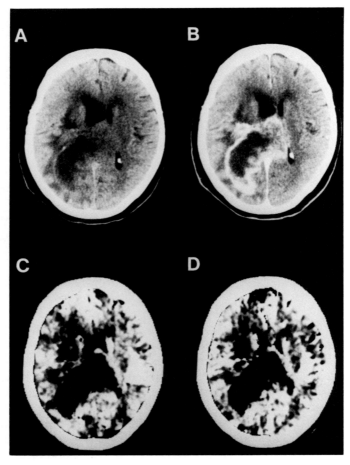

**FIG. 1.** (Patient 4) **A**: Plain CT. **B**: Intravenous iodine-enhanced CT. **C**: Blood flow map, resting state. **D**: Blood flow map, hypertensive state.

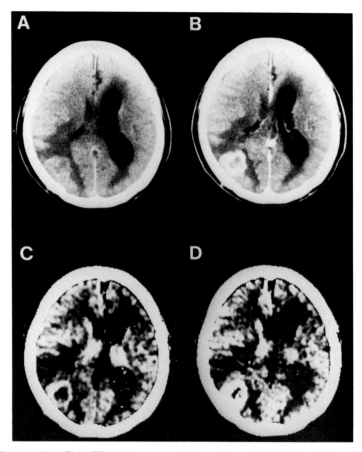

**FIG. 2.** (Patient 11) **A**: Plain CT. **B**: Intravenous iodine-enhanced CT. **C**: Blood flow map, resting state. **D**: Blood flow map, hypertensive state.

## DISCUSSION

Two factors defined the TBF changes that accompanied changes in blood pressure. The first was the vascularity of the tumor. Compared with hypovascular tumors, especially those with necrotic components, the TBF increased more in hypervascular tumors. Normal brain tissue can maintain blood flow because the autoregulation mechanism is functional. However, autoregulation is lacking in malignant tumors (2,3). Such tumors with high flow have more blood vessels that are responsive to blood pressure changes. Equally malignant low-flow tumors with necrotic components would be less responsive to blood pressure changes. Therefore, the increase in blood flow is greater in malignant tumors with already high flow.

The second factor that influenced TBF changes was the histologic composition of the tumor. The patient with the least malignant tumor (an ependymoma) had the smallest change in TBF. Perhaps the increase in tissue acidosis associated with increasing degrees of malignancy is responsible for a loss of autoregulation in the more malignant tumors.

## CONCLUSIONS

Our study showed that in some patients with malignant brain tumors, a marked increase in TBF accompanies a rise in the systemic arterial blood pressure. We therefore believe that chemotherapy under an induced hypertensive state will be more effective in patients with malignant tumors.

## REFERENCES

1. Arbit E, DiResta GR, Bedford RF, Shah NK, Galicich JH. Intraoperative measurement of cerebral and tumor blood flow with laser-Doppler flowmetry. *Neurosurgery* 1989;24:166–170.
2. Matsuura H, Ikeda I, Imaya H, Nakazawa S. Selective changes of blood flow in experimental brain tumor with induced hypertension. *Surg Neurol* 1987;27:433–436.
3. Suzuki M, Hori K, Abe I, Saito S, Sato H. A new approach to cancer chemotherapy: selective enhancement of tumor blood flow with angiotensin II. *J Natl Cancer Inst* 1981;67:663-669.

*Cerebral Blood Flow Measurement with Stable Xenon-Enhanced Computed Tomography,* edited by Howard Yonas. Raven Press, Ltd., New York © 1992.

# Cerebral Blood Flow Mapping in the Clinical Management of Gliomas

Osamu Nakamura and *Hiromu Segawa

*Department of Neurosurgery, Tokyo Metropolitan Komagome Hospital, 3–18–22 Honkomagome, Bunkyo-ku, Tokyo, Japan; and *Department of Neurosurgery, Fuji Brain Institute and Hospital, 270–12 Sugita, Fujinomiya, Shizuoka, Japan*

In the management of gliomas, it is important to know the extent and viability of the tumor. However, ordinary computed tomography (CT) with iodine enhancement has only limited ability to distinguish the tumor from surrounding normal tissue. Therefore, we used the xenon-enhanced CT method (Xe/CT) to investigate the cerebral blood flow (CBF) in tumors and the surrounding brain in 11 patients with gliomas and four with metastatic tumors. Xe/CT has several advantages over the conventional isotope method and enabled us to evaluate CBF maps with high spacial resolution.

## METHODS

The patient's head was firmly secured on the scanner table to avoid undesirable movement during scanning. After a baseline scan, patients inhaled 50% xenon mixed with oxygen for 25 minutes through a closed rebreathing ventilation system. During this saturation period, we performed a CT scan every 5 minutes. The expired air was sampled continually and passed through a mass spectrometer that determined the concentrations of xenon, oxygen, carbon dioxide, and nitrogen. We placed an arterial catheter in the patient's radial artery to permit blood gas determinations and to measure the xenon concentration in the arterial blood. A 5-ml syringe of blood was drawn after each scan and kept in a water bath for scanning after the procedure.

We analyzed the saturation curves using a program developed by Obrist. The regional (r) CBF can be derived from the time-dependent xenon concentrations in arterial blood and the tissue of interest: $f = \lambda \cdot k$, where $k$ is the flow rate constant and $f$ is blood flow. The spatial resolution of CT enables estimation of the blood-brain partition coefficient in small regions of the brain. If equilibrium is established between the arterial blood and the selected brain region, then $\lambda$ can be calculated. Equilibrium is confirmed by consistent CT enhancement in blood and brain on serial CT scans performed during inhalation. The maps of $k$, $\lambda$, and rCBF were displayed separately on a monitor (256 × 256 matrix) (1).

## RESULTS

The following five cases are presented to demonstrate the $k$, $\lambda$, and rCBF values of the brain tumors and to show their usefulness in clinical studies.

Case 1: a 53-year-old woman with a grade IV left-sided temporo-occipital astrocytoma. A routine CT scan demonstrated a ring-like region that enhanced with iodine contrast in the left occipital lobe. This area was consistent with a ring-like region of high rCBF defined by Xe/CT (Fig. 1).

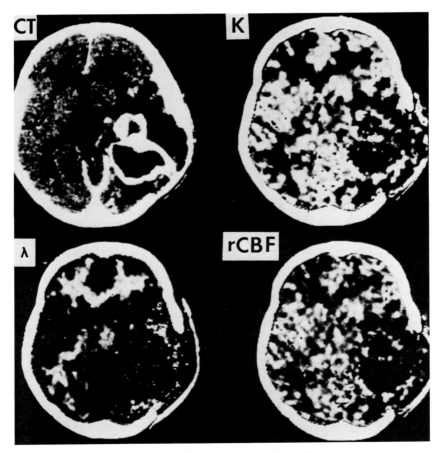

**FIG. 1.** Grade IV astrocytoma (case 1).

Case 2: a 68-year-old woman with a right frontal grade III astrocytoma. A routine CT scan showed an irregular iodine-enhanced area in the right frontal region, surrounded by a low-density area probably caused by brain edema. On the rCBF map, a larger ring-like zone of high rCBF surrounded the iodine-enhanced region on the CT scan (Fig. 2). Intraoperatively, the tumor was found to extend deeply into the right lateral ventricle. The area of high rCBF on the rCBF map helped to confirm the limit of the tumor.

Case 3: a 30-year-old man with a bilateral frontal gemistocytic astrocytoma. The CT scan demonstrated a low-density area in the frontal lobe that failed to enhance with iodine contrast. Bilaterally, the frontal lobes contained areas with

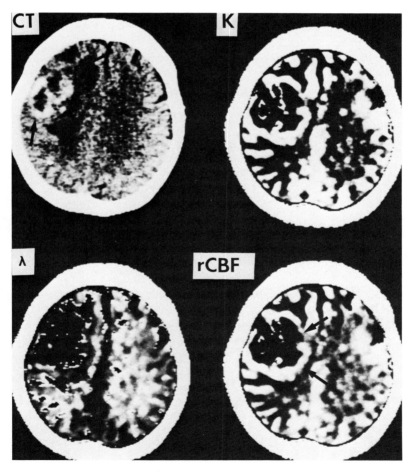

**FIG. 2.** Grade III astrocytoma (case 2). The extent of the tumor is indicated by arrows on the CT and rCBF images.

high flow (mean value: 69 ml/100 g/min) that extended posteriorly between the ventricles. These findings suggested extensive invasion of the tumor in the corpus callosum. Three months after radiation therapy, we again evaluated the CBF to study the effect of radiation. The CT and CBF findings before and after radiation are illustrated in Figure 3.

Case 4: a 36-year-old man with a right frontal grade III astrocytoma. CT showed a right frontal low-density area without iodine enhancement. However, it is difficult to distinguish gliomas from edema in CT images. In the rCBF image, we identified a region of increased rCBF, which was consistent with the CT findings. But in this case, a λ map was most useful in demarcating the lesion. The distinction between the tumor and white matter was demonstrated clearly as a difference in λ values (Fig. 4). After radiation therapy, the CBF study indicated that the extent of the tumor was reduced; the CBF value of the gray matter was also lower (Fig. 5). Thus, Xe/CT was useful in evaluating the therapeutic effect of radiation in both cases 3 and 4.

The mean gray-matter flow of the 15 patients with brain tumors was 55 ml/100 g/min, lower than that of normal subjects. We examined the rCBF in various

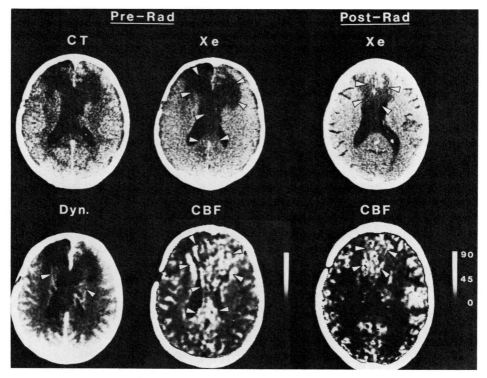

**FIG. 3.** Gemistocytic astrocytoma (case 3).

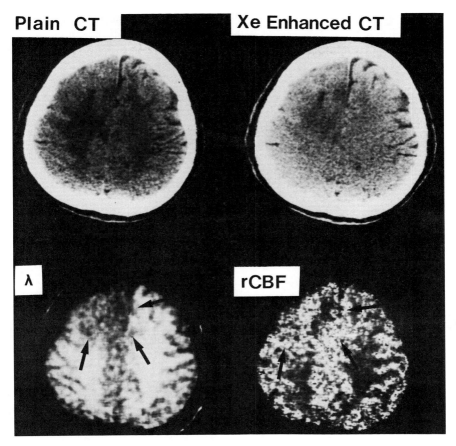

**FIG. 4.** Grade III astrocytoma (case 4). The extent of the tumor is indicated by arrows on the rCBF and λ maps.

parts of the tumors and found that it was almost zero in the cystic and necrotic areas. The mean rCBF value of the non-necrotic area in each brain tumor is listed in Table 1. In patients with glioblastoma, the average flow value in the tumor was a little lower than that of the gray matter in the same patient. In patients with gliomas, the mean λ value was 1.02 ± 0.06, almost the same as for gray matter. In contrast, the mean λ value of metastatic tumors was much lower, 0.72 ± 0.09 (see Table 1).

## DISCUSSION

Our analysis of the rCBF distribution in brain tumors has shown low flow values in the center because of necrosis or cysts and high values in a ring-like

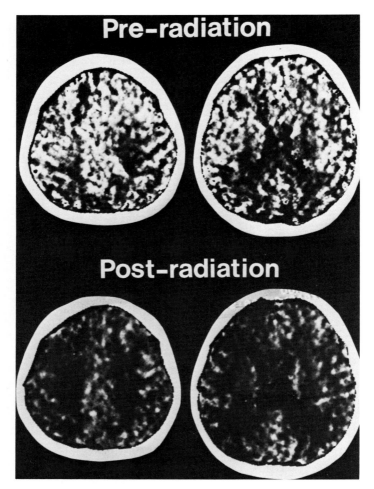

**FIG. 5.** Blood flow maps at two brain levels in a patient with a grade III astrocytoma (case 4).

peripheral region. The 55 ml/100 g/min rCBF value of this peripheral zone, which may indicate a proliferating tumor, was markedly higher than that of white matter. This was especially true when there were edematous changes in the white matter (below 10 ml/100 g/min). Thus, these tissues could easily be distinguished from one another. This difference displayed on the rCBF map enabled us to distinguish the boundaries of tumors showing low density and negative contrast enhancement on CT images, as in cases 3 and 4. Moreover, in case 2, we could identify a ring-like zone of increased rCBF around the contrast-enhanced region of the CT image, suggesting infiltration of the tumor. The contrast enhancement reflects the increased permeability of the blood-brain barrier

**TABLE 1.** *Blood flow and λ in the brain tumors*

| Patient | Age (yrs)/ sex | Histology | Gray matter | Tumor | Range | (Mean) |
|---------|------|-----------|-------------|-------|-------|--------|
| | | | Mean blood flow (ml/100 g/min) | | λ | |
| TU | 49/M | astrocytoma GII | 33 | 39 | 0.83–1.26 | (1.05) |
| TM | 30/M | astrocytoma GII | 54 | 69 | 0.87–1.22 | (1.05) |
| GN | 42/M | astrocytoma GII | 60 | 30 | 0.80–1.05 | (0.93) |
| FH | 32/M | astrocytoma GII | 95 | 24 | 1.09 | (1.09) |
| KG | 22/F | astrocytoma GI | 55 | 34 | 0.99–1.12 | (1.06) |
| MT | 47/M | astrocytoma GII | 75 | 48 | 0.87–1.36 | (1.12) |
| Group average | | | $62 \pm 19$ | $41 \pm 15$ | $1.05 \pm 0.06$ | |
| FA | 68/F | astrocytoma GIII | 45 | 35 | 0.92 | (0.92) |
| NH | 37/F | astrocytoma GIV | 32 | 24 | 0.82–1.12 | (0.97) |
| NK | 32/M | astrocytoma GIV | 59 | 38 | 1.04 | (1.04) |
| EN | 53/F | astrocytoma GIV | 68 | 57 | 0.88–1.00 | (0.94) |
| HF | 35/M | astrocytoma GIII | 45 | 35 | 0.99–1.01 | (1.00) |
| Group average | | | $50 \pm 12$ | $38 \pm 11$ | $0.97 \pm 0.04$ | |
| YS | 65/M | metastatic tumor | 40 | 50 | 0.71–0.81 | (0.76) |
| MK | 39/M | metastatic tumor | 51 | 60 | 0.55–0.67 | (0.61) |
| IM | 61/M | metastatic tumor | 42 | 43 | 0.66 | (0.66) |
| CK | 56/F | metastatic tumor | 76 | 33 | 0.79–0.88 | (0.84) |
| Group average | | | $52 \pm 14$ | $47 \pm 10$ | $0.72 \pm 0.09$ | |

G, grade.

and does not always show the extent of the tumor. Considering the fact that in most cases the contrast-enhanced region corresponded with the increased rCBF region, as in case 1, the ring-like area of increased rCBF does seem to indicate the extent of the tumor.

Another advantage of the Xe/CT method is that the λ maps can be calculated for each patient. Our finding that the λ value of gliomas was almost equal to that of gray matter but significantly lower in metastatic tumors is due to the different lipid contents in these two types of brain tumors. Because the λ value of gliomas is about 1.0, whereas that of white matter is 1.5, the λ map is also useful in distinguishing a glioma from surrounding white matter.

In conclusion, we found that through the evaluation of CT images, rCBF maps, and λ maps, brain tumors can be demarcated more precisely.

## REFERENCE

1. Segawa H, Wakai S, Nakamura O, et al. Computed tomographic measurement of local cerebral blood flow by xenon enhancement. *Stroke* 1983;14:356–362.

*Cerebral Blood Flow Measurement with Stable Xenon-Enhanced Computed Tomography,* edited by Howard Yonas. Raven Press, Ltd., New York © 1992.

# Cerebral Blood Flow in Patients with Normal Pressure Hydrocephalus

Ryuta Suzuki, Masaru Aoyagi, Kimiyoshi Hirakawa, and *Naomi Fukai

*Department of Neurosurgery, Tokyo Medical and Dental University, 1-5-45 Yushima Bunkyo-ku, Tokyo 113, Japan; and *Department of Neurosurgery, Tokyo Metropolitan Geriatric Medical Center, 35-2 Sakae-cho Itabashi-Ku, Tokyo 173, Japan*

Normal pressure hydrocephalus (NPH) is characterized by dementia, gait disturbance, and urinary incontinence. The therapy for this syndrome has focused on considering it a treatable dementia. Although many diagnostic methods have been introduced, none have yielded accurate, predictable data about the effectiveness of a cerebrospinal fluid (CSF) shunt (1). Now, as the human life span is prolonged and dementia among the elderly becomes a major sociomedical problem, the proper method of treating NPH and a more through understanding of its pathophysiology are more important than ever.

To aid in the quest for a reliable therapy, we measured the regional cerebral blood flow (rCBF) in patients with NPH using a stable xenon/computed tomography (Xe/CT) method. We also evaluated cognitive function with the Wechsler Adult Intelligence Scale (WAIS) before and after the patients underwent an effective CSF shunt.

## SUBJECTS AND METHODS

Our subjects were 18 patients with NPH, their ages ranging from 46 to 81 years. The diagnoses of NPH were based on clinical symptoms, a CT scan, and CT cisternography. All patients had undergone a CSF shunt and improved clinically after the operation. Table 1 shows their clinical presentations. To summarize, 11 patients with a mean age of 75 years were diagnosed as having idiopathic NPH. The others were diagnosed as having secondary NPH; their mean age was 71 years.

We graded the clinical symptoms from none (0) to most severe (III). The severity of dementia was categorized by the sum of the WAIS subtest scores, urinary incontinence by the frequency of occurrence, and gait disturbance by locomotive ability. Patients 15–18 demonstrated minimal or no dementia; their

**TABLE 1.** *Clinical summary of subjects*

| Subject | Age (yrs)/ sex | Etiology | Clinical grade[a] | | | Recovery |
|---|---|---|---|---|---|---|
| | | | Dementia | Incontinence | Gait | |
| 1 | 74/M | idiopathic | II | I | III | moderate |
| 2 | 71/F | idiopathic | III | III | II | excellent |
| 3 | 78/M | idiopathic | III | III | III | excellent |
| 4 | 81/F | idiopathic | III | II | II | good |
| 5 | 71/M | idiopathic | III | III | III | excellent |
| 6 | 72/F | idiopathic | III | I | II | slight |
| 7 | 78/M | idiopathic | III | III | III | excellent |
| 8 | 76/F | idiopathic | III | I | III | slight |
| 9 | 79/F | SAH | III | I | III | good |
| 10 | 67/F | SAH | II | | II | moderate |
| 11 | 64/M | SAH | III | II | III | moderate |
| 12 | 73/M | trauma | III | III | III | good |
| 13 | 67/F | trauma | II | I | I | moderate |
| 14 | 46/F | SAH | II | 0 | 0 | moderate |
| 15 | 81/F | idiopathic | 0 | II | II | good |
| 16 | 71/F | idiopathic | 0 | 0 | II | slight |
| 17 | 67/F | idiopathic | I | I | I | moderate |
| 18 | 60/M | SAH | I | III | II | excellent |

[a] Clinical grades ranged from 0 (none) to III (severe).
SAH, subarachnoid hemorrhage.

main manifestation was a gait disorder. We divided the patients into two groups: group A ($n = 14$), patients with severe dementia (grade II or III), and group B ($n = 4$), those with minimal or no dementia (grade 0 or 1) but with a prominent gait disturbance.

For the Xe/CT CBF studies, we used the method reported by Suzuki et al. (2,3). Briefly, after the baseline CT image was obtained, each patient inhaled a mixture of 40% xenon and 60% oxygen for 3 to 4 minutes while a series of 9-second scans was performed at 60-second intervals. Then a topographic rCBF map was constructed from the CT images. We previously had determined that the partition coefficient for the whole brain was 1.0 (2). We obtained the rCBF values for seven regions of interest in each cerebral hemisphere: the whole hemisphere, middle frontal gyrus, frontal white matter, superior temporal gyrus, occipital lobe, putamen, and thalamus. We then compared the values of the two groups.

## RESULTS

Figure 1 shows the WAIS scores for each group before and after the shunt operation. In group A, the verbal, performance, and total IQ scores were low preoperatively, but all improved significantly after the shunt. Group B had relatively high scores before the operation, and their performance and total scores were also significantly better postoperatively.

As shown in Fig. 2, the preoperative rCBF distribution patterns differed between

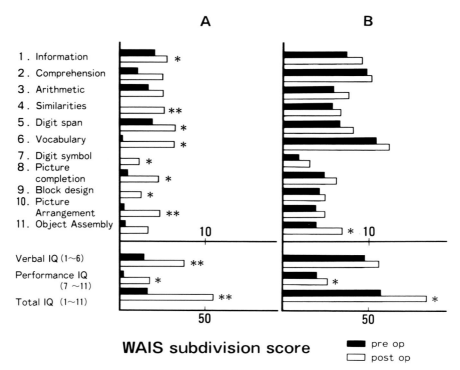

**WAIS subdivision score**   ■ pre op
                              □ post op

**FIG. 1.** Wechsler Adult Intelligence Scale (WAIS) scores before and after the shunt operation in groups A (severe dementia) and B (slight or no dementia).

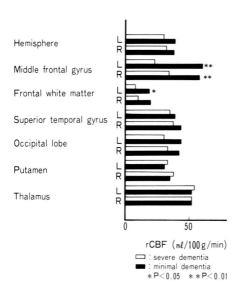

**FIG. 2.** Preoperative resting blood flow values in various brain regions in groups A and B. The differences in the values between the groups were prominent in the frontal regions.

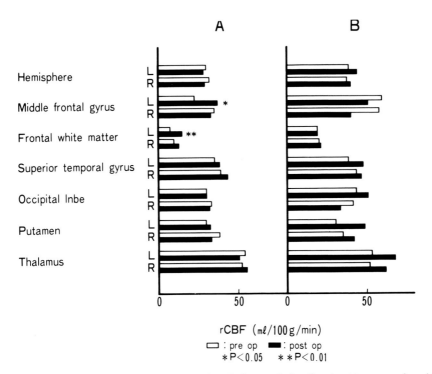

**FIG. 3.** Blood flow values in various brain regions before and after the shunt in groups A and B. Postoperative increases occurred in the frontal regions in group A but in the putamen and thalamus in group B.

the groups. The rCBF values in all regions except the putamen and thalamus were lower in group A than in group B, especially in the right and left middle frontal gyri and the left frontal white matter, where group A's values were significantly lower. After the shunt (Fig. 3), rCBF values in group A increased significantly in the left middle frontal gyrus and left frontal white matter. In contrast, differences in the pre- and postoperative rCBF values in group B varied among the brain regions, although values did increase postoperatively in the putamen and thalamus.

## DISCUSSION

Several researchers have studied CBF changes in patients with NPH. Tamaki et al. (4) found hypoperfusion in the frontal lobe in a study using [133]Xe, and Vorstrup et al. (5) reported findings of central brain hypoperfusion with [133]Xe single-photon emission tomography (SPECT). Meyer et al. (6) studied Xe/CT CBF measurements in patients with NPH and reported that CBF values and partition coefficients in the frontal lobe, frontal white matter, and putamen were higher after a shunt. Though controversial, the results of these studies suggest that both low flow in the frontal lobes and central hypoperfusion can occur in patients with NPH (7).

The discrepancies in these findings may have been due to limitations in the various methods of measuring rCBF. The $^{133}$Xe study does not provide CBF values in the deeper brain structures, and, because patients with NPH have dilated ventricles, the SPECT results may have been distorted by a partial volume effect in the periventricular regions. In contrast, the Xe/CT method produces results with high spatial resolution and good anatomical correlation (8). We therefore believe that Xe/CT is a more reliable clinically available method of measuring rCBF.

Our study suggests that the primary pathologic process of NPH involves ventricular enlargement and that the direction of the CSF pulse pressure may vary. Therefore, if the pressure were directed to the central brain structure, it could cause central hypoperfusion and result in an ataxic gait. Should the pressure escape from the frontal horn, especially the left frontal horn, it might cause low flow within the frontal lobes and result in dementia. Thus, NPH may be a combination of several phenomena, so that its clinical symptoms vary.

Our study also suggests that the CSF pressure in our subjects had escaped primarily toward the central brain. This may explain why good shunt responses were achieved in patients who had gait ataxia and minimal or no dementia as well as in those who had the classic triad. Several authors have asserted that a gait disturbance is a major indicator of shunt success (9,10). Additionally, Black et al. (7) reported that clinical symptoms improved after a shunt in 77% of their patients whose primary symptom of NPH had been gait ataxia. The findings of these researchers serve to confirm our hypothesis.

## REFERENCES

1. Symon L, Hinzpeter T. The enigma of normal pressure hydrocephalus: tests to select patients for surgery and to predict shunt function. *Clin Neurosurg* 1977;24:285–315.
2. Suzuki R, Matsushima Y, Hiratsuka H, Inaba Y. A simplified method of xenon-enhanced CT for regional cerebral blood flow (rCBF) measurement with reference to clinical experiences. *Bull Tokyo Med Dent Univ* 1986;33:107–116.
3. Suzuki R, Ohno K, Matsushima Y, Inaba Y. Serial changes in focal hyperemia associated with hypertensive putaminal hemorrhage. *Stroke* 1988;19:322–325.
4. Tamaki N, Kusunoki T, Wakabayashi T, Matsumoto S. Cerebral hemodynamics in normal-pressure hydrocephalus. Evaluation by $^{133}$Xe inhalation method and dynamic CT study. *J Neurosurg* 1984;61:510–514.
5. Vorstrup S, Christensen J, Gjerris F, Sørensen PS, Thomsen AM, Paulson OB. Cerebral blood flow in patients with normal-pressure hydrocephalus before and after shunting. *J Neurosurg* 1987;66:379–387.
6. Meyer JS, Kitagawa Y, Tanahashi N, et al. Pathogenesis of normal-pressure hydrocephalus—preliminary observations. *Surg Neurol* 1985;23:121–133.
7. Black PM, Ojemann RG, Tzouras A. CSF shunts for dementia, incontinence, and gait disturbance. *Clin Neurosurg* 1984;31:632–651.
8. Yonas H, Good WF, Gur D, et al. Mapping cerebral blood flow by xenon-enhanced computed tomography: clinical experience. *Radiology* 1984;152:435–442.
9. Fisher CM. The clinical picture in occult hydrocephalus. *Clin Neurosurg* 1977;24:270–284.
10. Laws ER Jr, Mokri B. Occult hydrocephalus: results of shunting correlated with diagnostic tests. *Clin Neurosurg* 1977;24:316–333.

*Cerebral Blood Flow Measurement with Stable Xenon-Enhanced Computed Tomography,*
edited by Howard Yonas. Raven Press, Ltd.,
New York © 1992.

# Measurements in Patients with Chronic Subdural Hematoma

## Akira Tanaka, Shinya Yoshinaga, and Masato Kimura

*Department of Neurosurgery, Fukuoka University, Chikushi Hospital,
377–1 Ohaza-Zokumyoin, Chikushino, Fukuoka 818, Japan*

Chronic subdural hematoma is a slowly expanding intracranial mass lesion that can cause reduction of cerebral function by compressing and displacing the brain. Although this effect is reversible, the exact mechanism remains unclear; cerebral blood flow (CBF) studies in these patients are quite few. We therefore studied CBF in patients with chronic subdural hematoma, performing quantitative and three-dimensional measurements using xenon-enhanced computed tomography (Xe/CT) scanning.

## MATERIALS AND METHODS

Our subjects were ten patients aged 23 to 79 years. We monitored their CBF before evacuation of their chronic subdural hematomas and again 3 to 4 weeks after, when all patients had improved clinically. The CBF studies were performed on an Xe/CT CBF analyzing system adapted to the Siemens Somatom DR-III scanner. A CBF map was created after each patient inhaled 30% xenon gas for 6 minutes. CBF values were derived for the following regions of interest on each side: the entire hemisphere, cortex, thalamus, and putamen.

## RESULTS

Table 1 presents the preoperative clinical symptoms and CT findings in these ten patients. All five patients in whom the hematoma had moderate or severe mass effect on CT had headache as well as hemiparesis, mental status disturbance, or both. Headache was the only clinical symptom in patients whose hematoma caused no or minimal mass effect.

Figure 1 compares average CBF values for the side of the hematoma, the opposite side, and previously obtained normal controls. We found that CBF in these patients was reduced not only ipsilateral to the hematoma, but also contralaterally. The reduction in cortical flow, however, was more marked on the

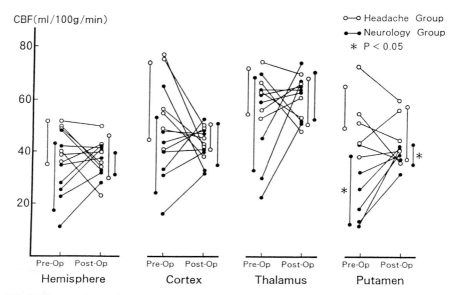

**FIG. 3.** Preoperative and postoperative cerebral blood flow (CBF) values in the hemisphere, cortex, thalamus, and putamen in each patient with chronic subdural hematoma. A vertical line indicates the mean CBF value with standard deviation for each group.

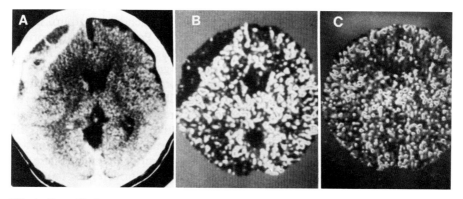

**FIG. 4.** Case 10. Preoperative (**A**) plain and (**B**) xenon-enhanced CT images. (**C**) Postoperative Xe/CT image.

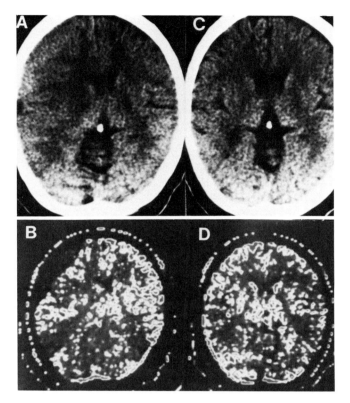

FIG. 5. Case 8. Preoperative (A) plain CT and (B) xenon-enhanced CT images. Postoperative (C) plain and (D) Xe/CT images.

Case 8: A 79-year-old man was admitted with headache, right-sided hemiparesis, and mental status disturbance. CT demonstrated a chronic subdural hematoma of high density in the left fronto-parietal region with severe brain shift (Fig. 5). A Xe/CT scan showed diffusely low CBF in the left hemisphere, including the cortex as well as the putamen and thalamus. Postoperatively, he was free of symptoms, and the hematoma had disappeared. His CBF recovered to nearly normal levels in both hemispheres.

Case 4: A 52-year-old man was admitted with headache, right-sided hemiparesis, and mental status disturbance. Plain CT revealed an isodense chronic subdural hematoma in the left fronto-parietal region with severe brain shift (Fig. 6). Xenon-enhanced CT showed a diffuse, severe reduction of CBF in both hemispheres. Postoperatively, he was symptom free and showed no evidence of the hematoma. His CBF had normalized on both sides.

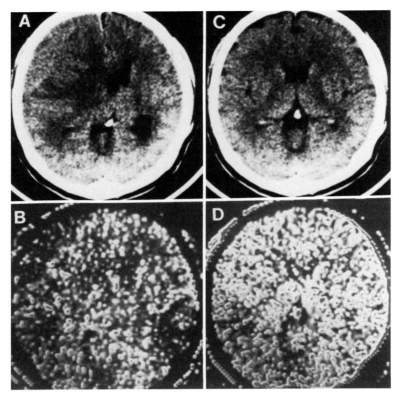

**FIG. 6.** Case 4. Preoperative (**A**) unenhanced and (**B**) xenon-enhanced CT images. Postoperative (**C**) plain CT and (**D**) Xe/CT images.

## DISCUSSION

Few CBF studies in patients with chronic subdural hematomas exit, and studies of quantitative CBF measurements with direct anatomical correlation are even more rare. Ueda et al. (1) used single-photon emission CT for this purpose, but the Xe/CT scan used by us and by Segawa et al. (2) is more accurate in its anatomical correlation.

In this study, we found that CBF was reduced more in the group with neurologic deficits than in the group with only headaches. We also found that flow reduction was greater in the putamen and thalamus than in the hemisphere and cortex. These results are compatible with those of Ueda et al. (1) and Segawa et al. (2) In our patients, CT showed mass effects to be moderate or severe in the neurology group and minimal or absent in the headache group. This suggests that decreased CBF in patients with chronic subdural hematoma occurs initially in the central cerebral areas, such as the basal ganglia and thalamus, then extends to the whole hemisphere, including the cortex, as brain compression and displacement progress. Therefore, the central cerebral areas might be more responsible than the cortex for clinical symptoms.

It is not clear whether CBF reduction is a cause of brain dysfunction or merely a result of a reduced metabolic demand in the dysfunctional brain. Nor do we know why the central cerebral areas are more susceptible than the cortex to pressure from a hematoma. Might the extent of brain displacement and distortion be more important reasons for damage in the central cerebral areas than is hematoma-induced pressure? These questions remain to be resolved.

## REFERENCES

1. Ueda M, Takahashi Y, Ohmiya N, et al. Single-photon emission CT-findings in chronic subdural hematoma. *Prog Comput Tomogr (Tokyo)* 1985;7:623–630.
2. Segawa H, Fujie K, Fujimaki T, et al. Effect of hematoma pressure on cerebral blood flow and function in chronic subdural hematoma. *Proc Jap Neurosurg* 1986;350.

*Cerebral Blood Flow Measurement with Stable Xenon-Enhanced Computed Tomography,* edited by Howard Yonas. Raven Press, Ltd., New York © 1992.

# Beneficial Effect of Stereotactic Hematoma Evacuation for the Small Putaminal Hemorrhage: Evaluation by Xenon-Enhanced Computed Tomography

Genhachi Hyotani, Tomoaki Terada, Mitsuharu Tsuura, Yoshinari Nakamura, Kazuki Miyamoto, Takashi Nishiguchi, Toru Itakura, Seiji Hayashi, and Norihiko Komai

*Department of Neurological Surgery, Wakayama Medical College, 7 bancho 27, Wakayama City 640, Japan*

Although stereotactic hematoma evacuation is a well-accepted operative procedure for a large hypertensive putaminal hemorrhage, controversy remains over its effectiveness in patients with a small hypertensive intracerebral hematoma. We thus examined how cerebral blood flow (CBF) is affected by stereotactic evacuation of hematomas associated with small hypertensive putaminal hemorrhages.

## SUBJECTS AND METHODS

We sequentially measured CBF 33 times in 11 patients with a small putaminal hemorrhage (volume < 25 ml). In six of these patients, the hematoma was evacuated stereotactically within 7 days after onset. The mean age in this group was 56 years, and the mean hematoma volume was 16 ml (Table 1). The other five patients were treated conservatively. Their mean age was 55 years, and their mean hematoma volume was 17 ml (Table 2). We examined CBF sequentially in the frontal and temporal lobes and thalamus in each group. These values were compared with the normal values measured at our institution (Table 3).

For the surgical procedures, we used the Komai computed tomography-guided (CT-guided) stereotactic apparatus, which is both accurate and easy to manipulate (1). We used stable xenon-enhanced CT to measure local CBF (2) with a Toshiba TCT 60-A scanner and a special head frame made by Anzai Company Limited for head fixation. CT images were obtained during 6-minute wash-in and 9-minute wash-out periods using 35% xenon gas. We selected two scan levels, each

**TABLE 1.** *Surgical cases of putaminal hemorrhage*

| Patient | Age (years) | Sex | Days from onset to operation | Hematoma volume (ml) |
|---------|-------------|-----|------------------------------|----------------------|
| 1 | 70 | F | 3 | 11 |
| 2 | 57 | M | 5 | 12 |
| 3 | 60 | F | 3 | 17 |
| 4 | 47 | F | 2 | 17 |
| 5 | 47 | M | 7 | 20 |
| 6 | 52 | M | 2 | 20 |
| mean | 56 | | 4 | 16 |

**TABLE 2.** *Conservatively treated cases of putaminal hemorrhage*

| Patient | Age (years) | Sex | Hematoma volume (ml) |
|---------|-------------|-----|----------------------|
| 1 | 58 | M | 25 |
| 2 | 49 | M | 15 |
| 3 | 52 | M | 15 |
| 4 | 66 | M | 14 |
| 5 | 50 | M | 14 |
| mean | 55 | | 17 |

**TABLE 3.** *Control cerebral blood flow values at our institution (n = 12)*

| Site | Mean CBF (±SD) (ml/100 g/min) |
|------|-------------------------------|
| Thalamus | 55.4 (8.9) |
| Putamen | 53.9 (11.0) |
| Internal capsule | 23.6 (5.1) |
| Frontal gray | 38.9 (7.5) |
| Frontal white | 17.5 (5.5) |
| Temporal gray | 41.1 (9.4) |
| Temporal white | 17.3 (4.3) |
| Occipital gray | 34.4 (6.7) |

SD, standard deviation.

10 mm thick, for the CBF study. The end-tidal xenon concentration was monitored continually, and the resulting data were used to derive the arterial blood gas concentration, with the Kety–Schmidt equation serving as the analytical method. The Xe/CT studies caused no adverse effects in our patients.

## RESULTS

The time course of CBF in the frontal lobe in both groups is shown in Fig. 1. During the third week after onset, CBF in the frontal lobe of the affected hemi-

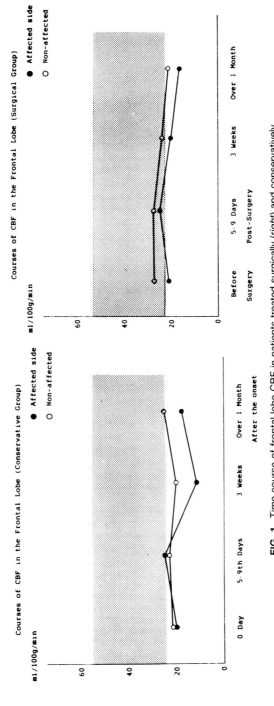

**FIG. 1.** Time course of frontal lobe CBF in patients treated surgically (*right*) and conservatively (*left*). The stippled areas show mean CBF values ± 2 SD in normal volunteers.

222

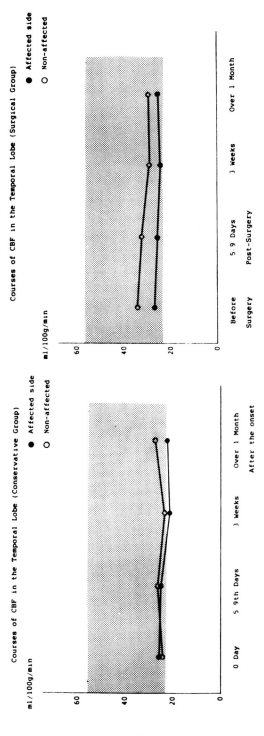

**FIG. 2.** Time course of CBF in the temporal lobe in both groups. There was no significant difference between the two.

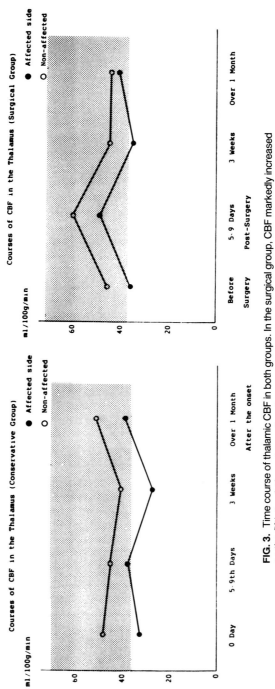

**FIG. 3.** Time course of thalamic CBF in both groups. In the surgical group, CBF markedly increased on the fifth to ninth postoperative day.

sphere decreased significantly in the conservatively treated group but only mildly in the surgical group. CBF in the temporal lobe did not differ significantly between these two groups (Fig. 2). On the fifth to ninth postoperative day, thalamic CBF markedly increased in both hemispheres in the surgical group. However, in the other group, CBF in the thalamus of the affected hemisphere remained low the third week after onset (Fig. 3). Although the surgical group had greater improvement in frontal lobe and thalamic CBF, there was no difference in neurological outcome between these two groups. The following are two representative cases.

Case 1: A 58-year-old man with mild left-sided hemiparesis received conservative treatment for a hematoma estimated to be 25 ml in volume. CT showed midline shift to be greatest in the third week after onset; the hematoma was absorbed 3 months after onset. The CBF study showed a continuous low-flow pattern, especially in the frontal lobe and thalamus of the affected hemisphere (Fig. 4).

Case 2: A 60-year-old woman had mild left-sided hemiparesis. CT indicated that the volume of her hematoma was 17 ml. Three days after onset, 80% of the hematoma volume was evacuated stereotactically. The hematoma had almost disappeared 1 month later. The CBF in the thalamus in the affected hemisphere improved 1 week after surgery (Fig. 5).

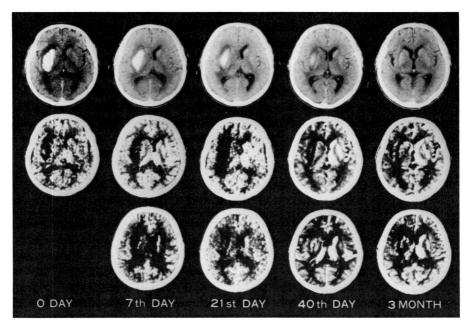

**FIG. 4.** Case 1. Serial CT scans (*top row*) and serial CBF maps (*middle and bottom rows*). The affected frontal lobe and thalamus showed continual low-flow patterns.

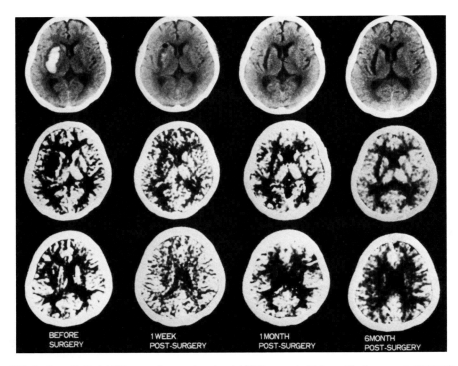

**FIG. 5.** Case 2. Serial CT scans (*top row*) and serial CBF maps (*middle and bottom rows*). Thalamic CBF in the affected hemisphere improved 1 week postoperatively.

## DISCUSSION

Recently, hypertensive intracerebral hemorrhage has been treated using the CT-guided stereotactic evacuation method (1). Although this method can improve the clinical outcome in patients with a large hematoma (3–5), there is less certainty about its effectiveness in patients with small hemorrhages.

Because the conventional neurological examination seemed inadequate for differentiating the true physiologic changes of the surgically and conservatively treated groups, we monitored CBF changes to evaluate the effectiveness of stereotactic evacuation for a small putaminal hemorrhage. Stereotactic evacuation led to increased CBF in the affected thalamus and frontal lobe, either because flow in these areas was influenced by the direct compression of the hematoma and/or because of damage to neural fibers surrounding the hematoma (diaschisis). Functional recovery in the thalamus and frontal lobes could not be evaluated by the usual neurological examination, which was useful only to assess motor function. Elevated CBF values in the frontal lobe and thalamus were consistent with improved cortical function. It is our impression that function improved after stereotactic evacuation of hematomas even in patients whose motor function was not notably better.

In summary, stereotactic aspiration of putaminal hematomas led to a marked increase in thalamic CBF in both hemispheres and a decrease in CBF in the affected frontal lobe. The frontal lobe decrease was smaller in the surgical group. Our findings indicate that stereotactic evacuation does contribute to improvements in local CBF in patients with a small putaminal hemorrhage.

## REFERENCES

1. Doi E, Moriwaki H, Komai N, Iwamoto M. Stereotactic evacuation of intracerebral hematoma. *Neurol Med Chir (Tokyo)* 1982;22:461–467.
2. Nakamura Y, Hyotani G, Terada T, et al. Regional cerebral blood flow measurement by stable xenon-enhanced CT. Methodology and problems. *J Wakayama Med Soc* 1990;41 (in press).
3. Komai N. Stereotactic evacuation of intracerebral hematomas using plasminogen activator. *Japanese Journal of Acute Medicine* 1990;14:47–59.
4. Matsumoto K, Hondo H. CT-guided stereotaxic evacuation of hypertensive intracerebral hematomas. *J Neurosurg* 1984;61:440–448.
5. Tanizaki Y. Improvement of cerebral blood flow following stereotactic surgery in patients with putaminal hemorrhage. *Acta Neurochir (Wien)* 1988;90:103–110.

*Cerebral Blood Flow Measurement with Stable Xenon-Enhanced Computed Tomography,* edited by Howard Yonas. Raven Press, Ltd., New York © 1992.

# Posterior Fossa Blood Flow in Cerebellopontine Angle Tumors

Shahram Mirzai, Marcos Tatagiba, and Madjid Samii

*Neurosurgical Clinic, Nordstadt Hospital, Hannover Medical School, Haltenhoffstr. 41, 3000 Hannover 1, Germany*

Although stable xenon-enhanced computed tomography (Xe/CT) has been widely and successfully applied to studies of the supratentorial circulation (1–3), it has been used less extensively to study blood flow in posterior fossa structures. The petrous and sphenoid bones sometimes hinder selection of a slice that clearly shows the cerebellum and brainstem with minimal artifacts.

Of the more than 500 Xe/CT blood flow studies performed in our clinic between 1984 and 1990, 62 were of the posterior fossa. We conducted the present study to assess the feasibility of Xe/CT studies in the posterior fossa and to determine the regional blood flow in tissue surrounding a tumor, particularly in the cerebellar hemispheres and brainstem. We also investigated whether regional blood flow alterations influence postoperative course and outcome and whether infratentorial mass lesions have remote depressive effects on the supratentorial flow.

## MATERIAL AND METHODS

A retrospective analysis of 62 posterior fossa blood flow measurements showed that, other than patient motion, bone artifacts were the most common cause of study failure. With increasing experience, however, it became possible to perform posterior fossa studies with a success rate of more than 90%. From these 62 investigations, we selected a homogeneous group of 11 patients with cerebellopontine angle (CPA) tumors to become the subjects of this study.

Selection criteria were as follows: (a) satisfactory visualization of cerebral and cerebellar hemispheres and brainstem, (b) absence of other morphologic brain alterations on routine CT images, and (c) tumor diameter larger than 3 cm. Five of the patients were men and six were women, with ages ranging from 27 to 73 years (mean: 54 ± 11 years). Table 1 summarizes their clinical presentations. We reviewed their CT and/or magnetic resonance imaging studies to establish the exact relationship of the neoplasms to surrounding structures and to determine the presence of perifocal edema.

**TABLE 1.** *Clinical presentation of 11 patients with cerebellopontine angle tumors*[a]

| Patient | Sex/age (yrs) | Tumor side | Right/left regional blood flow (ml/100 g/min) | | | Outcome |
|---|---|---|---|---|---|---|
| | | | Cerebral | Cerebellar | Brainstem | |
| 1 | M/49 | right | 68/57 | 68/64 | 53/83 | good |
| 2 | F/44 | left | 50/40 | 42/42 | 66/48 | good |
| 3 | F/57 | right | 73/69 | 66/72 | 57/71 | good |
| 4 | F/73 | right | 32/37 | 23/34 | 38/35 | fair[b] |
| 5 | F/61 | right | 73/70 | 46/71 | 67/70 | good |
| 6 | M/53 | right | 42/48 | 55/77 | 52/63 | fair[b] |
| 7 | F/27 | left | 57/46 | 47/31 | 51/41 | good |
| 8 | F/48 | left | 81/70 | 76/42 | 81/96 | good |
| 9 | M/67 | right | 57/45 | 41/48 | —/— | good |
| 10 | M/60 | right | 38/38 | 34/41 | 44/41 | good |
| 11 | F/55 | right | 56/67 | 56/67 | 68/65 | good |

[a] Histologically, all tumors were neurinomas.
[b] Transient hemiparesis.

The slice for the Xe/CT studies was selected to provide information not only from the cerebral hemispheres, but also from the cerebellar hemispheres, the brainstem, and in few cases, from the tumor. Because bone artifacts significantly degrade flow information, we obtained images over the petrous bone with a CT-gantry angle of approximately 25° to the orbitomeatal line (Fig. 1).

Regional blood flow was measured in the brainstem, cerebrum, and cerebellum (Fig. 2). We compared the flow values ipsilateral to the tumor with contralateral values. Brainstem and cerebellar blood flow values were evaluated in relation to the postoperative duration of hospitalization and outcome, which we categorized as either (a) unchanged, without additional neurological deficits or (b) worse, with transient hemiparesis and ataxia.

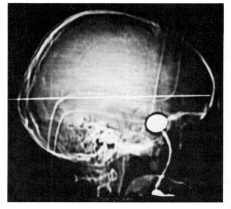
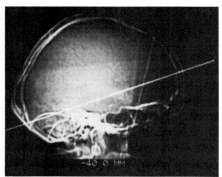

A                                                                                          B

**FIG. 1. (A)** Scout view showing standard slice for supratentorial Xe/CT cerebral blood flow studies. **(B)** Scout view with modified slice for studies of the posterior fossa.

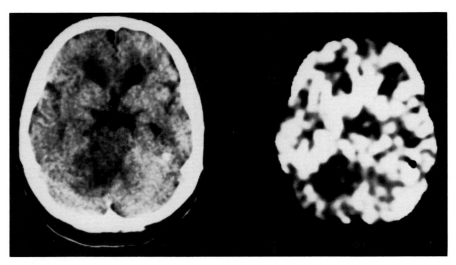

**FIG. 2.** CT image (*left*) and Xe/CT study (*right*) in patient 5 shows a hypodense area in the right cerebellar hemisphere and reduced blood flow in this region. Note that brainstem blood flow is not impaired.

## RESULTS

Table 2 presents the mean regional blood flow values obtained in the study. Blood flow was lowest in the cerebellum and highest in the brainstem. We noted no significant difference between hemispheric cerebral blood flow ipsilateral and contralateral to the tumor, nor did we find remote depressive effects on blood flow in any area of either cerebral hemisphere. The mean values for ipsilateral cerebellar blood flow were lower than those for the contralateral hemisphere. Regional blood flow was slightly reduced in the brainstem ipsilateral to the tumor.

**TABLE 2.** *Regional blood flow related to tumor side, postoperative course, and outcome in patients with cerebellopontine angle tumors*

| | Blood flow (ml/100 g/min) | | |
| --- | --- | --- | --- |
| | Brainstem | Cerebellum | Cerebrum |
| *Tumor side* | | | |
| Ipsilateral | 56 ± 16 | 45 ± 13 | 54 ± 15 |
| Contralateral | 61 ± 16 | 58 ± 15 | 56 ± 13 |
| *Hospital stay* | | | |
| ≤3 weeks | 62 ± 15 | 53 ± 11 | |
| >3 weeks | 54 ± 11 | 49 ± 14 | |
| *Outcome* | | | |
| Good | 62 ± 13 | 52 ± 11 | |
| Fair[a] | 46 ± 10 | 47 ± 19 | |

[a] Transient hemiparesis.

Lower preoperative brainstem blood flow values correlated more closely with a prolonged postoperative hospital stay than did cerebellar blood flow values. Patients needing more than 3 weeks of hospitalization had lower brainstem flows than those discharged earlier. Cerebellar blood flow did not correlate with postoperative clinical outcome. However, we found a direct correlation between preoperative brainstem blood flow values and postoperative outcome: Patients with additional neurologic deficits had lower brainstem flow values than did patients who were neurologically unchanged.

## DISCUSSION

Xe/CT blood flow measurements in the posterior fossa are rare (4–7), probably because of technical difficulties such as bone artifacts. With our modifications in the patient's position and the gantry angle, however, infratentorial Xe/CT flow investigations became feasible. We were thus able to find a relationship between new postoperative neurologic deficits and reduced brainstem blood flow. Findings of hypoperfusion in the cerebellar hemisphere and brainstem ipsilateral to the tumor could be explained by the presence of peritumoral edema in these regions. Consequently, preoperative determination of brainstem blood flow was of prognostic value in predicting the postoperative outcome in patients with posterior fossa tumors.

Crossed cerebellar diaschisis is a known phenomenon in patients with supratentorial infarction or tumors (8–11). Crossed cerebral diaschisis in patients with cerebellar infarction has also been described (12). However, little is yet known about whether such a remote effect also exists in which infratentorial tumors cause reduced cerebral blood flow. Our studies could not find any transtentorial remote effects on cerebral blood flow. Subsequent Xe/CT studies could be used to examine crossed cerebellar diaschisis.

Based on our experience with Xe/CT blood flow studies in the posterior fossa, we can draw the following conclusions. First, posterior fossa flow studies are feasible. Second, in some patients with CPA tumors, blood flow may be impaired in the cerebellar hemisphere and brainstem on the side of the tumor. Third, brainstem blood flow alterations caused by posterior fossa tumors might influence the postoperative outcome. Finally, no remote transtentorial effects such as a decrease in cerebral blood flow were evident in our investigations. We believe that a more detailed investigation of infratentorial brain function, including the measurement of brainstem and cerebellar blood flow, is necessary to understand pathophysiology of flow alterations in infratentorial lesions.

## ACKNOWLEDGMENT

This study was supported by a grant from DFG–Bonn/FRG (Sa 220/1–3).

## REFERENCES

1. Kohmura E, Gürtner P, Holl K, et al. Erfahrungen mit der Inhalation eines 33%igen Xenon-(stable-)-Sauerstoffgemisches im Zusammenhang mit einer neuen Methode zur lokalen Hirn-durchblutungsmessung. *RoFo* 1986;144:531-536.
2. Yonas H, Gur D, Latchaw RE, Wolfson SK. Stable xenon CT/CBF imaging: laboratory and clinical experience. *Adv Tech Stand Neurosurg* 1987;15:4-37.
3. Yonas H, Gur D, Latchaw RE, Wolfson SK. Xenon computed tomographic blood flow mapping. In: Wood JH, ed. *Cerebral blood flow: physiologic and clinical aspects.* New York: McGraw Hill, 1987;220-242.
4. Darby J, Yonas H, Brenner RP. Brainstem death with persistent EEG activity: evaluation by xenon-enhanced computed tomography. *Crit Care Med* 1987;15:519-521.
5. Darby J, Yonas H, Gur D, Latchaw RE. Xenon-enhanced computed tomography in brain death. *Arch Neurol* 1987;44:551-554.
6. Drayer B, Gur D, Wolfson S, Dujovny M. Regional blood flow in the posterior fossa: xenon enhanced CT scanning. *Acta Neurol Scand* 1979;Suppl 72:218-219.
7. Lerch KD, Nemati N, Kohmura E, Holl K, Samii M. Local cerebral blood flow measurements in the deep seated brain structures. In: Samii M, ed. *Surgery in and around the brain stem and the third ventricle.* Berlin: Springer-Verlag, 1986;200-206.
8. Baron JC, Bonsser MG, Comar D, Castaigne P. "Crossed cerebellar diaschisis" in human su-pratentorial brain infarction. *Trans Am Neurol Assoc* 1980;105:459-461.
9. Fukuyama H, Kameyama M, Harada K, et al. Thalamic tumours invading the brain stem produce crossed cerebellar diaschisis demonstrated by PET. *J Neurol Neurosurg Psychiatry* 1986;49:524-528.
10. Meneghetti G, Vorstrup S, Mickey B, Lindewald H, Lassen NA. Crossed cerebellar diaschisis in ischemic stroke. A study of regional cerebral blood flow by [133]Xe inhalation and single photon emission computerized tomography. *J Cereb Blood Flow Metab* 1984;4:235-240.
11. Martin WR, Raichle ME. Cerebellar blood flow and metabolism in cerebral hemisphere infarction. *Ann Neurol* 1983;14:168-176.
12. Broich K, Hartmann A, Biersack HJ, Horn R. Crossed cerebello-cerebral diaschisis in a patient with cerebellar infarction. *Neurosci Lett* 1987;83:7-12.

*Cerebral Blood Flow Measurement with Stable Xenon-Enhanced Computed Tomography,* edited by Howard Yonas. Raven Press, Ltd., New York © 1992.

# Correlation of Xenon-133 and Stable Xenon-Enhanced Computed Tomographic Cerebral Blood Flow Measurements in Patients with Severe Head Injury

Warren A. Stringer, *Donald W. Marion, *Gerrit J. Bouma, *J. Paul Muizelaar, Ira F. Braun, Panos P. Fatouros, and *Anthony Marmarou

*Departments of Radiology and *Neurosurgery, Medical College of Virginia, Virginia Commonwealth University, Box 615, MCV Station, Richmond, Virginia 23298*

For many years, the $^{133}$Xe method, involving either injection or inhalation of radioactive xenon gas, has been the clinical standard of cerebral blood flow (CBF) measurement. More recently, the stable xenon/computed tomography (Xe/CT) method has become available. Each of these studies has advantages and disadvantages relative to the other. The $^{133}$Xe methods require less patient cooperation, examine a larger amount of the brain, and can be done in the intensive care unit (ICU). The Xe/CT technique provides a better look at the deep structures of the brain, enables exact correlation of flow physiology and anatomy, and can be easily performed at the time of conventional CT. Because it may therefore be desirable to use both methods serially in the evaluation of patients with acute severe head trauma, we examined the correlation between flow values determined by these methods in head-injured patients.

## SUBJECTS AND METHODS

Our subjects were ten patients with acute severe closed head injury (Glasgow Coma Scale score 4–7) and without acute surgical lesions. We obtained the $^{133}$Xe and Xe/CT measurements within 6 hours of each other (mean: 3.4 hours). Because arterial $pCO_2$ could not be held constant between the studies, we corrected

---

Dr. Marion's present address is Department of Neurological Surgery, University of Pittsburgh, Presbyterian University Hospital, Room 9402, 230 Lothrop Street, Pittsburgh, Pennsylvania 15213.

Dr. Braun's present address is Department of Radiology, Baptist Hospital of Miami, 8900 N. Kendall Drive, Miami, Florida 33176-2197.

the measured flow values from each study to a $pCO_2$ value of 34 torr using a factor of 3% change in CBF per torr. In making this correction, we assumed that cerebrovascular reactivity was preserved in these patients, which was generally the case.

The Xe/CT studies were performed on a GE 9800 CT scanner using the standard hardware and software supplied by the manufacturer (GE Medical Systems, Milwaukee, WI). We chose to study three standard levels, encompassing the midbrain, basal ganglia, and centrum semiovale, and obtained two baseline and four enhanced scans at each level while patients inhaled 33% xenon in oxygen (Linde XeScan, stable xenon in oxygen USP, Union Carbide Rare Gases, Specialty Medical Products, Danbury, CT) for 4.5 minutes. End-tidal $CO_2$ concentrations, mean arterial pressure, and intracranial pressure (ICP) were monitored continually during the procedure, and arterial $pCO_2$ values were obtained just before and after xenon inhalation for correlation with the end-tidal measurements. All patients were mechanically ventilated and closely monitored for changes in vital signs or ICP.

We measured CBF in each hemisphere at each level using the standard "region of interest" (ROI) and "trace" functions of the GE 9800 system. We then weighted these measurements for the area included in each and averaged them to arrive at an approximate "global" CBF measurement.

We obtained the [133]Xe CBF measurements using the intravenous injection method. These studies were performed in the neurosurgical ICU using a portable system. Clearance of the xenon gas was monitored by five probes over each hemisphere; these probes were located over the frontal, parietal, occipital, high temporal, and low temporal lobes. To obtain global CBF, we averaged the CBF-15 (a noncompartmental index incorporating both gray- and white-matter flow [1]) index values from each probe. We then compared the resultant values to the "global" CBF values obtained with the Xe/CT method.

The results were analyzed by linear regression, with [133]Xe values acting as the independent variable and Xe/CT values acting as the dependent variable. Using the Student's $t$ test, we tested the regression lines against two hypothetical relationships: a line of unity (1:1 relationship, [133]Xe flow = Xe/CT flow) and a horizontal line (Xe/CT flow constant relative to [133]Xe flow), indicating no relationship between flow values determined by the two methods.

## RESULTS

Comparing "global" Xe/CT CBF with global [133]Xe CBF-15 values gave the regression

$$Q_{CT} = 13.07 + 0.65(Q_{Xe-133})$$

and a correlation coefficient $r = 0.785$ (Fig. 1). This regression line was significantly different from a horizontal line ($P < 0.01$ versus $Q_{CT}$ = constant) but was not significantly different from a line of unity ($P > 0.2$ versus $Q_{CT} = Q_{Xe-133}$).

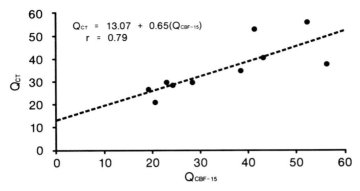

**FIG. 1.** Comparison of "global" CBF values obtained by stable xenon/computed tomography (Xe/CT) and intravenous radiolabeled [133]Xe methods.

## DISCUSSION

[133]Xe techniques, involving either injection or inhalation of small amounts of the radionuclide, have the advantage of being portable. They examine most of the brain surface and are repeatable after a few minutes, thus enabling measurement of the effects of physiological manipulations. However, unless special tomographic machines are used, the information provided by [133]Xe methods is weighted toward superficial structures in the brain; yet generally, the spatial resolution of the nontomographic methods is relatively poor. "Shine-through," in which photons from the opposite hemisphere are detected after passing through an area of low flow, is also a potential problem. Nevertheless, these techniques have been investigated thoroughly and have furnished much of the current knowledge about normal and pathological cerebral blood flow, reactivity, and autoregulation.

The newer Xe/CT method has also been investigated extensively. Several studies have shown good correlation between CBF values determined by Xe/CT and those determined by radiolabeled microspheres (2–4). More recently, the quantitative accuracy of this technique, even at low-flow levels, has been confirmed in comparison to CBF determination with [14]C-iodoantipyrine (5). The Xe/CT method is not portable and, therefore, is cumbersome to use unless the patient is already undergoing conventional CT. The technique affords an exact correlation between anatomy and flow physiology, although only a few levels of the brain can be examined.

As a tomographic method, Xe/CT provides flow measurements uncontaminated by flow in the calvarium or scalp. It can easily and accurately measure flow in deeper structures such as the midbrain and basal ganglia as well. Cortical flow must be measured carefully though, because cortical ROIs may inadvertently include cerebrospinal fluid in sulci as well as gyral white matter. CBF measurement can also be paired with "dynamic" CT during an intravenous bolus injection of iodinated contrast material to enable estimation of cerebral blood volume (CBV). Such data may have an important influence on the early management of head-injured patients (see Bouma et al. in this volume). And as with $^{133}$Xe techniques, Xe/CT measurements can be repeated after a few minutes to assess the effects of a physiological "challenge."

The relative advantages and disadvantages of these two methods make it desirable to use both in the early management of patients with head trauma. For example, a Xe/CT study can be obtained concurrently with the initial conventional CT scan to provide immediate assessment of local CBF, CBV, and vascular reactivity. This information may help to determine how best to manage the initial rise in ICP and can be re-evaluated whenever conventional CT is repeated. At other times, when exact anatomic correlation is not needed or a global assessment is preferred, CBF and vascular reactivity can be examined portably in the ICU by $^{133}$Xe methods.

Our results show a close linear correlation between the flow values measured by $^{133}$Xe and Xe/CT, particularly considering the diversity of clinical factors inherent in acutely head-injured patients. Such patients often have unstable vital signs (including arterial blood pressure) as well as elevated and highly fluctuating ICP. Associated injuries such as pulmonary contusions can lead to rapidly changing rates of ventilation and, consequently, arterial $pCO_2$ values. Indeed, as a result of either these effects or evolution of the cerebral injury, the CBF itself can be altered. The treatment required by these patients can also change the CBF substantially in a short time. These factors are difficult if not impossible to control for in a study of acutely injured patients. Obviously, this situation can lead to a significant discordance between individual CBF measurements, whether made by the same technique or by different techniques used sequentially. As more patients are studied, these factors should offset one another, and the relationship between flow values measured by these two techniques will become better defined.

At this time, our results do not support existence of a significant effect of flow activation from inhalation of 33% xenon for 4.5 minutes. If such an effect were present, Xe/CT-derived values would be expected to be consistently above $^{133}$Xe-derived values in higher flow states, rather than both above and below the regression line as we observed. In low-flow states, flow activation should be minimal in any case, because little xenon reaches the tissue.

In summary, Xe/CT and $^{133}$Xe flow measurements of global CBF showed a linear correlation under the conditions of this study. As more patients are studied, the nature of this correlation should become more clearly defined. Meanwhile, Xe/CT and $^{133}$Xe flow measurements obtained sequentially in these patients should be compared to the normal and pathological threshold flow values established for each technique. Our results did not show evidence that flow activation caused a significant error in the Xe/CT measurements.

# REFERENCES

1. Obrist WD, Wilkinson WE. The non-invasive xenon-133 method: evaluation of CBF indices. In: Bes A, ed. *Proceedings of the International Congress of Cerebral Circulation and Neurotransmitters.* International Congress Series #507. Amsterdam: Excerpta Medica;1980:119–124.
2. Gur D, Yonas H, Jackson DL, et al. Simultaneous measurements of cerebral blood flow by the xenon/CT method and the microsphere method. A comparison. *Invest Radiol* 1985;20:672–677.
3. Fatouros PP, Wist AO, Kishore PR, et al. Xenon/computed tomography cerebral blood flow measurements. Methods and accuracy. *Invest Radiol* 1987;22:705–712.
4. DeWitt DS, Fatouros PP, Wist AO, et al. Stable xenon versus radiolabelled microsphere cerebral blood flow measurements in baboons. *Stroke* 1989;20:1716–1723.
5. Wolfson SK, Clark J, Greenberg JH, et al. Xenon-enhanced computed tomography compared with [14C]-iodoantipyrine for normal and low cerebral blood flow states in baboons. *Stroke* 1990;21: 751–757.

Cerebral Blood Flow Measurement with Stable
Xenon-Enhanced Computed Tomography,
edited by Howard Yonas. Raven Press, Ltd.,
New York © 1992.

# $CO_2$ Reactivity and Cerebral Blood Flow in Comatose Survivors of Cardiac Arrest

James T. Love, *Howard Yonas, Joseph M. Darby,
and Edwin M. Nemoto

*Departments of Anesthesiology and Critical Care Medicine and *Neurological Surgery,
University of Pittsburgh School of Medicine,
Pittsburgh, Pennsylvania 15213*

Cerebral blood flow (CBF) is very sensitive to changes in arterial $pCO_2$, normally changing about 3% per torr change in $PaCO_2$ (1). Animal studies have suggested that $CO_2$ reactivity ($CO_2R$) is impaired early after transient global brain ischemia, such as occurs in patients comatose after cardiac arrest (2,3). However, there is a lack of data obtained in patients in this condition. The degree of $CO_2R$ impairment may have both therapeutic and prognostic implications for such patients. Therefore, $CO_2R$ should be considered in the interpretation of CBF studies performed in patients comatose after cardiac arrest.

## SUBJECTS AND METHODS

Patients eligible for our study were comatose adults resuscitated from cardiopulmonary arrest. We considered patients comatose if they had intact brainstem reflexes but exhibited no response to verbal command. All patients were mechanically ventilated and had a mean arterial pressure (MAP) of at least 60 torr. Patients in whom anesthetic or sedative agents were implicated as contributing to the coma were excluded from the study.

We performed a total of ten double CBF studies in eight patients, six men and two women, aged 24 to 66 years (mean: 53 years). Four of the patients were studied prospectively and four retrospectively. The length of cardiac arrest averaged 16.9 minutes (range: 6 to 30 minutes), and the average time from resuscitation to the first CBF study was 97.8 hours (range: 13.5–308 hours).

After stabilization and entry into the study, patients were transported to the computed tomography (CT) scanner for measurement of CBF by Xe/CT using the GE 9800 CT CBF system. The end-tidal $CO_2$ was monitored by capnography while the end-tidal xenon concentration was measured by a thermoconductivity analyzer. We obtained conventional 10-mm CT scans to select three levels for

CBF study. Following two baseline (unenhanced) images at each of these three levels, patients inhaled a mixture of 33% xenon and 67% oxygen (Linde XeScan, stable xenon in oxygen USP, Union Carbide Rare Gases, Specialty Medical Products, Danbury, CT) for approximately 4.5 minutes, during which four sequential scans were obtained at each level.

Using the arterial xenon build-up curve and the time-dependent tissue build-up of xenon, we calculated CBF for each CT voxel with a modification of the Kety–Schmidt equation. Details of this CBF method have been described previously (4,5). After the first measurement, we adjusted minute ventilation in an attempt to change PaCO$_2$ by 10 torr. In nine of the ten double CBF studies, PaCO$_2$ was raised from hypocapnic levels (CBF$_2$) to normocapnia (CBF$_1$). After allowing at least 15 minutes for xenon clearance, we measured CBF again.

Three regions were evaluated in each patient: the cortical hemispheres, basal ganglia, and brainstem. Hemispheric CBF was determined by placing contiguous 2-cm regions of interest (ROIs) over the cortical mantle at each CT level; we then averaged CBF values for all ROIs. We generated anatomically defined ROIs of CBF by tracing the basal ganglia and brainstem structures from the CT images and transferring the outline to the flow image. Absolute CO$_2$R was calculated as the change in CBF divided by the change in CO$_2$, and %CO$_2$R as the percentage change in CBF divided by the percentage change in CO$_2$.

## RESULTS

The average MAP at the time of CBF$_1$ (CBF at the higher PaCO$_2$ level for all ten patients) was 94.2 torr, which was not significantly different from the MAP of 90.3 torr during CBF$_2$. On the other hand, the change in CO$_2$ levels between CBF$_1$ and CBF$_2$ was statistically significant.

Table 1 shows CBF data for all patients. CBF$_2$ values were significantly lower than CBF$_1$ levels in the basal ganglia and brainstem; there was no significant difference in hemispheric values. We found significant changes in absolute CO$_2$R in the basal ganglia and brainstem and in %CO$_2$R for the basal ganglia.

**TABLE 1.** *CBF and CO$_2$ reactivity: pooled data[a]*

| | Mean (SD) values | | |
|---|---|---|---|
| | Hemispheres | Basal ganglia | Brainstem |
| CBF$_1$ (ml/100 g/min) | 54.3  (19.8) | 61.9  (21.2) | 56.6  (21.5) |
| CBF$_2$ (ml/100 g/min) | 47.7  (21.9) | 51.1  (21.1)** | 46.3  (18.3)** |
| Absolute CO$_2$R | 0.56 (0.93) | 1.12 (1.10)* | 1.15 (1.42)* |
| %CO$_2$R | 0.96 (1.93) | 1.72 (1.78)* | 1.59 (2.47) |

* $P < 0.05$; **$P < 0.05$ versus CBF$_1$.
[a] Mean PaCO$_2$ in CBF$_1$ was 39 ± 6 torr; in CBF$_2$, 29 ± 6 torr.
SD, standard deviation; CO$_2$R, CO$_2$ reactivity.

**TABLE 2.** Regional %CO₂ reactivity versus time to arrest and arousal

| Patient | Mins of arrest | Hrs to study | Regional %CO₂ reactivity | | | Days to awaken |
| | | | Hemispheres | Basal ganglia | Brainstem | |
|---|---|---|---|---|---|---|
| 4 | 6 | 308.0 | 3.48 | 2.57 | 5.33 | 46.5 |
| 7 | 20 | 138.3 | 3.31 | 5.76 | 0.72 | Never |
| 1 | 14 | 13.5 | 2.99 | 1.16 | 3.88 | 9.3 |
| 1 | | 80.5 | 3.18 | 3.51 | 2.84 | |
| 2 | 30 | 22.0 | 1.57 | 1.37 | — | Never |
| 8 | 10 | 65.0 | 1.03 | −0.29 | 0.39 | Never |
| 3 | 18 | 18.0 | −0.72 | 0.45 | 1.44 | Never |
| 3 | | 60.0 | 0.65 | 2.39 | 2.06 | |
| 5 | 30 | 82.5 | 0.20 | 0.07 | 1.19 | Never |
| 6 | 10 | 190.8 | −0.08 | 0.23 | 4.22 | Never |

Patients 1 and 3 underwent two studies.

Table 2 ranks patients in descending order according to hemispheric %CO₂R. Of the three patients whose %CO₂R was near that expected for normal brain, two awoke after resuscitation. None of those with %CO₂R < 3% regained consciousness. Brainstem %CO₂R was severely impaired in the only patient with hemispheric %CO₂R > 3% who failed to awaken. In the patients who had follow-up studies, CO₂R generally improved in the second evaluation.

We then analyzed the subgroup of patients who underwent Xe/CT examinations within 96 hours (mean: 44 hours) after resuscitation from cardiac arrest. To facilitate comparisons of CO₂R in different regions, we calculated mean conductance ($CBF_1/MAP_1$) for each region (Table 3). $PaCO_2$ was $35 \pm 4.8$ for $CBF_1$ versus $26.5 \pm 3.3$ for $CBF_2$ ($P < 0.05$). Although there was significant change in CBF in the cortex and basal ganglia, only the basal ganglia had significantly different CO₂R. We found no significant difference, however, between CO₂R in various regions (ANOVA), nor did we see a difference in conductance. The only region that demonstrated a preserved relationship between conductance and CO₂R was the brainstem ($r = 0.737$, $P < 0.024$).

**TABLE 3.** CBF, CO₂ reactivity, and conductance within 96 hours of arrest

| | Mean (SD) values | | |
| | Hemispheres | Basal ganglia | Brainstem |
|---|---|---|---|
| $CBF_1$ (ml/100 g/min) | 48.5  (18.4) | 60.3  (21.8) | 55.8  (22.2) |
| $CBF_2$ (ml/100 g/min) | 42.2  (20.1)** | 48.5  (20.2)** | 44.3  (18.6) |
| CO₂R | 0.63 (0.93) | 1.34 (1.32)* | 1.30 (2.07) |
| Conductance | 0.52 (0.17) | 0.64 (0.21) | 0.61 (0.24) |

*$P < 0.05$; **$P < 0.05$ versus $CBF_1$.
SD, standard deviation; CO₂R, CO₂ reactivity.

## DISCUSSION

Our study demonstrates that cerebrovascular $CO_2R$ is impaired in humans who are comatose after resuscitation from cardiac arrest. Moreover, $CO_2R$ appears to vary among individuals early after cardiac arrest and may change with time. During coma, controlled hyperventilation is often used in therapy because it is thought to reduce intracranial pressure, to help normalize the pH of the cerebrospinal fluid, and to better distribute CBF (6–9). Nevertheless, the variation in degree of $CO_2R$ impairment seen in patients comatose after cardiac arrest appears to limit, and sometimes even contraindicate, the applicability of hyperventilation therapy in this group.

The lack of correlation between conductance and $CO_2R$ in the cortex and basal ganglia suggests that vasomotor responsiveness to $CO_2$ is impaired in these structures but preserved in the brainstem. These findings are compatible with the theory that various brain structures differ in their sensitivity to ischemic insult. That the only patient with hemispheric $\%CO_2R$ above 3% who failed to awaken had severely impaired brainstem $CO_2R$ suggests that an abnormal $CO_2R$ may be of prognostic importance in comatose patients who have had cardiac arrest.

## REFERENCES

1. Grubb RL Jr, Raichle ME, Eichling JO, et al. The effects of changes in $PaCO_2$ on cerebral blood volume, blood flow, and vascular mean transit time. *Stroke* 1974;5:630–639.
2. Hossman KA, Lechtape-Grueter H, Hossman V. The role of cerebral blood flow for the recovery of the brain after prolonged ischemia. *J Neurol* 1973;204:281.
3. Nemoto EM, Snyder JV, Carroll RG, et al. Global ischemia in dogs: cerebrovascular $CO_2$ reactivity and autoregulation. *Stroke* 1975;6:425–431.
4. Gur D, Good WF, Wolfson SK Jr, et al. In vivo mapping of local cerebral blood flow by xenon-enhanced computed tomography. *Science* 1982;215:1267–1268.
5. Yonas H, Wolfson SK Jr, Gur D, et al. Clinical experience with the use of xenon-enhanced CT blood flow mapping in cerebral vascular disease. *Stroke* 1984;15:443–449.
6. Gisvold SE, Safar P, Rao G, et al. Prolonged immobilization and controlled ventilation after global brain ischemia in monkeys. *Crit Care Med* 1984;12:171.
7. Gordon E. Controlled respiration in the management of patients with traumatic brain injuries. *Acta Anaesthesiol Scand* 1971;15:193.
8. Snyder JV, Powner DJ, Grenvik A. Neurologic intensive care. In: Cottrell JE, Turndort H, eds. *Anesthesia and neurosurgery* 2nd ed. St. Louis: Mosby; 1978.
9. Bleyaert A, Safar P, Nemoto EM, et al. Effect of postcirculatory arrest life-support on neurological recovery in monkeys. *Crit Care Med* 1980;8:153.

*Cerebral Blood Flow Measurement with Stable Xenon-Enhanced Computed Tomography,* edited by Howard Yonas. Raven Press, Ltd., New York © 1992.

# Local $CO_2$ Reactivity and Autoregulation in the Normal Monkey Brain

Yukito Shinohara, Masahiro Yamamoto, Shigeharu Takagi, Munetaka Haida, Hitoshi Hamano, and Yutaka Kametsu

*Department of Neurology, Tokai University School of Medicine, Isehara, Kanagawa 259-11, Japan*

The responses of cerebral vessels and global or regional cerebral blood flow (CBF) to changes in arterial carbon dioxide tension and perfusion pressure are well known and have been confirmed by numerous experiments and clinical observations over many years (1,2). However, the actual mechanisms of the action of $CO_2$ ($CO_2$ reactivity) and perfusion pressure (autoregulation) on cerebral vessels remain somewhat an enigma (3,4). It is also still uncertain whether $CO_2$ reactivity and autoregulatory ability are uniform in different parts of the central nervous system. The purpose of this study was to determine whether there is inhomogeneity in regional cerebral $CO_2$ vasoreactivity and to compare these findings with those on regional autoregulatory ability.

## MATERIALS AND METHODS

Twenty-two monkeys of either sex weighing 3.5 to 9.0 kg were anesthetized with intramuscular ketamine hydrochloride (average: 7.2 mg/kg body weight) and intraperitoneal chloralose-urethan. Anesthesia was maintained by intravenous administration of ketamine throughout the procedure. Computed tomography (CT) performed in conjunction with 35% to 39% stable xenon inhalation was used to measure local CBF.

We investigated $CO_2$ reactivity by allowing the monkeys to inhale 5% $CO_2$ in air. We altered arterial blood pressure by exsanguination, varying the amount of blood withdrawn into a blood reservoir. As shown in Fig. 1, catheters were inserted into the femoral arteries and vein for continual blood pressure monitoring, arterial blood gas and hematocrit determinations, and connection to the blood reservoir. Following a tracheostomy, the monkeys were paralyzed with repeated doses of alcuronium dichloride (average: 1.4 mg/kg body weight) and artificially ventilated with a Harvard respirator.

After obtaining a baseline CT scan, we delivered a gas mixture of stable xenon and oxygen. We took images every 15 seconds for the first minute of inhalation and every 30 seconds thereafter until the end of inhalation. Resting local CBF was measured during the first 3 minutes of inhalation. Obtaining the partition

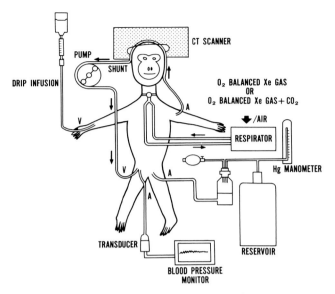

**FIG. 1.** Experimental schema of cold Xe/CT study.

coefficient ($\lambda$) required 20 to 30 minutes of inhalation. To obtain an arterial curve of xenon concentration, we created an extracorporeal circuit from artery to vein and used CT to repeatedly measure the xenon concentration in the arterial blood.

After smoothing the data by the moving average method, we calculated the local CBF and $\lambda$ of xenon in each four-pixel region (corresponding to a volume of $1.2 \times 1.2 \times 5$ mm), which then were displayed in colored maps. We selected 21 regions of interest (ROIs) for this study: the corpus callosum, cerebellar midline, midbrain and, bilaterally, the caudate nucleus; putamen; thalamus; frontal, parietal, and fusiform cortex; internal capsule; hippocampus; and the cerebellar hemispheres. One ROI consisted of 100 pixels corresponding to a volume of $6 \times 6 \times 5$ mm. We defined mean local blood flow as the average value of blood flow in these 21 regions. Additionally, we chose two other regions as watershed areas between the anterior and middle cerebral arteries and investigated their autoregulatory ability.

After obtaining these values, we began a 3-minute period of 5% $CO_2$ inhalation, followed by another 3 minutes of 5% $CO_2$, xenon, and oxygen.

## RESULTS

### CO₂ Reactivity

Local CBF values were symmetrically higher during hypercapnia (PaCO₂ $50.0 \pm 6.2$ mm Hg) than those measured during normocapnia (PaCO₂ $39.4 \pm$

6.8 mm Hg). The mean arterial blood pressure (MABP) rose from $123.8 \pm 18.8$ mm Hg to $130.6 \pm 15.8$ mm Hg during $CO_2$ inhalation, but this increase was not statistically significant. Figure 2 illustrates marked increases in local CBF in the basal ganglia (caudate, putamen, and thalamus).

In general, $CO_2$ responses were good in the basal ganglia, frontal cortex, and cerebellar midline; modest in the parietal and fusiform cerebral cortex and the cerebellar hemispheres; and low in the white matter. A rise in $PaCO_2$ of 1 mm Hg was accompanied by an average CBF increase of 6.6 ml/100 g/min in the basal ganglia, 4.7 ml/100 g/min in the cerebral cortex, and 4.8 ml/100 g/min in part of the cerebellum. These results indicate that higher resting CBF values seem to correspond to higher $CO_2$ reactivity. Therefore, we calculated the ratio of $CO_2$ reactivity per 1-mm-Hg rise in $PaCO_2$ and divided by the resting CBF value. This ratio ($CO_2$ reactivity/resting CBF) was almost the same throughout the various parts of the brain, ranging from 0.09 to 0.13.

## Autoregulatory Ability

Figure 3 shows the relationship between local CBF values and MABP in monkeys whose blood pressure was altered by hemorrhage (hemorrhagic hypotension). Each CBF value was obtained 3 to 5 minutes after blood pressure had stabilized. Local CBF values seemed well maintained when MABP ranged from 60 to 140 mm Hg, provided arterial $CO_2$ tension was stable. As shown in Fig. 3, we found a normal autoregulatory relationship, especially in higher blood-flow areas. But

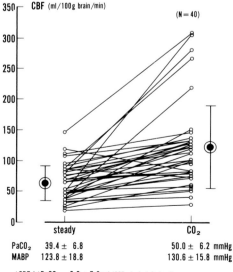

**FIG. 2.** Changes in local cerebral blood flow (CBF) in the basal ganglia before and after $CO_2$ inhalation.

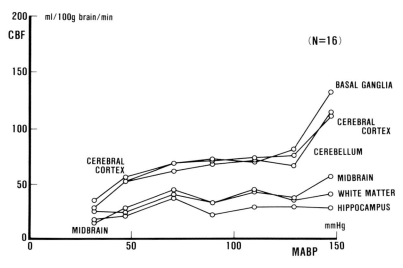

**FIG. 3.** Changes in local cerebral blood flow (CBF) with alteration of blood pressure (MABP).

in lower blood-flow areas such as the midbrain and hippocampus, we observed a slight elevation in blood flow at an MABP of 60 to 80 mm Hg.

We also investigated the relationship between MABP and CBF in the anterior watershed areas. The CBF values in these areas were low, but autoregulatory ability seemed to be maintained. The slight increase in CBF that we observed in the midbrain and hippocampus was not observed in these areas.

### Predysautoregulatory Overshoot of CBF

The slight elevation of blood flow in lower blood-flow areas such as the midbrain and hippocampus was not related to changes in arterial $CO_2$ tension or hematocrit. Because the blood pressure at which the elevation occurs is just above the lower limit of autoregulation, we designated this phenomenon as "predysautoregulatory overshoot of CBF" (5).

### DISCUSSION

The general shape of the response curve of CBF to changes in $PaCO_2$ has been well established, and most authors have successfully fitted a straight line or exponential function to their experimental data. In the present study, the basal ganglia and a part of cerebral cortex and cerebellum showed the greatest response to changes in $CO_2$ tension, while various other parts of the brain seemed to respond differently to $CO_2$. However, the ratio of $CO_2$ reactivity to resting CBF was almost the same throughout the brain, suggesting that $CO_2$ reactivity is related to the difference in microvascular density in the brain's various parts. This finding indicates that there is essentially no difference in regional $CO_2$ response in the brain. Our results are consistent with the proposal of Sato et al. (6) that large regulatory responses to $CO_2$ may be related to high levels of resting CBF. This was not, however, confirmed by Hata et al. (7) or Kanno et al. (8).

Although the mechanism of the observed "predysautoregulatory overshoot" is not known, the regions where the overshoot was seen coincide with those where an increase of glucose utilization has been found in hemorrhagic hypotension (9). Therefore, this phenomenon may be a kind of defense mechanism of brain tissue against hypoxia, especially in the lower-perfusion areas.

## REFERENCES

1. Kety SS, Schmidt CF. The effects of altered arterial tension of carbon dioxide and oxygen on cerebral blood flow and cerebral consumption of normal young men. *J Clin Invest* 1948;27:484–492.
2. Lassen NA. Cerebral blood flow and oxygen consumption in man. *Physiol Rev* 1959;39:183–238.
3. Shinohara Y. Mechanism of chemical control of cerebral vasomotor activity. *Neurology* 1973;23:186–195.
4. Gotoh F, Ebihara SI, Toyoda M, Shinohara Y. Role of autonomic nervous system in autoregulation of human cerebral circulation. *Eur Neurol* 1971–72;6:203–207.
5. Shinohara Y, Takagi S, Yamamoto M, et al. Predysautoregulatory overshoot of cerebral blood flow observed in hemorrhagic hypotension. The First International Stroke Congress, Kyoto, 1989.
6. Sato M, Pawlik G, Heis W-D. Comparative studies of regional CNS blood flow autoregulation and responses to $CO_2$ in the cat. Effects of altering arterial blood pressure and $PaCO_2$ on CBF of cerebrum, cerebellum, and spinal cord. *Stroke* 1984;15:91–97.
7. Hata T, Gotoh F, Ebihara S, et al. Three dimensional local cerebrovascular $CO_2$ responsiveness by cold xenon method. In: Meyer JS, et al., eds. *Cerebral vascular disease 5.* Amsterdam: Elsevier; 1985:141–146.
8. Kanno K, Uemura M, Murakami M, et al. Regional cerebrovascular reactivity to $PaCO_2$ change in man using $H_2^{15}O$ autoradiographic method and positron emission tomography. *J Cereb Blood Flow Metabol* 1985;5(Suppl 1):S659–660.
9. Savaki HE, Macpherson H, McCulloch J. Alterations in local cerebral glucose utilization during hemorrhagic hypotension in the rat. *Circ Res* 1982;50:633–644.

*Cerebral Blood Flow Measurement with Stable Xenon-Enhanced Computed Tomography,* edited by Howard Yonas. Raven Press, Ltd., New York © 1992.

# Prognostic Implications of Hyperglycemia and Reduced Cerebral Blood Flow in Near Drowning in Children

Stephen Ashwal, Sanford Schneider, Lawrence Tomasi, and *Joseph Thompson

*Departments of Pediatrics and *Radiation Sciences, Loma Linda University School of Medicine, Loma Linda, California 92350*

Drowning remains a common cause of death in children, and near drowning is associated with significant neurological morbidity (1). Many studies have attempted to categorize victims of near drowning into prognostic groups. Clinical rating scales, estimated immersion time, water temperature, initial pH, body temperature, occurrence of fixed and dilated pupils, coma, cardiac arrest—all have been used to group patients but have met with only limited success.

In this study of critically ill, nearly drowned children, we examined the predictive value of initial blood glucose concentration and cerebral blood flow (CBF) using stable xenon/computed tomography (Xe/CT). We chose these criteria because clinical studies in adults (2–4) and experimental studies in various animals (5–8) have suggested a correlation between initially high blood glucose levels or decreased CBF and poor neurologic outcome.

## METHODS

We retrospectively reviewed the clinical courses of 20 comatose, nearly drowned children aged 9 months to 10 years. Outcomes were categorized as normal ($n = 4$), persistent vegetative state (PVS) ($n = 9$), or dead ($n = 7$). Table 1 reports initial blood glucose values and those obtained during the first 3 days of hospitalization. We did not consistently obtain serum lactate or cerebrospinal fluid glucose levels.

The Xe/CT CBF determinations were made 24 to 48 hours after hospital admission using the General Electric 9800 xenon blood flow system while the patient breathed a 33% nonradioactive xenon-oxygen mixture (Linde XeScan stable xenon in oxygen USP, Union Carbide Rare Gases, Specialty Medical Products, Danbury, CT) (9). We routinely obtained images in three planes spaced

**TABLE 1.** *Blood glucose and outcome in 20 nearly drowned children*

| | Mean (±SD) blood glucose (mg %) | | |
| --- | --- | --- | --- |
| | Normal (n = 4) | Persistent vegetative state (n = 6) | Dead (n = 6) |
| Admission | 238 (170) | 465 (104)* | 511 (110)* |
| Day 1 | 209 (201) | 280 (129) | 331 (139) |
| Day 2 | 101 (—) | 254 (106) | 226 (43) |
| Day 3 | NA | 103 (8) | 111 (25) |

* P < 0.05 compared to normal group.
NA, data unavailable.

1 cm apart to include the upper brainstem, subcortical nuclei, and peripheral cortex in the lower and middle cerebrum. System software was used to analyze the xenon scan enhancement data. Once these data were combined with the estimated arterial concentrations of xenon, pixel-by-pixel data were calculated according to the Kety-Schmidt equation to derive the Xe/CT CBF map (10).

Flow values (ml/100 g/min) were determined with the system's region-of-interest cursor. We obtained CBF values for the right and left hemisphere of each brain section and regional flow values for the frontal gray and white matter; temporal, parietal, and occipital cortex; thalamus; lenticular nucleus; caudate nucleus; cerebellum; and midbrain. Flows through the medulla and pons could not be obtained routinely because of positioning and bone-induced CT artifacts.

Both analysis of variance and a stepwise discriminant function analysis were performed on the data using a SPSS software package (11). Data are reported as the mean ± standard deviation (SD) with significance at the $P < 0.05$ level.

## RESULTS

Initial blood glucose levels in the patients who died (511 ± 110 mg%) or survived in a PVS (465 ± 104 mg%) were significantly higher than those of children considered normal at follow-up (238 ± 170 mg%) (see Table 1). The elevation in blood glucose continued into day two; levels returned to normal by the third day of hospitalization.

Xe/CT CBF studies (Table 2) showed that global flows and those in the frontal gray and white matter and temporal and parietal gray matter were significantly lower in patients who later died than in those who were normal or survived in a PVS. Regression analysis of CBF and end-tidal $pCO_2$ for the patients who died showed no correlation, suggesting that CBF in these patients was not $pCO_2$ responsive. Although decreased CBF was correlated with increased intracranial pressure (ICP), no relationship was observed between ICP and elevated blood glucose.

Children who remained in a vegetative state had lower flows than those who completely recovered, but not significantly so. Preservation of diencephalic

**TABLE 2.** *Global and regional cerebral blood flow in 20 nearly drowned children*

| | Mean (±SD) blood flow (ml/100 g/min)[a] | | |
|---|---|---|---|
| | Normal (n = 4) | Persistent vegetative state (n = 9) | Dead (n = 7) |
| Global | 68.9 (24.1) | 57.9 (21.5) | 34.6 (17.3)* |
| Frontal gray | 74.0 (38.0) | 63.9 (22.9) | 34.3 (18.0)* |
| Frontal white | 55.5 (22.9) | 35.1 (15.0)* | 13.8 (8.8)* |
| Cortical gray | | | |
|   Temporal | 67.3 (24.2) | 62.2 (25.0) | 31.4 (15.2)* |
|   Parietal | 63.0 (35.9) | 63.0 (25.1) | 31.6 (16.7)* |
|   Occipital | 71.3 (15.7) | 62.4 (29.5) | 48.8 (37.7) |
| Thalamus | 112.0 (47.0) | 78.1 (43.1) | 63.3 (49.5) |
| Caudate nucleus | 73.3 (24.2) | 60.0 (24.9) | 37.8 (28.2) |
| Lenticular nucleus | 91.5 (29.3) | 71.6 (31.3) | 58.9 (42.5) |
| Cerebellum | 84.0 (26.8) | 52.4 (25.4) | 36.7 (31.5) |
| Midbrain | 75.8 (35.5) | 80.3 (52.7) | 34.7 (28.1) |

[a] Mean (SD) group end-tidal $pCO_2$ values (in torr): normal, 32.0 (8.5); persistent vegetative state, 31.2 (7.1); dead, 22.6 (7.9).
* $P < 0.05$, significantly different from normal group.

function in patients with vegetative survival was probably related to the preservation of CBF to such areas as the midbrain (80.3 ± 52.7 ml/100 g/min), thalamus (78.1 ± 43.2 ml/100 g/min), and deep frontal white matter (35.1 ± 15.0 ml/100 g/min).

A stepwise discriminant analysis of the different variables was predictive of death, PVS, or normal outcome as follows: immersion and resuscitation times, 55%; combined Conn, Orlowski, and Glasgow Coma Scale scores, 70%; initial pH, 50%; initial blood glucose, 68%; initial ICP, 64%; CBF, 50%; initial blood glucose and CBF 79%; and initial pH, blood glucose, and CBF, 74%.

## DISCUSSION

### Blood Glucose Determinations and Neurologic Outcome

Blood glucose levels were significantly higher in children who died or were PVS survivors than in those who recovered completely. None of the patients who died or were PVS survivors had blood glucose levels below 300 mg%. Only one of four children who completely recovered exceeded this threshold, with an initial value of 421 mg%. This child's clinical data and normal CBF were consistent with his good outcome, demonstrating that multiple criteria are required for prognostic guidelines.

In a variety of experimental models (6–8), elevated glucose levels increased the neurologic damage during hypoxic-ischemic injury. Some studies, however, have shown that hyperglycemia is either protective or has no deleterious effect (12–14). Yet in a recent study of 430 adults resuscitated after cardiac arrest, the mean admission blood glucose values were higher in those who remained comatose (341 mg%) than in those who awakened (252 mg%) (2). The mean glucose levels were also higher in subjects with a chronic neurologic deficit (286 mg%) than in those who recovered completely (251 mg%). Pulsinelli et al. (3) reported similar findings in patients with ischemic stroke. However, the greater cerebral injury associated with hyperglycemia could be an epiphenomenon manifesting a more profound generalized ischemic insult and stress response.

### Cerebral Blood Flow and Neurologic Outcome

Both global and regional flow to frontal gray and white matter and temporal and parietal gray matter were significantly lower in the patients who died than in the PVS or normal survivors. This was most likely due to elevation of ICP. When we compared CBF in normal and PVS survivors, there was no significant correlation. In fact, at least half the patients with vegetative survival had normal CBF. Although average flow in the remaining patients was reduced, it was still greater than the level thought necessary for tissue viability. Grotta (4) found only limited correlation between blood flow and neurologic outcome after acute ischemia or acute stroke, suggesting that although there may be subgroups of patients in whom either metabolic/flow or pressure/flow relations are disturbed, the effect on neuronal recovery is related to other phenomena intrinsic to neuronal function and activity.

### Predictors of Outcome in Near Drownings in Children

Estimated CBF and initial blood glucose determinations are useful predictors of outcome and should be included in the criteria used for prognosis. Perhaps more importantly, they are predictors that are independent of the history and variables of cardiopulmonary resuscitation and, like the Glasgow Coma Scale, are objective measurements that can be repeated or quantified. In addition, the variables of CBF and blood glucose measurements can be refined for greater significance in predicting future recovery.

### ACKNOWLEDGMENTS

The authors wish to thank Dr. Grenith Zimmerman and Dr. Douglas Deming for assistance in statistical analysis and Ann Elliott for secretarial assistance.

### REFERENCES

1. Orlowski JP. Drowning, near-drowning, and ice-water submersions. *Pediatr Clin North Am* 1987;34:75–92.

2. Longstreth WT Jr, Inui TS. High blood glucose level on hospital admission and poor neurological recovery after cardiac arrest. *Ann Neurol* 1984;15:59–63.
3. Pulsinelli WA, Levy DE, Sigsbee B, et al. Increased damage after ischemic stroke in patients with hyperglycemia with or without established diabetes mellitus. *Am J Med* 1983;74:540–544.
4. Grotta JC. Can raising cerebral blood flow improve outcome after acute cerebral infarction? *Stroke* 1987;18:264–267.
5. Crockard HA, Gadian DG, Frackowiak SJ, et al. Acute cerebral ischemia: concurrent changes in cerebral blood flow, energy metabolites, pH, and lactate measured with hydrogen clearance and $^{31}$P and $^1$H nuclear magnetic resonance spectroscopy. II. Changes during ischemia. *J Cereb Blood Flow Metab* 1987;7:394–402.
6. Myers RE, Yamaguchi S. Nervous system effects of cardiac arrest in monkeys. *Arch Neurol* 1977;34:65–74.
7. Pulsinelli WA, Waldman S, Rawlinson D, et al. Moderate hyperglycemia augments ischemic brain damage: a neuropathologic study in the rat. *Neurology* 1982;32:1239-1246.
8. Bloomstrand S, Hrbek A, Karlsson K, et al. Does glucose administration affect the cerebral response to fetal asphyxia? *Acta Obstet Gynecol Scand* 1984;63:345–353.
9. Ashwal S, Schneider S, Thompson J. Xenon computed tomography cerebral blood flow in the determination of brain death in children. *Ann Neurol* 1989;25:539–546.
10. Gur D, Yonas H, Good WF. Local cerebral blood flow by xenon-enhanced CT: current status, potential improvements, and future directions. *Cerebrovascular and Brain Metabolism Reviews* 1989;1:68–86.
11. Noruss MJ. *Advanced statistics SPSS/PCT for the IBM PC/XT/AT.* Chicago: SPSS Inc; 1986: B1–39.
12. Ginsberg MD, Prado R, Dietrich WD, et al. Hyperglycemia reduces the extent of cerebral infarction in rats. *Stroke* 1987;18:570–574.
13. Ibayashi S, Fujishima M, Sadoshima S, et al. Cerebral blood flow and tissue metabolism in experimental cerebral ischemia of spontaneously hypertensive rats with hyper-, normo- and hypoglycemia. *Stroke* 1986;7:261–266.
14. Vannucci RC, Vasta F, Vannucci SJ. Cerebral metabolic responses of hyperglycemic immature rats to hypoxia-ischemia. *Pediatr Res* 1987;21:524–529.

*Cerebral Blood Flow Measurement with Stable
Xenon-Enhanced Computed Tomography,*
edited by Howard Yonas. Raven Press, Ltd.,
New York © 1992.

# Heterogeneity of Cerebral Reperfusion after Prolonged Cardiac Arrest in Dogs

*†Sidney K. Wolfson Jr, **Peter Safar, **Harvey Reich,
†Joni M. Clark, ***David Gur, **William Stezoski,
†Eugene E. Cook, †Mary Ann Krupper,
and ***Richard Latchaw

*International Resuscitation Research Center; Departments of *Neurological Surgery,
**Anesthesiology, and ***Radiology; and †Montefiore University Hospital,
University Health Center of Pittsburgh, Pittsburgh, Pennsylvania 15213*

Global cerebral ischemia following cardiac arrest is associated with a complex sequence of neurocirculatory disarray, producing a number of discernible dysfunctions during recovery (1,2). This effect has been called "reperfusion syndrome" (1). It includes aberrations of reperfusion, neural cell injury, and injury to other body organs that then have secondary effects on cerebral function. Such reperfusion leads to an immediate global hyperemic phase followed by globally low flow. It ultimately leads to recovery or brain damage, depending on several factors, some unknown. Our prior work has led to the hypothesis that this syndrome has four interacting components: impaired perfusion, reoxygenation injury, toxic effects of damage to extracerebral organs, and blood abnormalities due to stasis (2).

We studied local cerebral blood flow (LCBF) to determine the pattern of reperfusion during the early post-resuscitation period in a ventricular fibrillation, cardiac-arrest, long-term outcome model in dogs. We compared this pattern with perfusion patterns before arrest and in longer-term sham experiments. Although the model permits long-term survival, in this preliminary study we limited our observations to the first 6 to 8 hours after arrest.

Though these reperfusion phenomena have been much-studied, a problem has been the lack of a method suited to multiple, noninvasive measurement of LCBF that has high resolution and good anatomic specificity and that is capable of extending to all levels of the brain. Xenon-enhanced computed tomography (Xe/CT) is such a method (3–7). Functional integrity depends on maintaining some minimal flow level in every tissue region (>20 ml 100 g min has been suggested [8]). Thus, because it represents the average flow of all regions, the global flow cannot predict functional outcome or viability. In addition to providing local flow values, the Xe/CT method offers resolution exceeded only by invasive techniques such as the $H_2$ electrode or methods such as autoradiography that require death of the subject after a few measurements.

We designed experiments using the Xe/CT method specifically to test the hypothesis that there are multiple small tissue regions without reperfusion ("multifocal no-reflow") after cardiac arrest. This hypothesis, proposed by Safar in 1984, includes the following three propositions. First, re-establishment of normotension after prolonged cardiac arrest is accompanied by multifocal no-reflow or trickle flow foci, which extend through the hyperemic phase and "mature" into global hypoperfusion (9,10). Second, global CBF measured after arrest, even when values are >20% of normal, includes gray matter foci in which flow is <20% of normal, potentially preventing both the recovery of neurons and the beneficial actions of resuscitative drugs. And finally, noninvasive monitoring of multifocal CBF after arrest can help in the development of treatments to optimize CBF distribution and thereby improve outcome.

## MATERIALS AND METHODS

We performed five experiments in coon hounds. All procedures observed the guidelines of the Institutional Animal Care and Use Committee of Montefiore University Hospital and the University of Pittsburgh. Three animals received endotracheal anesthesia with 10 mg/kg ketamine, 0.5% halothane, and 10 mg/kg fentanyl. They were immobilized with 0.2 mg/kg pancuronium bromide and connected to mechanical positive-pressure ventilation. We then subjected the animals to a standard cardiac arrest protocol (no flow for 10 minutes). This was followed within 5 minutes by restoration of spontaneous circulation with cardiopulmonary resuscitation and advanced life support and then by standardized life support to maintain normotension, $PaO_2$, $PaCO_2$, base excess, and temperature. The model leads to survival with brain damage. Two controls had sham procedures. The $PaCO_2$ was 30 to 35 torr before arrest and 25 to 30 torr after.

We monitored the LCBF in all experimental animals before and for 6 hours after cardiac arrest. In sham animals, LCBF was monitored throughout the 6- to 8-hour period of observation. To do this, we used the Xe/CT CBF software/hardware system integrated within the GE 9800 scanner (General Electric Medical Systems Division, Milwaukee, WI). The contrast agent was a mixture of 33%

**TABLE 1.** *Brain regions included in the three CT levels studied*[a]

| Level | Structures |
|---|---|
| 1 | Pons, mesencephalon, temporal lobe, hippocampus |
| 2 | Temporal lobe, basal ganglia, parietal lobe, hippocampus |
| 3 | Thalamus, hippocampus, cingulate gyri, substantia nigra, lateral geniculate body, parietal lobe |

[a] Coronal cuts, 5, 10, and 15 mm rostral to the interaural zero plane.

xenon in oxygen (Linde XeScan®, stable xenon in oxygen USP, Union Carbide Rare Gases, Specialty Medical Products, Danbury, CT).

We measured the data in several ways. Computer-generated LCBF values were compiled voxel by voxel (1 × 1 × 5 mm) in coronal CT slices. Global flow was defined as the mean of all voxels in all slices. We chose a limited number of regions of interest (ROIs) in structures identified in the CT slices used for CBF measurement (Table 1).

Gray-scale flow images were viewed alongside the CT images. An appropriately sized and shaped cursor (square or elliptical) was used to sample flow in structures of interest on the CT slice; then, the coordinates and dimensions of the ROI

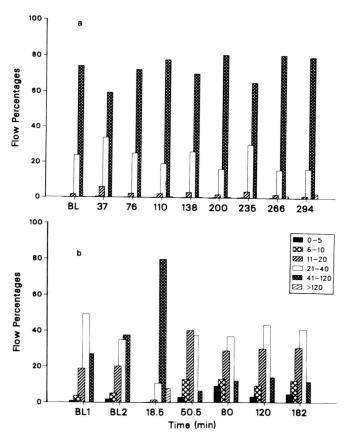

**FIG. 1.** Fractional cerebral blood flow for a control (**a**) and an experimental (**b**) animal. Note the relatively uniform flows that were restricted to high fractions > 20 ml/100 g min for the control animal. For the experimental animal, flows were more widely distributed after arrest. With the exception of the hyperemic phase (18.5 minutes), flows after arrest were lower, including the very lowest fractions (0–5 ml/100 g min). There was also more temporal variability, which correlated with the geographic (anatomic) variability described in the text. BL, baseline.

were recorded for subsequent placement on the corresponding LCBF map. These cursors were never smaller than the expected resolution of the method (125–350 mm$^3$). We constructed anatomical masks and bar graphs of fractional flow for these ROIs and for whole slices (Fig. 1). Fractional flow was calculated by measuring the percentage of voxels in each ROI that fell into each of the following ranges: 0–5, 6–10, 11–20, 21–40, 41–120, or >120 ml/100 g/min.

## RESULTS

Our results clearly demonstrated both the immediate post-resuscitative hyperemic phase and the general global reduction in flow over the next 5 to 6 hours. Of greatest interest were the migrating regions of very low flow scattered among regions of low, normal, or high flow, depending on the post-resuscitative interval. These were 125- to 500-mm$^3$ regions of CBF < 10 ml/(100 cm$^3 \cdot$ min) in different areas at varying times and involved many different deep and superficial structures. We also saw similarly sized migratory regions of high flow that persisted into the late period of generally lower flow (4 to 6 hours; see Fig. 1).

## COMMENT

The presence of different flows in small regions is suggested by the varying fractional flow quantities in Fig. 1. Flow masks, which represented geographic zones of fractional flow as listed above (0–5, 6–10, and so forth), were computer generated and laid over the anatomical CT image. Masks obtained over time were also superimposed on each other. This process clearly indicated the migratory nature and small size of the regions, an observation also supported by the data from the various ROIs.

## ACKNOWLEDGMENTS

Timothy Kerr, Henry Alexander, Frank Houghton, Leslie Scarborough, David Snyder, Patricia Streppa, and Donna Wojciechowsky contributed their technical expertise. Dr. Manfred Boehnke provided the CT facility. Drs. Mark Angelos, Fritz Sterz, Yuvel Leonov, Erga Cerchiari, Stephen Hecht, and David Johnson helped with protocol preparation or experiments. Drs. Walter Obrist and Howard Yonas served as consultants. This research was supported in part by the Asmund S. Laerdal Foundation and USPHS grants 27208 (Dr. Wolfson) and NS24446 (Dr. Safar).

## REFERENCES

1. Negovsky VA, Gurvitch AM, Zolotokrylina ES. *Post-resuscitation disease.* Amsterdam: Elsevier; 1983.

2. Safar P. Cerebral resuscitation after cardiac arrest: a review. *Circulation* 1986;74:138–153.
3. Drayer BP, Wolfson SK Jr, Reinmuth OM, Dujovny M, Boehnke M, Cook EE. Xenon enhanced computed tomography for the analysis of cerebral integrity, perfusion, and blood flow. *Stroke* 1978;9:123–130.
4. Wolfson SK Jr, Drayer BP, Boehnke M, Dujovny M, Cook EE. Regional cerebral blood flow by xenon enhanced computed tomography. *Proceedings of the Annual Meeting of the American Association of Neurological Surgeons*, New Orleans; Chicago: AANS 1978:1–3.
5. Yonas H, Wolfson SK Jr, Dujovny M, Boehnke M, Cook EE. Selective lenticulostriate occlusion in the primate; a highly focal cerebral ischemia model. *Stroke* 1981;12:567–572.
6. Gur D, Good WF, Wolfson SK Jr, Yonas H, Shabason L. In vivo mapping of local cerebral blood flow by xenon enhanced CT. *Science* 1982;215:1267–1268.
7. Gur D, Wolfson SK, Yonas H, Good WF, Shabason L. Cerebral blood flow by xenon CT. *Stroke* 1983;14:108.
8. Symon L. Flow thresholds in ischemia and the effects of damages. *Br J Anaesth* 1985;57:34.
9. Vaagenes P, Cantador R, Safar P, et al. Amelioration of brain damage by lidoflazine after prolonged ventricular fibrillation cardiac arrest in dogs. *Crit Care Med* 1984;12:846–855.
10. Safar P, Cantadore R, Vaagones P. Prolonged cardiovascular system failure after cardiac arrest and cardiopulmonary resuscitation in dogs. *Circ Shock* 1984;13:70 (abst).

*Cerebral Blood Flow Measurement with Stable Xenon-Enhanced Computed Tomography,* edited by Howard Yonas. Raven Press, Ltd., New York © 1992.

# Spinal Cord Blood Flow Measurement: Nimodipine in the Treatment of Experimental Injury of the Spinal Cord in Monkeys

Denis Gense de Beaufort, Anne M. Bidabé, Vincent Pointillart, Anne M. Gin, and Jean M. Caillé

*Service de Neuroradiologie, CHR-33076 Bordeaux, France*

There are more than 1,500 new cases of vertebromedullar trauma in France every year, leaving victims with serious neurologic sequelae. The purpose of our study was twofold: to evaluate spinal cord blood flow (SCBF) using the stable xenon computed tomography (Xe/CT) method and to test the effectiveness of a calcium channel blocker on SCBF after experimental injury of the spinal cord in monkeys. In this model, the final medullar lesion was the result of the initial contusion; secondary aggravation resulted from ischemia, edema, and biochemical and/or enzymatic reactions.

## MATERIALS AND METHODS

We divided ten monkeys (Papio type) weighing 10 kg ± 300 g into two groups: five untreated and five treated with nimodipine. Each animal was premedicated with 10 mg/kg of ketamine hydrochloride and 0.05 mg/kg of atropine administered intramuscularly 15 minutes before starting the manipulations. We then implanted a deep venous catheter in one of the lower limbs and withdrew a blood sample to measure the hematocrit. Anesthesia was started and then maintained with thiopental sodium (Nesdonal). A balloonless tube was placed intratracheally with pharyngeal packing to prevent aspiration of secretions and to obtain a closed respiratory circuit. The animal breathed spontaneously. We recorded the blood pressure and pulse rate every 10 minutes using a blood pressure monitor (Dinamap). An electric blanket was used to maintain the core temperature at 38° C.

### Protocol for Each Animal

Day 1: (a) implantation of balloon catheter; (b) reference somatosensory-evoked potentials (SEP); (c) reference SCBF; (d) trauma; (e) SCBF registration, 30, 90, 150, and 210 minutes after trauma; (f) post-traumatic SEP; (g) magnetic resonance imaging (MRI), 5 hours after injury

Day 7: (a) SEP; (b) SCBF of the lesion area; (c) MRI; (d) removal of cord for histologic analysis

The treated group received 0.02 mg/kg/hour nimodipine (Nimotop, Bayer Laboratories) over the 2 hours beginning immediately after the trauma and 0.04 mg/kg/hour during the next 7 days. Both groups received a standard glucose and electrolyte infusion.

### Trauma Model

A laminectomy was performed at the L-5 vertebral level, and a 4-French Fogarty catheter was inserted into the epidural space to L-1. We induced the trauma by inflating the catheter balloon with 2 ml of Ringer's solution, producing a pressure of 2 bars for 5 seconds.

### Measurement of SCBF

We measured the SCBF according to the same principle used to measure cerebral blood flow with Xe/CT. Examinations were performed with a Siemens Somatom DRH scanner (Fig. 1). The animal was positioned on the scanner table with a bag of flour under the lumbar region to ensure uniform x-ray absorption. The animal initially breathed 40% room air with 60% oxygen, causing the reduction of nitrogen from the alveolar air and improving the uptake of xenon by blood at the pulmonary interface. A scout view was performed to localize the catheter tip and determine the level at which to obtain the reference slice (Fig. 2). The animal then breathed a mixture of 38% xenon with 62% oxygen for 10 minutes while 8-mm-thick slices were imaged every 50 seconds for a total of 12 slices. We used the following technical factors in our study. Tube feeding tension was 96 kVp, 560 mA-s and the kernel, 5. The image matrix was 256 × 256; the zoom factor, 5; and the calculation time for image reconstruction, 5 seconds. The end-tidal air was analyzed by sensors that evaluated the percentages of $CO_2$ and xenon.

We obtained the first SCBF measurement 3 hours after positioning the balloon (1). We allowed at least 30 minutes between measurements to permit the tissue to eliminate the xenon (thus the scheduling of subsequent measurements as noted in the protocol).

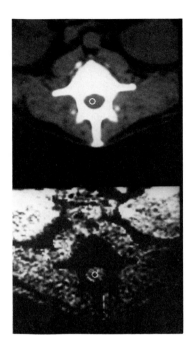

**FIG. 1.** CT scan of spinal cord (*top*) and spinal cord blood flow image (*bottom*) for a 0.07-cm$^2$ region of interest.

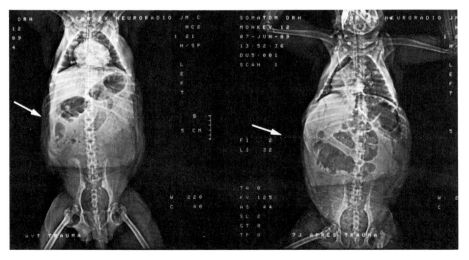

**FIG. 2.** Monkey 12. Scout view at J0 (*left*) and J7 (*right*) to locate the same slices at the level of spinal cord injury. J0, scout view before trauma; J7, scout view 7 days after trauma.

For each animal, we selected three regions of interest (ROIs): one centro-medullar and two contiguous (to avoid partial volumes in the subarachnoid space). The surfaces studied were $\geq 0.07$ cm$^2$, based on the assumption that these zones included both white and gray matter. The mean blood flow of these three ROIs yielded the mean SCBF. The same ROIs were selected for each measurement.

### Recording the SEP

We chose the posterior tibial nerve of the free lower limb for stimulation. The signal was recorded on the contralateral parietal cortex. An SEP was recorded immediately after introduction of the Fogarty catheter to verify the integrity of the posterior column of the spinal cord and was used for reference (with amplitudes of waves N 13, P 22, N 26 recorded using a Racia 21P) (2–5).

### Magnetic Resonance Study

We performed MRI using a Thomson-CGR 0.5-tesla Magniscan with a cervical spinal surface coil. The sequence parameters were as follows: sagittal $T_1$-weighted (TR, 300–500 msec; TE, 28 msec) and $T_2$-weighted slices (TR, 2000 msec; TE, 35–90 msec, three echoes), $256 \times 256$ matrix, 4-mm slice thickness, and 10% interslice gap.

### Histological Study

Animals were killed 7 days after the injury, and their spines and spinal cords were removed and fixed in a 10% formalin solution for 8 days. After macroscopic examination of the spinal cord, the histological study was performed in a blinded manner using 2-$\mu$m-thick slices with a trichrome stain.

### Statistical Analysis

For statistical analysis of the data, we used the Student's $t$ test for small samples.

## RESULTS

### Spinal Cord Blood Flow

Table 1 shows the results for each animal in the untreated and treated groups. The heart rate and mean blood pressure were held constant during all SCBF measurements in the same animal. The spinal injury induced a 38% average

**TABLE 1.** *Mean spinal cord blood flow (SCBF) in the untreated and treated groups*

| Monkey | Pretrauma SCBF (ml/100 g/min) | Post-trauma SCBF (% change from baseline) (ml/100 g/min) | | | | |
|--------|--------|--------|--------|--------|--------|--------|
| | | 30 min | 90 min | 150 min | 210 min | 7 days |
| *Treated group* | | | | | | |
| 1 | 69 | 127 (+84) | 10 (−86) | unmeasurable | unmeasurable | 10 (−86) |
| 2 | 30 | 80 (+170) | ~0 (−100) | unmeasurable | unmeasurable | 7 (−77) |
| 3 | 31 | 39 (+26) | ~0 (−100) | unmeasurable | unmeasurable | 3 (−90) |
| 4 | 45 | 68 (+51) | 10 (−78) | unmeasurable | unmeasurable | 5 (−89) |
| 5 | 34 | 42 (+23) | 5 (−86) | unmeasurable | unmeasurable | 8 (−77) |
| Mean | 41 | 71 (+71) | 5 (−90) | | | 7 (−83) |
| SD | 16 | 36 (+61) | 5 (10) | | | 3 (6) |
| *Untreated group* | | | | | | |
| 6 | 64 | 158 (+146) | 27 (−58) | 34 (−47) | 35 (−45) | 40 (−38) |
| 7 | 26 | 67 (+157) | 10 (−61) | 13 (−50) | 13 (−51) | 14 (−47) |
| 10 | 25 | 40 (+40) | 17 (−32) | 17 (−34) | 16 (−35) | 14 (−44) |
| 11 | 41 | 60 (+46) | 30 (−27) | 28 (−32) | 27 (−33) | 30 (−27) |
| 12 | 43 | 60 (+39) | 35 (−19) | 33 (−25) | 30 (−30) | 33 (−24) |
| Mean | 40 | 77 (+86) | 24 (−39) | 25 (−38) | 24 (−39) | 26 (−36) |
| SD | 16 | 46 (60) | 10 (19) | 10 (11) | 9 (9) | 12 (10) |

increase in mean blood pressure, which normalized after 20 minutes. The infusion of 0.02 mg/kg/hour of nimodipine during the first 2 hours did not change any of the hemodynamic variables.

There was no significant difference in baseline SCBF values for the two groups. Because of the great variation in individual flow values in both groups, results were expressed as a percentage of baseline values. Table 2 shows the mean changes in SCBF in both groups. The SCBF in the groups differed significantly ($P < 0.001$) beginning 90 minutes after the injury until the seventh day. Figure 3 illustrates these results, and Fig. 4 shows the results in a single animal (#12).

### Electrophysiology

The SEP recorded 4 hours after trauma showed no evidence of a functional pathway in either group. On the seventh day, the SEP of the untreated group

**TABLE 2.** *Summary of the significant differences between the treated and untreated groups*

| | Mean % change (SD) in SCBF post-injury | | | SEP after injury | | Lesion size (mm) | |
|---|--------|--------|--------|--------|--------|--------|--------|
| | | | | | | White matter | Gray matter |
| | 30 min | 90 min | 7 days | Day 0 | Day 7 | | |
| Untreated | +70 (60.6) | −90 (9.7) | −8.4 (6.4) | abolished | abolished | 45.2 (6.1) | 31.6 (3.1) |
| Treated | +86 (60.3) | −39 (18.9) | −36 (10.2) | abolished | present in 2 animals | 26.4 (4.3) | 14 (4.3) |
| P | 0.709 | <0.001 | <0.001 | | | <0.001 | <0.001 |

SCBF, spinal cord blood flow; SEP, somatosensory-evoked potentials.

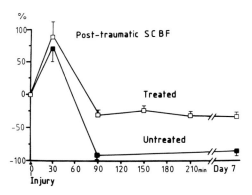

**FIG. 3.** Evolution of spinal cord blood flow at the lesion site in the treated and untreated groups for the first 210 minutes and on the seventh day. Results are expressed as a percentage of control flow values.

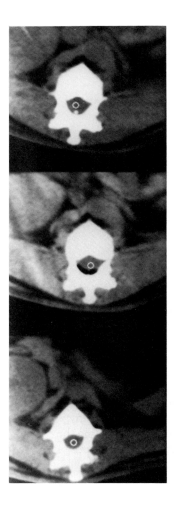

**FIG. 4.** Monkey 12 (treated). **Top**: SCBF before trauma. Note catheter tip in the spinal canal. **Middle**: SCBF 210 minutes after trauma. **Bottom**: SCBF 7 days after trauma.

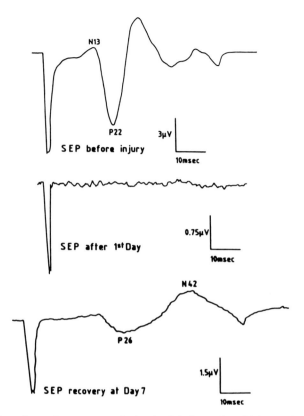

**FIG. 5.** Evolution of somatosensory evoked potentials in monkey 11 (treated), who showed an electrical improvement.

remained abolished (no recognizable electric variation on the recorded tracks). In the treated group, the SEP began to recover in two animals (#7 and #11), with one positive wave at 26 msec and one negative wave at 42 msec at 10% of the pretraumatic amplitude (Fig. 5).

## Magnetic Resonance Imaging

On the first day, a heterogeneous signal on the $T_1$-weighted images prevented measurement of the lesion. In the $T_2$-weighted images, an area of high signal intensity was visible (Fig. 6). On the seventh day, there were two hyperintense zones in both $T_1$- and $T_2$-weighted images. The difficulty in delimiting the contour of the lesions with MRI made the lesion measurements unreliable and prohibited comparison of the two groups. The only constant obtainable with MRI was verification of the medullar trauma in vivo (6,7).

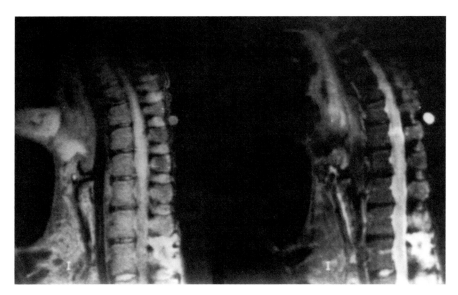

**FIG. 6.** Magnetic resonance images, monkey 4, four hours after trauma. **Left**: $T_1$-weighted (TR 360, TE 26, 4-mm thickness). Note the mild and heterogeneous hyperintensity of the spinal cord in the hyperacute stage. The location of the trauma is visualized by a glass tube on the skin of the monkey, 5 vertebrae from the site of intervention. **Right**: $T_2$-weighted (TR 2000; TE 50, 100, 150; 4-mm thickness). Note the clearly increased signal encompassing the entire cord section.

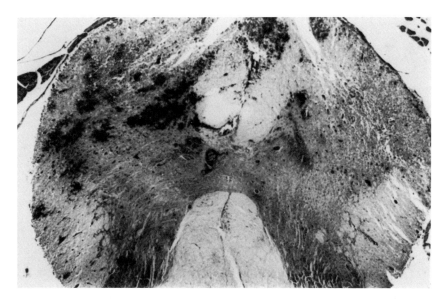

**FIG. 7.** This histological slice shows hemorrhagic suffusions in the interstitium of the white and gray matter with unilateral focus and on the anterior tracts.

### Histology

The lesions appeared diffuse with hemorrhagic suffusion of varying intensity, ranging from small hemorrhages to zones of hemorrhagic contusion (Fig. 7). These were situated in both gray and white matter, and histological slices showed that they extended from one side of the spinal cord to the other. The gray matter was more hemorrhagic than the white matter. The smallest lesion in the untreated group was 37 mm (monkey 2); the largest lesion in the treated group was 32 mm (monkey 11). We found a significant difference between the two groups in the size of both white- and gray-matter lesions (see Table 2).

## DISCUSSION

The method for calculating SCBF has three drawbacks: low signal-to-noise ratio, tissular heterogeneity, and animal movement. For these reasons, we combined 38% xenon with the inhaled air for 10 minutes to increase the attenuation coefficient and improve the signal. Although the Xe/CT method allows for the repeated examinations, a rather long (30-minute) delay is necessary between each study to allow for the elimination of xenon from the tissue, because blood flows are often low, and xenon "wash-out" time depends on the rate of flow.

Determining the tissue volume in which blood flow could be analyzed depended on a balance between the quality of spatial resolution and the likelihood for error caused by tissular heterogeneity. We thus considered the mixture of white and gray matter in ROIs $7 \times 7 \times 8$ mm$^3$. Moreover, because their size was too similar to the voxel noise, we excluded from our analysis ROIs with a smaller volume. Expressing the SCBF results as the percentage of change from initial levels also takes these problems into account, especially the heterogeneity of the measurements and the partial volumes between white and gray matter.

The SCBF increased in all animals 30 minutes after the injury and fell 60 minutes after injury. In the treated group, flow was maintained at a level equal to half of the initial flow through the seventh day, whereas the flow in the untreated group was either almost nonexistent or unmeasurable. Our results agree with those of other studies using other animals and methods such as hydrogen clearance or radiolabeled microspheres (8–11).

SCBF measurements (12–14) and microangiographic studies (11,15) have shown that ischemia is largely responsible for the secondary aggravation seen after injury. Similarly, Fehlings et al. (16) showed a linear relationship between SCBF and axonal function after experimental spinal cord injury. SCBF decreases in the hour after the medullar injury, possibly because of an arterial spasm in which the role of calcium is well known (8,17). This is why, like many other investigators (9,18,19), we used nimodipine to try to diminish the arterial spasm.

All monkeys were clinically paraplegic after 7 days. Two nimodipine-treated monkeys, however, initially showed electrical signs of recovery. As indicated in the literature, SEP was the most sensitive study for evaluating spinal cord lesions, especially those involving the level of the posterior column (5). The histological study was also very important, showing a significant difference between the two groups in the size of the white- and gray-matter lesions.

In conclusion, we found nimodipine to have a beneficial effect. The threshold value of functional perfusion was maintained in three of the five treated animals. These results were highly correlated with those of the histological analysis, which found smaller spinal cord lesions in the treated group than in the untreated group.

## REFERENCES

1. Hitchon PW, Lobosky JM, Yamada T, et al. Effect of laminectomy and anesthesia upon spinal cord blood flow. *J Neurosurg* 1984;61:545–549.
2. Dimitrijevic MR. Neurophysiology in spinal cord injury. *Paraplegia* 1987;25:205–208.
3. Dullberg JJ, Koeppen S. Diagnostic value of segmental somatosensory evoked potentials in cases with chronic progressive para- or tetraspastic syndromes. In: Courjon J, Mauguiere F, Revol M, eds. *Clinical applications of evoked potentials in neurology. Advances in neurology*, vol. 32. New York: Raven Press; 1982.
4. Levy WJ, McCaffrey M, Hagichi S. Motor evoked potentials as a predictor of recovery in chronic spinal cord injury. *Neurosurgery* 1987;20:138–142.
5. Li CH, Houlden DA, Rowed DW. Somatosensory evoked potentials and neurological grades as predictors of outcome in acute spinal cord injury. *J Neurosurg* 1990;72:600–609.
6. Hackney D, Asato R, Joseph P. Hemorrhage and edema in acute spinal cord compression: demonstration by MR imaging. *Radiology* 1986;161:387–390.
7. Kulkarni MV, Bondurant FJ, Rose SL, Narayana PA. 1.5 tesla magnetic resonance imaging of acute spinal trauma. *Radiographics* 1988;8:1059–1081.
8. Bingham WG, Goldmann H, Friedmann S, et al. Blood flow in normal and injured monkey spinal cord. *J Neurosurg* 1975;43:162–171.
9. Fehlings MG, Tator CH, Linden RD. The effect of nimodipine and dextran on axonal function and blood flow following experimental spinal cord injury. *J Neurosurg* 1989;71:403–416.
10. Sandler AN, Tator CH. Effect of acute spinal cord compression injury on regional spinal cord blood flow in primates. *J Neurosurg* 1976;45:660–676.
11. Wallace MC, Tator CH. Spinal cord blood flow measured with microspheres following spinal cord injury in the rat. *Can J Neurol Sci* 1976;13:91–96.
12. Griffith IR. Spinal cord blood flow after acute experimental cord injury in dogs. *J Neurol Sci* 1976;27:247–259.
13. Guha A, Tator C, Rochon J. Spinal cord blood flow and systemic blood pressure after experimental cord injury in rats. *Stroke* 1989;20:372–377.
14. Rivlin AS, Tator CH. Regional spinal cord blood flow in rats after severe cord trauma. *J Neurosurg* 1978;49:844–853.
15. Fairholm DJ, Turnbull IM. Microangiographic study of experimental spinal cord injuries. *J Neurosurg* 1971;35:277–286.
16. Fehlings MG, Tator CH, Linden RD, et al. Relationship between spinal cord blood flow and axonal function in the motor and sensory tracts of the cord after experimental spinal cord injury. *Surgical Forum* 1987;38:508–509.
17. Balentine JD, Hogan EL, Banik NL, et al. Calcium and the pathogenesis of spinal cord injury. In: Dacey RG Jr et al., eds. *Trauma to the central nervous system.* New York: Raven Press, 1985.
18. Guha A, Tator C, Piper I. Effect of a calcium channel blocker on post-traumatic spinal cord blood-flow. *J Neurosurg* 1987;66:423–430.
19. Hitchon PW, Hansen T, McKay T, et al. Nicardipine after spinal cord compression in the lamb. *Surg Neurol* 1989;31:101–110.

*Cerebral Blood Flow Measurement with Stable Xenon-Enhanced Computed Tomography,* edited by Howard Yonas. Raven Press, Ltd., New York © 1992.

# Effect of 33% Xenon Inhalation on Intracranial Pressure in a Primate Model of Head Injury

Joseph M. Darby, Edwin M. Nemoto, *Howard Yonas, and John A. Melick

*Departments of Anesthesiology and Critical Care Medicine and*
**Neurological Surgery, University of Pittsburgh*
*School of Medicine, Pittsburgh, Pennsylvania 15261*

Several reports have suggested that stable xenon causes cerebrovascular dilation (1–3) and may increase intracranial pressure (ICP) (4,5). Xenon inhalation, therefore, might have detrimental effects on ICP, especially when brain compliance is low, as it is in head injury. We evaluated the ICP response to 33% stable Xenon inhalation in a primate model of closed-skull head injury produced by liquid nitrogen.

## MATERIALS AND METHODS

Our protocol was approved by the Institutional Animal Care and Use Committee of the University of Pittsburgh. Eight rhesus monkeys (*Macaca mulatta*) of both sexes and weighing 4 to 6 kg were fasted overnight with free access to water. On the day of the experiment, we anesthetized the animals with ketamine (10 mg/kg administered intramuscularly) and transported them to the laboratory.

There we intubated their tracheas and mechanically ventilated their lungs with a Harvard ventilator set at 15 to 20 ml/kg, adjusting minute ventilation to maintain end-tidal $CO_2$ at 5%. Intravenous (IV) pancuronium bromide (0.05–0.10 mg/kg) was used intermittently for immobilization. We inserted femoral artery catheters and made small burr holes bilaterally over the parietal cortex; Silastic-tipped catheters were inserted into the subdural space to monitor ICP. The dura and burr holes were sealed with cyanoacrylate glue and methylmethacrylate cement. We monitored all pressures using a Grass polygraph (Grass Instruments, Quincy, MA). For the cortical freeze injury, a 1.5-cm-diameter area of the outer table of the right parietal bone was removed with a high-speed drill, leaving the inner table intact. After surgical preparation, we maintained anesthesia with fentanyl, 25 $\mu$g/kg IV initially, and hourly doses of 25 to 50 $\mu$g thereafter.

The monkeys were then moved to the computed tomography facility, where they inhaled a mixture of 67% $O_2$/33% nitrogen and were allowed to equilibrate for 20 to 30 minutes. After this period of stabilization, we made two to three baseline cerebral blood flow (CBF) measurements during 5-minute inhalation of 33% Xe/67% $O_2$ (Linde XeScan, stable xenon in oxygen USP, Union Carbide Rare Gases, Specialty Medical Products, Danbury, CT) delivered via a Harvard ventilator. Peak xenon concentration (30–31%) in end-tidal air was reached 1 to 2 minutes after inhalation began. Once we had obtained baseline measurements of physiological parameters and CBF, a 5-cc plastic syringe with its distal tip cut off was inserted into the right parietal skull defect and sealed to it. We then poured liquid nitrogen into the syringe for 10 minutes. After the freeze injury, the skull was rewarmed with 37°C tap water. Physiologic measurements were repeated after multiple inhalations of the gas mixture over 6 hours. We measured arterial blood gases and pH at the end of each CBF determination. At the conclusion of the experiment, the monkeys were killed with IV saturated potassium chloride.

The strip chart recordings for each animal were used to obtain values of physiologic variables before xenon delivery and at 1-minute intervals throughout the inhalation period. All pre-injury (control) and post-injury (freeze) observations were pooled. We compared the baseline physiologic measurements with those during xenon inhalation using repeated measures of analysis of variance. Posthoc tests for statistical significance were obtained using the Student-Newman-Keuls test; $P$ values < 0.05 were considered significant. Data are presented as the mean ± standard deviation.

## RESULTS

Table 1 presents the physiological data measured in the control and post-injury periods. Because of ICP instability, we discarded physiological data from

**TABLE 1.** *Intracranial pressure and blood pressure during 5-minute inhalation of 33% xenon/67% oxygen*

| | N | Baseline | 1 Min | 2 Min | 3 Min | 4 Min | 5 Min |
|---|---|---|---|---|---|---|---|
| **MAP** | | | | | | | |
| Control | 17 (8) | 116 ± 14 | 113 ± 14 | 113 ± 15 | 113 ± 19 | 114 ± 20 | 114 ± 21 |
| Freeze | 50 (7) | 117 ± 20 | 115 ± 20 | 115 ± 20 | 109 ± 18* | 107 ± 18* | 105 ± 16* |
| **R ICP** | | | | | | | |
| Control | 14 (8) | 8.2 ± 5.2 | 8.3 ± 5.4 | 8.5 ± 6.1 | 8.4 ± 6.1 | 8.0 ± 5.5 | 8.0 ± 5.8 |
| Freeze | 45 (7) | 19.1 ± 10.6 | 21.3 ± 16.1 | 20.6 ± 17.3 | 20.2 ± 16.6 | 20.3 ± 16 | 19.3 ± 14 |
| **L ICP** | | | | | | | |
| Control | 17 (8) | 5.2 ± 2.4 | 5.1 ± 2.5 | 4.8 ± 2.5 | 4.8 ± 2.4 | 4.7 ± 2.2 | 4.6 ± 2.4* |
| Freeze | 49 (7) | 16.2 ± 13.5 | 18.9 ± 19.6 | 17.5 ± 19.5 | 17.5 ± 19.6 | 17.9 ± 19.4 | 16.9 ± 16.9 |

* $P$ < 0.05 compared to baseline values.
Control indicates data obtained before injury; freeze, data obtained after injury. $PaCO_2$ control = 31.6 ± 5.5 mm Hg; freeze = 32.7 ± 4.5 mm Hg (not significantly different). MAP, mean arterial pressure; R ICP, right-sided intracranial pressure; L ICP, left-sided ICP; N, number of observations (number of monkeys).

one monkey in the post-injury period. Overall, ICP did not increase significantly during the 5 minutes of xenon inhalation, either in the control or post-injury period. PaCO$_2$ levels were similar in the control (31.6 ± 5.5 mm Hg) and post-injury observations (32.7 ± 4.5 mm Hg).

Blood pressure was unchanged during xenon inhalation in the control period. After injury, however, arterial blood pressure decreased significantly ($P < 0.05$) at 3, 4, and 5 minutes of inhalation, compared to baseline values.

## DISCUSSION

Under both normal and injured conditions, ICP does not appear to increase in association with 33% Xe/67% O$_2$ inhalation administered over 5 minutes. These findings are consistent with our previous report that xenon had little or no effect on ICP in a group of patients with severe head injury (6). If xenon inhalation does cause cerebrovascular dilation, as some have claimed, both the narcotic anesthesia and mild hyperventilation used in our studies are possible explanations for the lack of significant ICP increase during xenon inhalation.

Although ICP was unaffected by xenon inhalation, post-injury arterial blood pressure decreased late in the inhalation period. It is likely that, under the conditions of head injury, the combined effects of narcotics and subanesthetic doses of xenon caused this reduction in blood pressure.

It thus appears that stable xenon can be administered safely to head-injured patients without raising ICP significantly, as long as pCO$_2$ is well controlled. Arterial blood pressure must be monitored closely to avoid large drops in cerebral perfusion pressure.

## ACKNOWLEDGMENTS

This work was supported in part by grants from the Departments of Anesthesiology, Neurological Surgery, and Radiology, University of Pittsburgh, and NIH grant 2 R01 HL27208–07A1.

## REFERENCES

1. Gur D, Yonas H, Jackson DL, et al. Measurement of cerebral blood flow during xenon inhalation as measured by the microspheres method. *Stroke* 1985;16:871–874.
2. Junck L, Dhawan V, Thaler HT, Rottenberg CA. Effects of xenon and krypton on regional cerebral blood flow in the rat. *J Cereb Blood Flow Metab* 1985;5:126–132.
3. Obrist WD, Jaggi J, Harel D, Smith DS. Effect of stable xenon inhalation on human CBF. *J Cereb Blood Flow Metab* 1985;5(Suppl 1):557–558.
4. Gur D, Wolfson SK, Yonas H, et al. Progress in cerebrovascular disease: local cerebral blood flow by xenon enhanced CT. *Stroke* 1982;13:750–758.
5. Harrington TR, Manwaring K, Hodak J. Local basal ganglion and brain stem blood flow in the head-injured patient using stable xenon-enhanced CT scanning. In: Miller JD, Teasdale GM, Rowan JO, eds. *Intracranial Pressure VI.* Berlin: Springer-Verlag; 1986:680–686.
6. Darby JM, Yonas H, Pentheny S, Marion D. Intracranial pressure response to stable xenon inhalation in patients with head injury. *Surg Neurol* 1989;32:343–345.

*Cerebral Blood Flow Measurement with Stable Xenon-Enhanced Computed Tomography,*
edited by Howard Yonas. Raven Press, Ltd.,
New York © 1992.

# Discussion

Participants:
Dr. Anthony Marmarou (Richmond, Virginia, USA)
Dr. Joseph Darby (Pittsburgh, Pennsylvania, USA)
Dr. Walter Obrist (Pittsburgh, Pennsylvania, USA)
Dr. Jens Astrup (Aarhus, Denmark)
Dr. Jan Ploughmann (Aarhus, Denmark)
Dr. Howard Yonas (Pittsburgh, Pennsylvania, USA)

The need to exercise caution in interpreting blood flow changes that follow flow elevation was stressed by Dr. Marmarou. He questioned whether that the highly variable cerebral blood flow (CBF) responses to hypertension reported by Dr. Darby might have been influenced by elevated intracranial pressure (ICP), which could have caused a reduction in local blood flow. Dr. Darby responded that because his patients usually had little mass effect, a direct vasoconstrictive response to dopamine would best explain the occasional dopamine-induced fall in CBF.

The presentations concerning the effects of xenon inhalation on ICP in head-trauma victims (see also Section IV) provoked misgivings in Dr. Obrist, Dr. Marmarou, and Dr. Astrup. They were concerned that xenon-induced flow activation and a resultant increase in ICP could be a serious problem if the patient had severely compromised brain compliance. Dr. Marmarou wondered whether the University of Pittsburgh studies excluded patients who were more unstable and therefore unable to leave the intensive care unit to undergo CBF studies. To this, Dr. Darby responded that xenon-enhanced computed tomographic (Xe/CT) CBF studies were a standard part of their head-injury treatment and were obtained at the time of CT imaging with no bias in patient selection. Dr. Obrist commented that information from conventional CT scans should aid in identifying patients who would benefit from additional hyperventilation therapy before undergoing Xe/CT CBF studies. Dr. Ploughmann added that ICP elevation does usually occurr after about 7 to 8 minutes of 30% to 40% xenon inhalation.

Finally, Dr. Yonas remarked that a discussion of Xe/CT effects on ICP and, more generally, the safety of these studies, should consider the differences in the concentrations of xenon and the duration of inhalation used at various centers. The system developed at the University of Pittsburgh uses 33% xenon for no longer than 4.5 minutes. If the fear of raising ICP exists, studies can be further shortened to 3 minutes while still yielding accurate flow information. Because flow activation tends to be delayed, he believes that brief inhalation is unlikely to cause any significant effect on ICP or cerebral perfusion.

*Cerebral Blood Flow Measurement with Stable Xenon-Enhanced Computed Tomography,* edited by Howard Yonas. Raven Press, Ltd., New York © 1992.

# Complications and Problems

## Teiichi Takasago, Tetsuo Yamashita, Shigeki Nakano, Shiro Kashiwagi, Seisho Abiko, and Haruhide Ito

*Department of Neurosurgery, Yamaguchi University School of Medicine, 1144 Kogushi Ube, Yamaguchi 755, Japan*

Since 1985, 450 subjects have undergone xenon-enhanced computed tomographic cerebral blood flow (Xe/CT CBF) studies in our institution. This chapter evaluates the incidence of complications and problems associated with the procedures.

### SUBJECTS AND METHODS

The subjects were 348 men and 102 women, their ages ranging from 1 to 75 years (average: $51.8 \pm 15.4$ years). Of this total, 400 were patients with various intracranial diseases, including ischemic cerebrovascular disease (290 cases), brain tumors (23 cases), aneurysms (6 cases), Moya Moya disease (30 cases), arteriovenous malformations (28 cases), intracerebral bleeding (10 cases), and others (13 cases). The remaining 50 subjects were normal volunteers.

We conducted the Xe/CT CBF studies using a Somatom DR3 CT scanner and a Xetron III closed rebreathing xenon inhalator (1). Subjects inhaled 30% stable xenon for 3 to 10 minutes, during which time we obtained CT scans once a minute. We continually monitored the end-tidal $CO_2$, electrocardiogram, blood pressure, and electroencephalogram (in some cases) and observed the subjects carefully.

### RESULTS

There were no side effects significant enough to necessitate termination of the study. Respiration slowed in 17 subjects (3.8%), three subjects (0.7%) experienced nausea or vomiting, and one subject (0.2%) had a seizure immediately after the procedure. This patient had a brain tumor, and the seizure was not well controlled.

The slowing of respiration was a major side effect in this study. The incidence gradually increased during the first 5 minutes of inhalation (Fig. 1). Nevertheless, all subjects regained a normal respiratory pattern, either spontaneously or in response to a verbal command to take a breath.

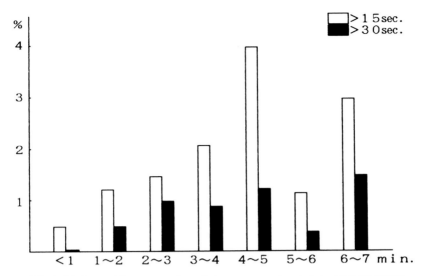

**FIG. 1.** Timing and frequency of respiratory suppression during xenon inhalation.

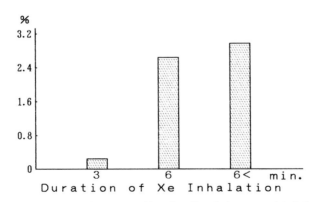

**FIG. 2.** Timing and frequency of head motion during xenon inhalation.

A total of 96.7% of the studies were successful. Nondiagnostic studies resulted from head motion in 2.7% (12 subjects) and from anxiety and/or claustrophobia in 0.7% (3 subjects). Figure 2 shows the timing and incidence of head motion during xenon inhalation.

## DISCUSSION

Most of the subjects experienced no significant side effects during the stable Xe/CT CBF study. Although the incidence of intolerance to xenon inhalation appeared to be low, some people were very sensitive to xenon and manifested early anesthetic effects. Therefore, scrupulous observation of patients, especially during the first few minutes of xenon inhalation, is very important to earmark those who are intolerant.

Other reports have noted respiratory suppression caused by xenon inhalation (2–4). Latchaw et al. (3) reported that 3.6% of 1,830 examinations were associated with apneic episodes of longer than 10 seconds; 0.6% were apneic for longer than 15 seconds. Kobayashi et al. (2) reported a 2.2% incidence of respiratory suppression in 137 examinations. Our study found respiratory apnea of longer than 30 seconds in 3.8% of subjects. When respiratory suppression is prolonged, the patient should be commanded to take a breath. If a normal respiratory pattern does not return, the procedure should be terminated.

Head motion was the major cause of nondiagnostic studies. Although the importance of preventing head motion has been emphasized, its incidence has not been reported. To prevent head motion, a new head holder was developed and tested in recent CBF studies. In addition, carefully explaining the procedure to the patient seemed to be important in minimizing inadvertent movement under the light anesthetic effect of xenon. It is evident that the longer the inhalation time, the more frequent the head motion, even if a low concentration (27–35%) of xenon is inhaled. If the success rate is to be more than 90%, the time limit seems to be 4–5 minutes (5–6). We therefore advocate a shorter inhalation period, which is also more economical.

A transcranial Doppler study of hemodynamic changes during xenon inhalation showed that flow velocity increased relatively rapidly 2 to 4 minutes after xenon inhalation started and returned to former levels with its discontinuation (7). It is interesting that the timing of the CBF increase seems to coincide with that of the increase in the incidence of head motion and other practical problems such as respiratory slowing. This suggests that the effect of xenon begins to change the cerebral hemodynamic state and central nervous system function in about 2 to 4 minutes. Therefore, technical improvements should be sought that will enable satisfactory CBF measurements within 2 to 4 minutes of xenon inhalation.

## REFERENCES

1. Kashiwagi S, Yamashita T, Abiko S, et al. Measurement and imaging of cerebral blood flow with stable xenon and computed tomography (Xe-CT). *Electromedica* 1986;54:136-144.
2. Kobayashi N, Ono Y, Kakinoki Y, et al. Usefulness of xenon inhalation CT lCBF study. From the points of view of the clinical effectiveness and safety. *Journal of Medical Imaging* 1990;10: 1120–1131.
3. Latchaw RE, Yonas H, Pentheny SL, Gur D. Adverse reactions to xenon-enhanced CT cerebral blood flow determination. *Radiology* 1987;163:251–254.
4. Winkler S, Turski P, Holden J, Koeppe R, Rusy B, Garber E. Xenon effects on CNS control of respiratory rate and tidal volume: the danger of apnea. In: Hartmann A, Hoyer S, eds. *Cerebral blood flow and metabolism measurement*. New York: Springer; 1985:356–360.
5. Meyer JS, Hayman LA, Amano T, et al. Mapping local blood flow of human brain by CT scanning during stable xenon inhalation. *Stroke* 1981;12:426–436.
6. Yonas H, Grundy B, Gur D, Shabason L, Wolfson SK Jr, Cook EE. Side effects of xenon inhalation. *J Comput Assist Tomogr* 1981;5:591–592.
7. Giller CA, Purdy P, Lindstrom WW. Effect of inhaled stable xenon on cerebral blood flow velocity. *AJNR* 1990;11:177–182.

*Cerebral Blood Flow Measurement with Stable Xenon-Enhanced Computed Tomography,* edited by Howard Yonas. Raven Press, Ltd., New York © 1992.

# Patient Motion: Prevention and Correction

Willi Kalender, Heidi Brestowsky, *Laszlo Solymosi, and **Alexander Hartmann

*Siemens Medical Systems, Henkestr. 127, 8520 Erlangen, Germany; and Departments of *Neuroradiology and **Neurology, University of Bonn, Sigmund Freud Str. 25, D-5300 Bonn 1, Germany*

Patient motion is one of the most serious problems in clinical studies of regional cerebral blood flow (rCBF) with the xenon/computed tomography (CT) method. There have been no reports of objective quantitative evaluations indicating how often and with which amplitude motion occurs. Investigators experienced in this field estimate that failure rates due to motion range from 3% to 15%. Moreover, these figures do not imply that the remaining studies are unaffected. Close examination of bone contours and similar structures in subtraction images shows that very few studies do not suffer from some degree of patient motion. We tried to estimate both the frequency and amplitude of this motion. More importantly, we investigated approaches to alleviate the problem.

Preventing motion is certainly the most desirable approach. We examined several systems for patient immobilization. These included standard fixation materials, modified head holders, thermoplastic face masks, and different types of vacuum bags.

Although a less ideal approach, rCBF values can be corrected for patient motion. We designed software algorithms to detect motion and subsequently correct for it by image transformations. To quantify possible improvements in flow calculations, we evaluated the confidence image. For every pixel, this image would present the squared sum of the deviation, $\chi^2$, between the measured data and the assumed model, the Kety equation. The $\chi^2$ will be large—and the rCBF values accordingly uncertain—whenever the data is very noisy. Nonetheless, even the slightest patient motion during the study will disturb the data and lead to errors in the curve fit. Thus, a study of the motion-induced effect on the confidence image would be a reasonable approach for improving the Xe/CT CBF method.

## ALGORITHMS TO DETECT AND CORRECT FOR MOTION

Our algorithms to correct for patient motion between CT scans are based on determining the skull contour and using an anatomy-oriented brain coordinate

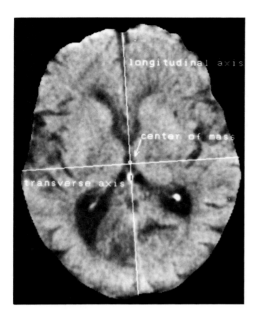

**FIG. 1.** Definition of an anatomy-oriented brain coordinate system. After isolation of the brain parenchyma, the center of mass of the brain and a symmetry axis are calculated.

system (BCS) in the initial and succeeding scans. The BCS is defined by the center of mass $(X, Y)$ of the isolated brain tissue and its symmetry axis, which passes through $(X, Y)$ and subtends an angle $\alpha$ with the $x$-axis (Fig. 1). The symmetry axis is calculated in an iterative manner as that line along which the distances to the skull, measured perpendicular to the axis, differ the least between left and right.

Knowing the skull contour and the geometric parameters of every scan makes it possible to determine if motion has occurred. Changes in the size of the total area enclosed by the skull or the lengths of the longitudinal and transverse axes indicate motion out of the image plane, which cannot be corrected in single-slice studies. Changes in the BCS parameters $X, Y$, and $\alpha$ indicate motion within the image plane only. Translation in the image plane is derived simply by $\Delta X_i = X_i - X_0$ and $\Delta Y_i = Y_i - Y_0$; the corresponding distance $d_i$ is calculated as the square root of $\Delta X_i^2 + \Delta Y_i^2$. Rotation can be determined in two ways. Using the above definitions, $\Delta\alpha = \alpha_i - \alpha_0$ follows immediately; we term this approach the "symmetry axis method."

Because the iterative approximation of the symmetry axis did not converge in all cases, we also investigated an alternative that we call the "radial method." In the radial method, the distances $R_{i,k}$ from the center of the brain to skull-contour points k for any scan i, measured at fixed-angle intervals $\Delta\beta$, are taken to build up a "radial map" for every scan. The map of scan i is moved relative to that of the reference scan such that the squared sum of differences is minimized.

That is, we determine $n$ for which $\Sigma\,(R_{i,k} - R_{0,k+n})^2 = \min$; $\Delta\alpha = n \cdot \Delta\beta$ follows immediately. Knowing the parameters $\Delta X_i$, $\Delta Y_i$, and $\Delta\alpha_i$, scan i can be transformed into the coordinate system of the initial scan.

## RESULTS

### Frequency and Amplitude of Motion

We analyzed motion in a total of 30 studies (eight of these were in volunteers). For each subject, we obtained two reference scans and then ten scans at 1-minute intervals after subjects inhaled a gas mixture containing 28% xenon. The motion parameters translation distance $d$, rotation angle $\Delta\alpha$, and change in cross-sectional area $\Delta A$ are plotted in Fig. 2 as a function of time, averaged over all studies. Mean values for the maximal changes were $d = 2.8$ mm (range: 0.1–6.7 mm), $\Delta\alpha = 1.1°$ (range: 0.2–3.4°), and $\Delta A = 1890$ mm$^2$ (range: 53–12,078 mm$^2$).

### Prevention of Motion

The most favorable response among the volunteers was to the use of thermoplastic face masks and a dedicated vacuum system. Patients reacted differently, however, generally preferring to be less constrained. Too tight a fixation seemed to cause adverse reactions. In any case, fixation systems did not prevent movement of a few millimeters.

### Correction of Motion

The accuracy of the algorithms was tested in simulation studies. Clinical images were rotated artificially by arbitrary degrees $\Delta\alpha$ (by permutating the original measured projection data and reconstructing the images again) and translated by arbitrary distances $\Delta X$ and $\Delta Y$. We applied both algorithms to determine the motion parameters. After motion correction, $\Delta X$ and $\Delta Y$ had errors of less than 0.1 mm; $\Delta\alpha$, less than 0.1°.

We evaluated the effects of the two motion correction algorithms in our 30 clinical studies by determining the percentage change in the $\chi^2$ error of the rCBF calculation. The symmetry axis method caused greater inaccuracy ($\Delta\chi^2 < -5\%$) in five cases, had insignificant effects ($\Delta\chi^2 < 5\%$) in ten cases, and improved the "goodness of fit" by 6% to 51% (mean: 23.4%) in 15 cases. Motion correction by the radial method caused worse errors in one case, had insignificant effects in 11 cases, and improved the goodness of fit by 6% to 46% (mean: 28.1%) in 18 cases.

Motion parameters

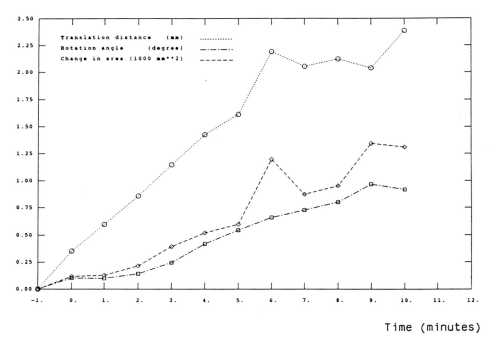

Time (minutes)

**FIG. 2.** Motion parameters. Values are averaged over 30 patient studies. The two reference scans are arbitrarily assigned scan times -1 and 0 minutes on the time scale. The xenon-enhanced images 1 to 10 were within ±10 seconds of the nominal scan times in 1-minute intervals.

## DISCUSSION AND CONCLUSIONS

The accuracy of rCBF measurements using dynamic CT and the quality of the resulting blood flow maps partially depend on the prevention of motion by patient fixation. After experimenting with several devices, we found that patient constraint was most efficient with the thermoplastic face mask, a system used in radiation therapy, which we adapted to Xe/CT CBF studies. Because of the limited number of studies in patients, we cannot offer a final recommendation yet. Alternatives for motion prevention include the use of sedatives and wash-in/wash-out measurement strategies. The former are considered only as a last resort. Yet, the latter constitute a very promising new approach, because these methods avoid long inhalation times (more than 4 to 6 minutes) that increase the likelihood of patient motion (see Kashiwagi et al. in this volume).

An analysis of motion by digital image processing algorithms and subsequent image transformation for motion correction are efficacious in a great number of rCBF studies. The radial method for determination of rotation proved to be the better method. The axial method failed to converge in a number of cases in which the subject's skull contour tended to be circular. We continue to work with the radial method for motion correction purposes.

Our analysis of this relatively small number of studies does not establish that patient motion occurs only after a certain duration of xenon inhalation. It merely confirms that motion becomes more severe with prolonged inhalation. Corrections for motion can be expected to be highly successful if the motion occurs predominantly within the plane of the CT image; they cannot improve the situation if motion occurs out of the plane. We have yet to establish criteria for the different types of motion. These criteria would be used to determine whether attempts to correct for motion would be productive.

*Cerebral Blood Flow Measurement with Stable Xenon-Enhanced Computed Tomography,* edited by Howard Yonas. Raven Press, Ltd., New York © 1992.

# Stable Xenon Inhalation Does Not Change Internal Carotid Artery Blood Flow in Awake Monkeys

James T. Love, Edwin M. Nemoto, *Howard Yonas, Joseph M. Darby, and John A. Melick

*Departments of Anesthesiology and Critical Care Medicine and *Neurological Surgery, University of Pittsburgh School of Medicine, Pittsburgh, Pennsylvania 15261*

Xenon-enhanced computed tomography (Xe/CT) overcomes the limitations of many other technologies used to measure cerebral blood flow (CBF) (1–4). Despite substantial evidence that Xe/CT-derived CBF values correlate closely with those obtained by radiolabeled microspheres and [133]Xe (4–7), their validity has been questioned due to reports of large, unpredictable increases in CBF accompanying stable xenon inhalation (8,9). Although xenon-induced CBF activation would introduce an error into the resultant CBF measurement, concern would be lessened if this effect were small or occurred late in the inhalation sequence. Therefore, determining the time course and magnitude of CBF activation during the inhalation of 33% stable xenon is critical. We thus studied the effect of 33% xenon inhalation on bilateral internal carotid artery (ICA) blood flow in unanesthetized rhesus monkeys to detect even rapid and transient changes in CBF.

## MATERIALS AND METHODS

Using standard sterile surgical technique, we placed Doppler ultrasonic transit-time 2-mm blood flow probes (Transonic Systems, Ithaca, NY) bilaterally around the ICA of five female rhesus monkeys in a nonocclusive fashion. The probe leads were then tunneled subcutaneously and externalized posteriorly. We dressed the monkeys in a special jacket with interior pockets into which the flow-probe leads were secured to prevent access by the animal.

After 2 weeks, the validity of the flow-probe measurements was verified by connecting the leads to a Transonic T201D dual channel flowmeter with direct digital display of signal strength. Arterial and nasopharyngeal catheters were inserted in each animal. Then a clear plastic helmet was placed over (but not touching) the animal's head and sealed to the top deck of the restraining chair, leaving the neck hole as an exhalation port. The adapter at the top of the helmet was connected to a source of 33% $N_2$/67% $O_2$ (control gas) administered at 10 L/min to prevent rebreathing. The ultrasonic flow probes were connected to the flowmeter. One nasopharyngeal catheter was connected to a capnograph (LB-2, Beckman Instruments, Fullerton, CA) and the other to a thermal conductivity analyzer (Gow-MAC Instruments, Bridgewater, NJ). Heart rate, mean arterial pressure (MAP), end-tidal $CO_2$, end-tidal xenon, and ICA blood flow were recorded continually.

We obtained baseline arterial blood gas measurements after administering the control gas for 15 minutes. We then randomly assigned the animals to receive either 33% Xe/67% $O_2$ (Linde Xe/Scan, stable xenon in oxygen USP, Union Carbide Rare Gases, Specialty Medical Products, Danbury, CT) or 10% $CO_2$/23% $N_2$/67% $O_2$ for 5 minutes, after which we again obtained arterial blood gases. Both gas mixtures were administered at least three randomly chosen times. Each test gas exposure was separated by 15 minutes of control gas inhalation, followed by an arterial blood gas measurement to document the return to baseline blood gas levels.

## RESULTS

The ICA flow values, MAP, and $PaCO_2$ data for the five monkeys during control, xenon/oxygen, and $CO_2$/oxygen inhalation periods are presented in Table 1. Inhalation of 33% Xe/67% $O_2$ did not cause any of the three variables to change from control values. Inhalation of 10% $CO_2$ in oxygen, however, increased ICA blood flow by nearly 70%, from 23 ± 10 ml/100 g/min to 39 ± 15 ml/100 g/min ($P < 0.001$). The MAP ($P < 0.05$) and $PaCO_2$ ($P < 0.001$) were also significantly higher in animals during inhalation of $CO_2$ in oxygen.

## DISCUSSION

Inhalation of stable xenon did not change blood flow values in the ICA of the awake, unsedated, spontaneously breathing rhesus monkey. We recognize that

**TABLE 1.** *Effects of different gas combinations*

| Gas tested[a] | Mean values (SD) | | |
|---|---|---|---|
| | ICA blood flow (ml/100 g/min) | $PaCO_2$ (mm Hg) | Mean arterial pressure (mm Hg) |
| Control | 23 (10) (n = 43) | 34 (6) (n = 30) | 101 (13) (n = 42) |
| 33% Xe | 22 (12) (n = 23) | 34 (7) (n = 17) | 98 (16) (n = 21) |
| 10% $CO_2$ | 39 (15) (n = 13)* | 54 (5) (n = 9)* | 112 (16) (n = 12)** |

[a] Forced inspiratory oxygen was 67% in all study groups.
* $P < 0.001$; ** $P < 0.05$.
SD, standard deviation; ICA, internal carotid artery.

CBF can change regionally without variation in flow through large conductance vessels such as the ICA. Nonetheless, any significant global variation in CBF should have been reflected in ICA blood flow.

The reported CBF response to xenon has varied widely (5,6,8-10). Most reports indicate that xenon increases CBF, but there is little documentation of the time course of xenon-induced effects on CBF and disagreement on pattern and magnitude. The only report of such an observation in humans was contained in an abstract published in 1985 (9). Normal volunteers inhaled a mixture containing 35% xenon while $^{133}$Xe CBF measurements were made, and the area under the $^{133}$Xe wash-out curve was averaged over 15 minutes. The CBF increased 17% to 28% if the end-tidal $CO_2$ was allowed to fall during xenon inhalation, but increased 30% to 50% if the end-tidal $CO_2$ was controlled by adding $CO_2$ to the mixture. In our study in monkeys, we did not observe the decrease in end-tidal $CO_2$ with xenon inhalation that these investigators reported finding in humans. We do not know whether this is because of the differences in the species studied, but the minimum anesthetic concentration for xenon is similar in humans and monkeys (11,12).

We used Doppler ultrasonic measurements of ICA flow to monitor the rapid flow changes upon exposure to xenon that would be missed by other methods. However, this technique does not measure global CBF. Thus, it is conceivable, although unlikely, that CBF may have increased via the vertebral arteries without altering flow in the ICA.

We used the same concentration of oxygen in all three gas mixtures to avoid any possible effect of hyperoxia on cerebrovasculature, whereas room air was used in several of the studies that found CBF changes. In addition, we used 33% xenon, the same mixture most often used clinically, the other investigators used 35% to 80%. These higher concentrations presumably would have a greater effect. The lack of change in ICA blood flow and $PaCO_2$ with inhalation of 33% stable xenon in oxygen suggests that a clinically relevant change in CBF is unlikely to result from the inhalation of this mixture.

## ACKNOWLEDGMENTS

This work was supported in part by a grant from the National Institutes of Health #2ROI HL 27208-07A1. Linde Xe/Scan stable xenon in oxygen USP was provided by Union Carbide Rare Gases, Specialty Medical Products, 39 Old Ridgebury Road, Danbury, CT 06817-0001. Dr. Robert Boston provided invaluable assistance with the statistical analysis of the data.

## REFERENCES

1. Gur D, Wolfson SK Jr, Yonas H, et al. Progress in cerebrovascular disease: local cerebral blood flow by xenon-enhanced CT. *Stroke* 1982;13:750–758.

2. Gur D, Good WF, Wolfson SK Jr, et al. In vivo mapping of local cerebral blood flow by xenon-enhanced computed tomography. *Science* 1982;215:1267–1268.

3. Kishore PRS, Rao GU, Fernandez RE, et al. Regional cerebral blood flow measurements using stable xenon-enhanced computed tomography: a theoretical and experimental evaluation. *J Comput Assist Tomogr* 1984;8:619–630.

4. Meyer JS, Hayman LA, Yamamoto M, et al. Local cerebral blood flow measured by CT after stable xenon inhalation. *AJR* 1980;135:239–251.

5. Gur D, Yonas H, Jackson DL, et al. Measurements of cerebral blood flow during xenon inhalation as measured by the microspheres method. *Stroke* 1985;16:871–874.

6. Fatouros PP, Wist AO, Kishore PRS, et al. Xenon/computed tomography cerebral blood flow measurements: methods and accuracy. *Invest Radiol* 1987;22:705–712.

7. Segawa H. Tomographic cerebral blood flow measurement using xenon inhalation and serial CT scanning: normal values and its validity. *Neurosurg Rev* 1985;8:27–33.

8. Junck L, Dhawan V, Thaler HT, et al. Effects of xenon and krypton on regional cerebral blood flow in the rat. *J Cereb Blood Flow Metab* 1985;5:126–132.

9. Obrist WD, Jaggi JL, Harel D, et al. Effect of stable xenon inhalation on human CBF. *J Cereb Blood Flow Metab* 1985;5(Suppl):557–558.

10. Hartman A, Wassman H, Czernicki Z, et al. Effect of stable xenon in room air on regional cerebral blood flow and electroencephalogram in normal baboons. *Stroke* 1987;18:643-648.

11. Cullen SC, Gross EG. The anesthetic properties of xenon in animals and human beings, with additional observations on krypton. *Science* 1951;113:580–582.

12. Pittinger CB, Faulconer A, Knott JR, et al. Electroencephalographic and other observations in monkeys during anesthesia at elevated pressures. *Anesthesiology* 1955;16:551–563.

*Cerebral Blood Flow Measurement with Stable Xenon-Enhanced Computed Tomography,* edited by Howard Yonas. Raven Press, Ltd., New York © 1992.

# Effects of Xenon and $CO_2$ Inhalation on Flow Velocity Measured with Transcranial Doppler

Elizabeth C. Marks, Howard Yonas, *Mark H. Sanders, and **James T. Love

*Departments of Neurological Surgery, *Pulmonary Medicine, and **Critical Care Medicine, University of Pittsburgh School of Medicine, Pittsburgh, Pennsylvania 15261*

Despite an increasing number of papers describing clinical and laboratory applications of the stable xenon-enhanced computed tomography cerebral blood flow (Xe/CT CBF) method (1,2) several questions about xenon's ability to alter baseline physiology have not been fully resolved. The high probability that the pharmacological effects of xenon are accompanied by flow alteration raises concerns regarding the calculation of CBF using the Xe/CT technique (3).

To better understand the extent and time course of the pharmacological effects of the inhalation of 33% xenon on CBF, we indirectly measured CBF with transcranial Doppler (TCD). Our investigation included repeated studies with varying concentrations of $CO_2$ (0, 0.4%, 0.8%, and 1.2%) in an attempt to stabilize the expected decrease in $PCO_2$ that commonly accompanies xenon inhalation.

## SUBJECTS AND METHODS

We recruited 15 healthy adults over the age of 30 for our study. Our subjects were 8 men and 7 women ranging in age from 33 to 69 years (average: 49 ± 12 years). All subjects gave informed consent in accordance with the guidelines of the University of Pittsburgh Institutional Review Board. None had a history of head injury; hypertension; migraine; or cerebrovascular, heart, or lung disease.

During the study, patients were monitored with electrocardiography and 12-lead electroencephalography. We also continually measured hemoglobin oxygen saturation, end-tidal xenon concentration, end-tidal carbon dioxide tension, and the ventilatory pattern. Blood pressure and CBF velocities were recorded every minute (Table 1). Once the subjects' breathing pattern stabilized, we recorded their baseline data while they inhaled room air. Then we began delivery of the

**TABLE 1.** *Study design*

| Physiologic variable | Minutes of xenon inhalation | | | | | | | | | | | | | |
|---|---|---|---|---|---|---|---|---|---|---|---|---|---|---|
| | BL | 1.0 | 1.5 | 2.0 | 2.5 | 3.0 | 3.5 | 4.0 | 4.5 | 5.0 | 5.5 | 6.0 | 6.5 | 7.0 |
| End-tidal Xe (%) | × | × | × | × | × | × | × | × | × | × | × | × | × | × |
| End-tidal CO$_2$ (%) | × | × | × | × | × | × | × | × | × | × | × | × | × | × |
| TCD | × | × | | × | | × | | × | | × | | × | | × |
| Blood pressure | × | × | | × | | × | | × | | × | | × | | × |
| EEG | × | × | × | × | × | × | × | × | × | × | × | × | × | × |
| SaO$_2$ | × | × | × | × | × | × | × | × | × | × | × | × | × | × |
| Ventilation | × | × | × | × | × | × | × | × | × | × | × | × | × | × |
| Tidal volume | × | × | × | × | × | × | × | × | × | × | × | × | × | × |
| Respiratory rate | × | × | × | × | × | × | × | × | × | × | × | × | × | × |
| EKG | × | × | × | × | × | × | × | × | × | × | × | × | × | × |

BL, baseline; TCD, transcranial Doppler; EEG, electroencephalogram; SaO$_2$, hemoglobin oxygen saturation; EKG, electrocardiogram.

Xe/O$_2$/CO$_2$ gas mixture (Linde XeScan stable xenon in oxygen USP, Union Carbide Rare Gases, Specialty Medical Products, Danbury, CT), and flow data were collected for 7 minutes. Each subject underwent a total of four xenon inhalation periods, with a 30-minute rest period between each trial. We monitored the subjects closely at all times, and if they experienced any unpleasant side effects, the inhalation of room air was restored immediately. After each trial, we questioned the subjects about their response to xenon.

## RESULTS

Three subjects could not participate in the fourth trial due to nausea, and several others could not breathe xenon for the full 7 minutes because they were unable to keep a tight seal around the mouthpiece. Therefore, data are reported for only the first 5 minutes of inhalation. Using a scale of 1 to 10 (most to least favorable) to rate the inhalation experience, only two subjects reported a worse-than-neutral experience (Table 2).

End-tidal xenon concentration during trial 1 steadily increased from time zero, reaching an equilibrium of 28 ± 4% (growth curve analysis) in 2.5 minutes. There were no end-tidal xenon differences between the four trials (Fig. 1).

During the first trial, flow velocities measured by TCD increased significantly over time from, 51 ± 16 to 61 ± 23 cm/sec (MANOVA, $P < 0.0001$). Flow velocity increased less than 5% in the first 2.5 minutes of xenon inhalation and had changed 20% by 5 minutes (Table 3). For the first 5 minutes of inhalation, there were no significant differences between TCD measurements in subjects who were able to complete xenon inhalation for 5 ($n = 2$), 6 ($n = 7$), and 7

**TABLE 2.** *Subject responses to xenon inhalation*

| Subject | Age (yrs) | Rating[a] | | | |
|---|---|---|---|---|---|
| | | Trial 1 | Trial 2 | Trial 3 | Trial 4 |
| 1 | 41 | 3 | 3 | 6 | sick |
| 2 | 44 | 1 | 1 | 1 | 1 |
| 3 | 61 | 2 | 2 | 2 | 2 |
| 4 | 34 | — | — | — | sick |
| 5 | 56 | 1 | 1 | 1 | 1 |
| 6 | 62 | 2 | 1 | 1 | 1 |
| 7 | 35 | 10 | 10 | 10 | 10 |
| 8 | 33 | 2 | 2 | 2 | 1 |
| 9 | 55 | 3 | 3 | 3 | 3 |
| 10 | 62 | 5 | 4 | 4 | 4 |
| 11 | 64 | 5 | 5 | sick | — |
| 12 | 69 | 1 | 1 | 1 | 1 |
| 13 | 39 | 1 | 1 | 1 | 1 |
| 14 | 42 | 3 | 3 | 3 | 3 |
| 15 | 43 | 1 | 1 | 1 | 1 |

[a] Numbers correspond to scale of 1 to 10, respectively indicating most to least favorable experience.

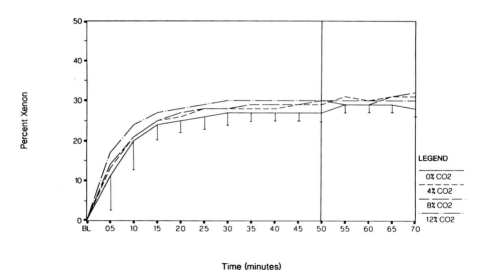

**FIG. 1.** End-tidal xenon curves for each of the four gas mixtures.

**TABLE 3.** *Change in Doppler velocity in response to xenon inhalation*

| | Direction and extent of velocity change $(cm \cdot sec^{-1})$ at | |
|---|---|---|
| Subject | 2 min | 5 min |
| 1 | −2 | −2 |
| 2 | −24 | 4 |
| 3 | 3 | 26 |
| 4 | 8 | 24 |
| 5 | 27 | 70 |
| 6 | 0 | −22 |
| 7 | 9 | 20 |
| 8 | −2 | −21 |
| 9 | −5 | 18 |
| 10 | 24 | 59 |
| 11 | 15 | 24 |
| 12 | 19 | 43 |
| 13 | −10 | 14 |
| 14 | −5 | — |
| 15 | 9 | 23 |

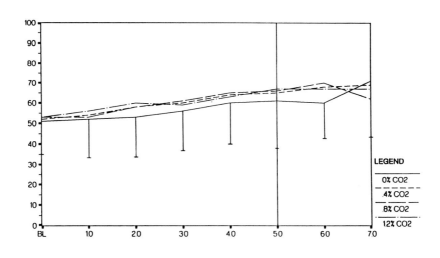

**FIG. 2.** Transcranial Doppler recordings for each of the four gas mixtures.

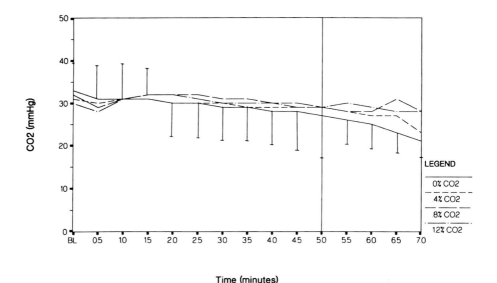

**FIG. 3.** End-tidal carbon dioxide curves for each of the four gas mixtures.

($n$ = 6) minutes, and there were no velocity differences between breathing trials (Fig. 2).

End-tidal CO$_2$ decreased from 33 ± 6 to 29 ± 8 mm Hg during the first 5 minutes of xenon inhalation in trial 1 (MANOVA, $P < 0.0001$). This measurement did not change significantly when we used different gas mixtures (Fig. 3). There was no relationship between flow velocities and end-tidal CO$_2$.

Mean arterial blood pressure did not increase over the course of inhalation. Pressures recorded during the various trials did not differ significantly.

## DISCUSSION

The effect of xenon inhalation on TCD-gauged velocity, although not a direct measure of CBF, should serve as a useful indirect measure of the time course and extent of flow activation that accompanies xenon inhalation. The average time at which gray matter becomes maximally saturated with xenon is at 2.5 minutes of inhalation. The fact that TCD at that time showed only a 5% mean increase in flow velocity in our subjects suggests that the Xe/CT CBF method acquires vital gray-matter information before xenon can cause any significant flow alteration.

Giller et al. (3) recently demonstrated that individual flow velocity, as measured by TCD, is highly variable in response to 5 minutes of xenon inhalation. In 78% (18/23) of the studies they reported, flow velocity increased; another 4% (1/23) had no change; 17% (4/23) had a decrease in velocity. Our data revealed similar trends. After 5 minutes of xenon inhalation during trial 1, flow velocity increased in 79% of our subjects and decreased in 21%. The magnitude of changes we saw at 2 minutes, however, were consistently smaller: velocity had increased in 53%, remained the same in 6%, and decreased in 40%.

The lack of a relationship between flow velocity and end-tidal CO$_2$ and the wide variation in the response of velocity to xenon leaves several questions unanswered. For example, is TCD-monitored flow velocity an appropriate measure of CBF? Sorteberg et al. (4) reported that although several authors have found a significant relationship between Doppler-measured velocity and CBF, others found no significant relationship between the two. Vriens et al. (5) proposed that CBF velocity in the middle cerebral artery is a complicated measure and that age, sex, and resting pCO$_2$ must be considered, as all of these variables affect blood velocity.

## ACKNOWLEDGMENT

This work was supported by a grant from Union Carbide Rare Gases, Specialty Medical Products, Danbury, Connecticut.

## REFERENCES

1. Yonas H, Good WF, Gur D, et al. Mapping cerebral blood flow by xenon-enhanced computed tomography: clinical experience. *Radiology* 1984;152:435–442.
2. Yonas H, Gur D, Latchaw R, Wolfson SK Jr. Stable xenon CT/CBF imaging: laboratory and clinical experience. In: Symon L, Brihaye J, Cohadon F, et al., eds. *Advances and technical standards in neurosurgery*, Vol 15. Vienna: Springer-Verlag; 1987:3–39.
3. Giller CA, Purdy P, Lindstrom WW. Effects of inhaled stable xenon on cerebral blood flow velocity. *AJNR* 1990;11:177-182.
4. Sorteberg W, Lindegaard KF, Rootwelt K, et al. Blood velocity and regional blood flow in defined cerebral artery systems. *Acta Neurochir (Wien)* 1989;97:47–52.
5. Vriens EM, Kraaier V, Musbach M, Wieneke GH, van Huffelen AC. Transcranial pulsed Doppler measurements of blood velocity in the middle cerebral artery: reference values at rest and during hyperventilation in healthy volunteers in relation to age and sex. *Ultrasound Med Biol* 1989;15: 1–8.

*Cerebral Blood Flow Measurement with Stable Xenon-Enhanced Computed Tomography,*
edited by Howard Yonas. Raven Press, Ltd.,
New York © 1992.

# The Effect of Stable Xenon Inhalation on Cerebral Blood Flow Velocities and Topographic Electroencephalography in Normal Volunteers

Karl Broich, *Peter Bülau, Alexander Hartmann,
**Laszlo Solymosi, Christian Dettmers, Fernand Ries,
*Sigrid Poersch, and ***Willi Kalender

*Departments of Neurology, *Epileptology, and **Neuroradiology, University of Bonn,
Sigmund Freud Str. 25, D-5300 Bonn 1, Germany; and ***Siemens Medical Systems,
Henkestr. 127, 8520 Erlangen, Germany*

Studies using the inhalation of stable xenon gas and recording of its increasing concentration in brain tissue by computed tomography (CT) have made it possible to calculate local cerebral blood flow (CBF) with high spatial resolution and to use these data in a variety of clinical applications (1,2). Currently, xenon concentrations of 28% to 35% are used with conflicting findings about side effects (3). Our experience in anesthetized normal baboons and normal volunteers (4) and the results of other groups indicate that stable xenon itself alters CBF. Most authors have described increases of up to 30% in CBF during stable xenon inhalation (5–7). This effect must be a concern in interpreting flow values derived from xenon-enhanced CT.

We undertook the following study to determine which effect of stable xenon inhalation is responsible for the CBF increase. We used transcranial Doppler sonography (TCD) in conjunction with Xe/CT. With the TCD, blood flow velocities of the basal intracranial arteries can be measured noninvasively and continually for prolonged periods (8). A further purpose of the study was to investigate simultaneous electroencephalographic changes and side effects during xenon inhalation.

## SUBJECTS AND METHODS

Our subjects were 11 volunteers (9 men and 2 women) between 24 and 45 years of age (mean age: 28.3 ± 6.3 years). None had a history of neurologic or vascular disease affecting function of the central nervous system, and none took any medication. Conventional electroencephalograms (EEG)—including those under hyperventilation and flashlight stimulation—showed no significant abnormalities in any of these subjects.

We measured TCD velocities in the M1 segment of the middle cerebral artery (MCA) with a TC 2–64 Doppler (EME, Überlingen, Germany), which has a 2-MHz emitted ultrasonic frequency, 100-mW total emitted ultrasound energy, and a 1.5-cm$^2$ emitting area. The highest signals were sought at a depth of 45 to 55 mm, with care taken to avoid interference from other vessels. We measured TCD velocities every minute beginning 10 minutes before inhalation (26% stable Xe in 30% oxygen and room air) and ending 10 minutes after inhalation was completed. For each measurement, the Gosling pulsatility index was estimated as the systolic minus diastolic velocities divided by the mean velocities. This index is a measure of the pulsatile energy of the velocity wave-form and is known to reflect an estimation of the peripheral resistance. An increase of the index accompanies vasoconstriction, and a decrease accompanies vasodilation. For statistical evaluation, we used Fisher's $z$ test.

Using the international 10–20 System and Goldmann references, topographical EEG activity was recorded by a Picker-Schwarzer electroencephalograph equipped with the Brain Surveyor BS 2400. Records were amplified and filtered with the band-pass filter set at 0.5–50 Hz. In addition to automatic artifact elimination, EEG artifacts were removed after visual inspection by a board-certified electroencephalographer. Using a standard fast Fourier transformation, power spectra of the delta, theta, alpha, and beta bands were calculated, as were peak frequencies and ratios of the different bands (alpha/theta and alpha/beta index) and regional patterns (frontoparietal and temporoparietal theta index). Statistical analysis was performed using a paired Student's $t$ test.

## RESULTS

There was no significant change in blood pressure or heart rate with 26% stable xenon inhalation, and we detected no significant breathing irregularities with changes in end-tidal carbon dioxide. Inhalation of the xenon mixture was tolerated well by all subjects, who reported feelings of only slight excitation and euphoria. Mean TCD velocity at rest was 62.5 ± 8.2 cm/sec at a mean depth of 45 to 55 mm. Because we and others have found that interindividual resting values vary significantly (8), the changes in TCD velocities during xenon inhalation are reported as percentage changes.

We found a significant increase in flow the velocity in the MCA in all 11 subjects ($z$ test, $P \leq 0.01$). In two subjects, however, an initial small (10%) decrease in velocity was followed by a significant increase after 5 minutes of xenon inhalation. Figure 1 shows percentage changes in mean and maximal flow velocities, demonstrating that velocities began to increase within 60 seconds. After 2 minutes of xenon inhalation, the percentage change in mean, minimal, and maximal velocities exceeded three standard deviations of the baseline recordings and

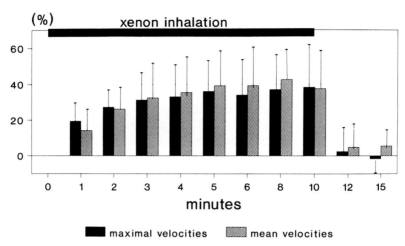

**FIG. 1.** Percentage increase in blood flow velocities measured by transcranial Doppler sonography during 26% stable xenon inhalation.

reached a plateau of about 38–40% ± 18–20% (range: 20–95%) after 5 minutes, stabilizing thereafter. When xenon inhalation ended, velocities rapidly fell to resting values. There were no significant differences between either the maximal (systolic), minimal (diastolic), or mean velocities before and during xenon inhalation. The Gosling pulsatility index decreased significantly to a mean of 14% ± 6.9% ($z$ test, $P \leq 0.05$); the return to baseline values differed interindividually from 0 to 5 minutes after ending xenon inhalation.

About 10 to 20 seconds after xenon inhalation began, EEG changes were obvious; slow-wave activity was increased on visual inspection. Instead of a decrease in alpha power and an increase in theta power, there was no statistically significant change in absolute alpha, beta, or theta power. Nevertheless, a significant decrease in the alpha/beta and alpha/theta indices was seen, indicating a significant reduction in alpha activity. Whereas the physiological maximum of occipital alpha activity was stable during xenon inhalation, we found a marked increase in slow-wave activity in the frontal and temporal areas (frontoparietal and temporoparietal theta index). In three subjects, xenon-induced diffuse paroxysmal and dysrhythmic as well as focal (theta/delta) EEG abnormalities (of the temporal lobes) were recorded. Normalization of the EEG pattern after xenon inhalation was variable, requiring from 0.5 to 10 minutes (mean: 1.7 minute), with no parallel normalization of flow velocities.

## DISCUSSION

Our results suggest that there is a statistically significant rise in flow velocity during 26% stable xenon inhalation. This is paralleled by a decrease in the pulsatility index resulting from dilation of the small-resistance cerebral vessels. These effects were detectable 1 to 2 minutes after xenon inhalation began and remained stable after 5 minutes of inhalation. We detected no changes in heart rate, blood pressure, or end-tidal carbon dioxide pressure. Other investigators have reported similar results (9), and it is known that other anesthetic agents such as halothane cause vasodilatory effects in the initial phases of anesthesia (10). The elevation of CBF can be heightened further by the slight xenon-induced excitation corresponding to the small increase in beta and theta activity observed on EEG. Therefore, the observed rise in cerebral blood velocity and flow can result from the combined vasodilatory and excitatory properties of stable xenon, even in the low concentration we used.

## REFERENCES

1. Yonas H. Xenon-enhanced CT: evaluating cerebral blood flow. *Diagnostic Imaging* 1988;57: 88–94.
2. Yonas H, Gur D, Latchaw RE, Wolfson SK. Xenon computed tomographic blood flow mapping. In: Wood JH, ed. *Cerebral blood flow: physiologic and clinical aspects.* New York: McGraw Hill, 1987:220–242.
3. Yonas H, Grundy B, Gur D, Shabason L, Wolfson SK, Cook EE. Side effects of xenon inhalation. *J Comput Assist Tomogr* 1981;5:591–592.
4. Dettmers C, Hartmann A, Tsuda Y, et al. Stable xenon effects on regional cerebral blood flow and EEG in normal baboons and volunteers. In: Wüllenweber R, Klinger M, Brock M, eds. *Advances in Neurosurgery*, Vol 15. Berlin: Springer-Verlag; 1987:67–71.
5. Gur D, Yonas H, Jackson DL, et al. Measurement of cerebral blood flow during xenon inhalation as measured by the microspheres method. *Stroke* 1985;16:871–874.
6. Obrist WD, Jaggi JL, Smith DS. Effect of stable xenon inhalation on human CBF. *J Cereb Blood Flow Metab* 1985;5(Suppl 1):S557–558.
7. Hartmann A, Wassmann H, Czernicki Z, et al. Effect of stable xenon in room air on rCBF and electroencephalogram in normal baboons. *Stroke* 1987;18:643–648.
8. Aaslid R. *Transcranial Doppler sonography.* New York: Springer Verlag, 1986.
9. Giller CA, Purdy P, Lindstrom WW. Effects of inhaled stable xenon on cerebral blood flow velocity. *AJNR* 1990;11:177-182.
10. Albrecht RF, Miletich DJ, Rosenberg R, Zahed B. Cerebral blood flow and metabolic changes from induction to onset of anesthesia with halothane or pentobarbital. *Anesthesiology* 1977;47: 252–256.

*Cerebral Blood Flow Measurement with Stable Xenon-Enhanced Computed Tomography,* edited by Howard Yonas. Raven Press, Ltd., New York © 1992.

# Concomitant Effect of Acetazolamide and Xenon on Cerebral Blood Flow, Intracranial Pressure, Flow Velocity, and Electroencephalogram: Possible Risk for the Patient?

Mohammad-Nabi Nemati, Hermann Dietz, Kurt Holl, Michael Gaab, Ernst Rzesacz, Jens P. Witt, *Bernd Haubitz, and *Hartmut Becker

*Departments of Neurosurgery and *Neuroradiology, Hannover School of Medicine, Konstanty-Gutschow-Str. 8, D-3000 Hannover 61, Germany*

Motivated by the clinical need for an effective, accurate, and accessible method to measure cerebral blood flow (CBF), we began using the xenon computed tomography (Xe/CT) technique in 1987 (1–4). Because of our success with this method, we began using Xe/CT in conjunction with a stimulation test involving the intravenous injection of 1 g of acetazolamide (Diamox) to evaluate cerebrovascular reserve capacity.

In this chapter, we examine both the Xe/CT CBF method and the implications of the combined administration of xenon and acetazolamide. Some have questioned not only the validity of the Xe/CT CBF method, but its clinical safety as well. The Kety-Schmidt theory (5) requires that the tracer used in CBF analysis be biologically and chemically inert. It remains important to determine whether the inhalation of 33% xenon, alone or combined with the use of acetazolamide, endangers patients by producing a significant narcotic effect (6), increases the cerebral tendency toward seizures, or elevates CBF enough to invalidate its use as a CBF tracer. Based on studies in rats (7), primates (8), and humans (9), we can conclude that the xenon concentration necessary for CBF studies does increase CBF. Both the inhalation of xenon and the introduction of acetazolamide can induce a vasodilative stimulus (10–12), which theoretically could increase intracranial blood volume and, in turn, intracranial pressure (ICP) (13–14).

We sought to address these potential problems by recording clinical, electroencephalographic, and ICP responses to xenon inhalation, both with and without acetazolamide administration. We also assessed the validity of the Xe/CT CBF technique by examining intracranial velocities before, during, and after administering xenon and xenon plus acetazolamide.

## MATERIAL AND METHODS

### Electroencephalography

We performed electroencephalography (EEG) in 58 patients (35 men and 23 women with a mean age of 56.6 ± 12 years) with various clinical syndromes (tumors in 27, cerebrovascular insufficiency in 26, subarachnoid hemorrhage in one, arteriovenous angiomas in two, and cranial cerebral trauma in two). Subjects were selected randomly for EEG recordings from among patients undergoing CBF studies for clinical indications.

Electrode placement corresponded to the 10–20 System and included ten positions in the frontocentral and parietotemporal regions. The EEG recordings lasted at least 3 minutes during each of the following designated periods: (a) before, (b) during, and (c) after xenon inhalation; (d) beginning 10 minutes after acetazolamide injection; (e) during xenon inhalation; and (f) after xenon inhalation. The xenon concentration was at a minimum end-tidal value of 21% for all studies. The EEG data were evaluated both visually and by statistical analysis with the help of an eight-channel power spectral analytical package run on an Epson personal computer. The significance-probability ($P$) of the mean levels for the group as a whole was assessed with the Wilcoxon test.

### The Effect of Xenon and Acetazolamide on ICP

To monitor suspected disturbances of cerebrospinal fluid (CSF) dynamics, we implanted epidural ICP monitors (Gaeltec ICT-6 Transducer, Gaeltec Ltd., Dunvagen, Scotland) in 16 patients. Based on continuous ICP recordings for at least 24 hours prior to CBF studies, patients were assigned to either group I, those with disturbed ICP dynamics, or group II, those with undisturbed dynamics. Group I included four men and four women whose mean age was 42 ± 16 years. The major pathologic ICP finding in this group was beta waves during sleep. Group II included three men and five women with a mean age of 57 ± 12 years. ICP was recorded for all 16 patients before and during a baseline Xe/CT CBF study and a post-acetazolamide-administration study. Statistical analysis was performed with the programming package SAS 6.03 (SAS Institute Inc.).

### Effect of Acetazolamide on Transcranial Doppler (TCD) Sonography

We defined 72 patients (45 men and 27 women with a mean age of 47 ± 12 years) as control subjects. These were patients with minor abnormalities identified on CT whose clinical conditions were not expected to affect CBF. To evaluate the effect of acetazolamide on flow velocities, we continuously monitored the Doppler signal of the middle cerebral artery, starting before and ending 3 hours after acetazolamide administration. The signal was recorded by a standard clinical

Group I had a mean baseline ICP of 13.6 ± 7.6 mm Hg and, an average of 13.1 ± 4.5 minutes after acetazolamide injection, reached a maximum of 36.4 ± 19.1 mm Hg. This represented a significant increase of 168% ($P < 0.01$). In group II, the mean baseline ICP was 6.3 ± 4.2 mm Hg. The mean ICP for this group reached a peak of 11.9 ± 4.8 mm Hg, occurring an average of 13.6 ± 1.1 minutes after receiving acetazolamide ($P < 0.01$).

### TCD and the Effect of Acetazolamide

After the administration of 1 g of acetazolamide, flow velocity peaked at 13.5 minutes; the half-life of this effect was 85 minutes. In approximately 6 hours, velocities returned to baseline levels. When individual velocities were examined, we determined that acetazolamide's maximal effects occurred 15 ± 5 minutes after injection began. We found a negative linear correlation ($r = -0.65$) between the initial CBF at rest ($rCBF_R$) and the rise in blood flow after acetazolamide administration ($\Delta rCBF$). The higher the $rCBF_R$, the lower the reserve capacity (Fig. 3). The mean velocity increase after acetazolamide was 43%.

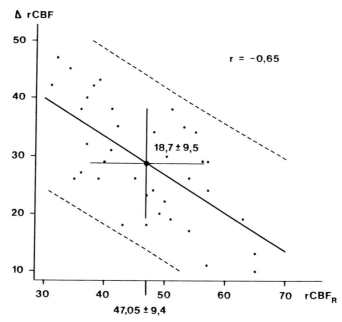

**FIG. 3.** Normal range of cerebrovascular reserve capacity demonstrated by Xe/CT: $rCBF_R$ (CBF at rest)/$\Delta rCBF$ (CBF rise after Diamox) in ml/100 g/min ($n = 72$). A reciprocal linear correlation ($r = -0.65$) was found between $rCBF_R$ and $\Delta rCBF$. The distance to the regression degrees drawn in slopes demonstrates the 95% reliability region.

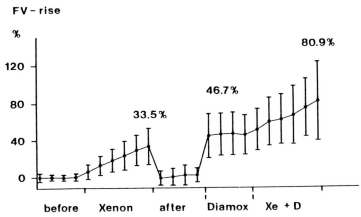

**FIG. 4.** Mean flow velocity in the middle cerebral artery (*n* = 69) during a baseline Xe/CT study and then during another study after Diamox administration.

## TCD for Validation of the Xe/CT Method

We measured the following mean percentage changes in flow velocities for each study segment (Fig. 4). Xenon inhalation alone resulted in a 33.5% increase in flow velocity. Xenon inhalation under the effect of acetazolamide produced an 80.9% increase of flow velocity, 47.4% more than observed after xenon alone. The mean increase in CBF measured with Xe/CT before and after acetazolamide administration was 47.3%.

## DISCUSSION

Despite the use of relatively low concentrations of stable xenon (30–35%) for Xe/CT CBF studies (3,4,16), a significant number of patients have said that inhalation caused changes in sensation. Xenon does cause a tendency toward respiratory depression (6,17,18), and we believe that xenon inhalation also significantly increases CBF. The literature suggests that xenon affects the central nervous system, even in concentrations that have no narcotic effect. Our studies have shown marked decreases in beta-power during xenon inhalation in 50% of 18 healthy subjects (19). Sclabassi et al. (20) found an increase of the alpha-1 power in 75% and of the alpha-2 power in 32% of studies in ten healthy subjects. Results closest to ours were reported by Hartmann et al. (21) in a study in young, healthy monkeys. Approximately 10 to 20 seconds after beginning xenon inhalation, alpha and beta activity decreased significantly in association with a mild increase in theta and delta activity. Within 60 seconds after discontinuing xenon inhalation, the EEG had returned to baseline levels. During xenon-induced anesthesia in humans, such EEG changes were also observed by Morris et al. (22), which correlates with our findings and suggests a very light stage of anesthesia.

The literature has lacked reports of EEG findings in patients who received both acetazolamide and xenon. Our research indicates that the inhalation of 33% xenon, either alone or combined with acetazolamide administration, does not lead to a state of anesthesia. The inhalation of 33% xenon combined with the effect of acetazolamide, however, produces a marked decrease in the absolute alpha power. At most, this type of EEG change correlates with an early stage of anesthesia. Because of this sedative effect, a tendency for xenon inhalation to induce seizures would be very unlikely, even in patients predisposed to epilepsy.

We and others have observed that 1 g of acetazolamide leads to a rapid increase in CBF (10,12,23–26). Gotoh and Shinohara (11) and Kreisig et al. (27) found the mean increase to be approximately 30%. Though our results were a little higher (mean increase: 43%), this difference can be explained by the fact that our studies were not obtained in neurologically normal persons. Like others, we have observed a linear reciprocal relationship between the rCBF at rest and the acetazolamide-induced rCBF increase. This supports the conclusion that the lower the initial value, the greater the activation with acetazolamide. Various authors have described increases in CBF caused by the drug that range from 25% to 70% (10–12,25–28). The 47% elevation in Xe/CT-derived CBF measurements in both of our groups, occurring 23.7 ± 5.5 minutes after the injection of 1 g of acetazolamide, thus fell within the expected limits.

There was no statistically significant difference between the ICP increases in the group with disturbed CSF circulation and in the group without. In 1976, Knopp et al. (14) described increased ICP following acetazolamide administration and assumed that the drug had caused an increased intracranial blood volume. Wilkinson's study (29) found that dogs with an artificially decreased intracranial reserve volume had severe ICP levels after receiving acetazolamide intravenously. We cannot find similar data regarding humans. Our results tend to confirm this observation, but, nevertheless, lead to a different view of the problem. Like Darby et al. (30), we did not find any clinically relevant increase in ICP after xenon inhalation alone. We did, however, record ICP elevations after administering acetazolamide and noted that the highest ICP levels were in the group with impaired CSF dynamics. Although the increase in ICP was considerable in some patients in this group, the clinical response observed was mild (nausea in only one case). Compared to ICP increases resulting from other pathologic mechanisms (15), the relatively short-term elevation produced by vasodilation appeared to be well-tolerated. In our experience, patients who are entered into CBF studies are more likely to have undisturbed CSF dynamics, and the post-acetazolamide changes in such a group are not clinically relevant.

Furthermore, we have concluded that the inhalation of 33% xenon leads to an increase in blood flow velocity, which must result from an increased blood supply. Our results regarding this effect agree with data reported in the literature (7–9). The administration of acetazolamide has a relatively stronger influence on the circulation. The combined effect of xenon and this drug results in a further increase in blood flow, the effect of both substances being cumulative. When we combined the velocity changes induced by xenon inhalation with those induced by acetazolamide, flow velocities averaged 40% higher than during xenon inhalation alone. This corresponds with the 41% increase in hemispheric circulatory levels manifested in the flow maps after acetazolamide injection. Such a strong degree of correlation justifies the conclusion that the effect on CBF attributed to acetazolamide is a reproducible physiological stimulation that can be measured by the high-resolution Xe/CT method.

Overall, we conclude that there is no risk to patients from the inhalation of 33% xenon in conjunction with the administration of acetazolamide to evaluate cerebrovascular reserve capacity. Both TCD studies and our clinical experience in 1,100 Xe/CT examinations verify the high reproducibility of Xe/CT CBF measurements and the validity of the Xe/CT technique.

## ACKNOWLEDGMENTS

The authors thank Mrs. Gertrud Kirschstein, U.S. Military Hospital, Bremerhaven, Germany, for her editorial assistance, and Mrs. Swanhild Fischer, Department of Neurosurgery, Hannover School of Medicine, for preparing this manuscript.

## REFERENCES

1. Meyer JS, Hayman LA, Yamamoto M, Sakai F, Nakajima S. Local cerebral blood flow measured by CT after stable xenon inhalation. *AJNR* 1980;1:213–215.
2. Meyer JS, Hayman LA, Takahira A, et al. Mapping local blood flow of human brain by CT scanning during stable xenon inhalation. *Stroke* 1981;12:426–436.
3. Gur D, Wolfson SK, Yonas H, et al. Progress in cerebrovascular disease: local cerebral blood flow by xenon enhanced CT. *Stroke* 1982;13:750–759.
4. Gur D, Good WF, Wolfson SK Jr, Yonas H, Shabason L. In vivo mapping of local cerebral blood flow by xenon enhanced computed tomography. *Science* 1982;215:1267–1268.
5. Kety SS, Schmidt CF. The nitrous oxide method for the quantitative determination of cerebral blood flow in man. Theory, procedure, and normal values. *J Clin Invest* 1948;27:478–483.
6. Lawrence JH, Loomis WF, Tobias CA, Turpin FH. Preliminary observations on the narcotic effect of xenon with a review of values for solubilities of gases in water and oils. *J Physiol* 1946;105:197–204.
7. Junck L, Dhawan V, Thaler HT, Rottenberg DA. Effects of xenon and krypton on regional cerebral blood flow in the rat. *J Cereb Blood Flow Metab* 1985;5:126–132.
8. Gur D, Yonas H, Jackson DL, et al. Measurements of cerebral blood flow during xenon inhalation as measured by the microsphere method. *Stroke* 1985;16:871–874.
9. Obrist WD, Jaggi J, Harel D, Smith DS. Effect of stable xenon inhalation on human CBF. *J Cereb Blood Flow Metab* 1985;5:557–558.
10. Ehrenreich DL, Burns RA, Alman RW, Fazekas JF. Influence of acetazolamide on cerebral blood flow. *Arch Neurol* 1961;5:227–232.
11. Gotoh F, Shinohara Y. Role of carbonic anhydrase in chemical control and autoregulation of cerebral circulation. *Int J Neurol* 1977;11:219–227.
12. Hauge A, Nicolaysen G, Thoresen M. Acute effects of acetazolamide on cerebral blood flow in man. *Acta Physiol Scand* 1983;117:233–239.

13. Coppen AJ, Russel GFM. Effect of intravenous acetazolamide on cerebrospinal fluid pressure. *Lancet* 1957;1:926–927.
14. Knopp LM, Atkinson JR, Ward AA Jr. Effect of Diamox on cerebrospinal fluid pressure of cat and monkey. *Neurology* 1967;7:119–123.
15. Marshall LF, Smith RW, Shapiro HM. The influence of diurnal rhythm in patients with intracranial hypertension: implications for management. *Neurosurgery* 1978;2:100–102.
16. Drayer BP, Wolfson SK, Reinmuth OM, Dujovny M, Boehnke H, Cook EE. Xenon enhanced CT for analysis of cerebral integrity, perfusion, and blood flow. *Stroke* 1978;9:123–130.
17. Winkler SS, Turski P. Potential hazards of xenon inhalation. *AJNR* 1985;6:974–975.
18. Winkler SS, Nielsen A, Mesina J. Respiratory depression in goats by stable xenon: implications for CT studies. *J Comput Assist Tomogr* 1987;11:496–498.
19. Holl K, Nemati N, Kohmura E, Gaab MR, Samii M. Stable-xenon-CT: effects of xenon inhalation on EEG and cardio-respiratory parameters in the human. *Acta Neurochir (Wien)* 1987;87:129–133.
20. Sclabassi RJ, Lofink RM, Guthkelch AN, Gur D, Yonas H. Effect of low concentration stable xenon on the EEG power spectrum. *Electroencephalogr Clin Neurophysiol* 1987;67:340-347.
21. Hartmann A, Wassman H, Czernicvki Z, Dettmers C, Schumacher HW, Tsuda Y. Effect of stable xenon in room air on regional cerebral blood flow and electroencephalogram in normal baboons. *Stroke* 1987;18:634–638.
22. Morris LE, Knott JR, Pittinger CB. Electroencephalographic and blood gas observations in human surgical patients during xenon anesthesia. *Anesthesiology* 1955;12:312–319.
23. Laux BE, Raichle ME. The effect of acetazolamide on cerebral blood flow and oxygen utilization in the rhesus monkeys. *J Clin Invest* 1978;62:585–592.
24. Severinghaus JW, Cotev S. Carbonic acidosis and cerebral vasodilatation after Diamox. *Scand J Clin Lab Invest* 1968;22:(Suppl 102):I.E.
25. Sullivan HG, Kingsbury TB, Morgan ME, et al. The rCBF response to Diamox in normal subjects and cerebrovascular disease patients. *J Neurosurg* 1987;67:525–534.
26. Vorstrup S, Henriksen L, Paulson OB. Effect of acetazolamide on cerebral blood flow and cerebral metabolic rate for oxygen. *J Clin Invest* 1984;74:1634–1639.
27. Kreisig T, Schmiedek P, Leisinger G, Einhäupl K, Moser E. [133]Xe-DSPECT: Normalwerte von zerebraler Ruhedurchblutung und Reservekapazität. *Nuklearmedizin* 1987;26:192–197.
28. Sorteberg W, Lindegaard KF, Rottwell K, et al. Effect of acetazolamide on cerebral artery blood velocity and regional cerebral blood flow in normal subjects. *Acta Neurochir (Wien)* 1989;97:139–145.
29. Wilkinson HA. Cerebral blood flow response to acetazolamide. *J Neurosurg* 1989;70:156.
30. Darby JM, Yonas H, Pentheny SL, Marion D. Intracranial pressure response to stable xenon inhalation in patients with head injury. *Surg Neurol* 1989;32:343–345.

*Cerebral Blood Flow Measurement with Stable Xenon-Enhanced Computed Tomography,* edited by Howard Yonas. Raven Press, Ltd., New York © 1992.

# Microsphere Cerebral Blood Flow Measurements During Xenon Inhalation in a Model of Focal Ischemia

Christian Dettmers, Alexander Hartmann, *Thomas Rommel, Sandra Hartmann, **Jean C. Baron, **Sabina Pappata, and **Marco Fiorelli

*Department of Neurology, University of Bonn, Sigmund Freud Str. 25, D-5300 Bonn 1, Germany; *Department of Neurosurgery, University of Köln, Köln, Germany; and **Frederic Joliot Hospital, Orsay, France*

It is well known from studies in animals (1–5) and humans (5–7) that stable xenon increases cerebral blood flow (CBF). Most investigators agree that gray-matter flow increases about 12% to 28% during inhalation of 30% to 35% xenon (1,3,5–7). We hypothesized that after infarction, a xenon-induced increase in CBF might be greater in the unaffected tissue than in the infarcted tissue. To test this hypothesis, we used the microsphere technique to compare CBF changes during xenon inhalation in infarcted tissue with those in normal tissue.

## MATERIALS AND METHODS

### Animal Preparation

After an initial intraperitoneal injection of ketamine, six male adult baboons weighing 10 kg were intubated, relaxed with alcuronium, and ventilated with nitrous oxide and oxygen (3:1 ratio) by a Harvard respirator. One femoral vein was cannulated for administration of medication and fluids, and a femoral artery was cannulated for continuous recording of arterial pressure, sampling of blood gases, and withdrawal of reference blood for the microsphere measurements. We continually monitored the electrocardiogram and electroencephalogram and kept body temperature constant with an electric heating system. Focal ischemia was produced by enucleating the left eye, opening the dura, and clipping the middle cerebral artery (MCA) via the transorbital approach (8). For injection of the microspheres, we performed a thoracotomy and inserted a balloon catheter into the left atrium of the heart.

## Local Blood Flow Measurements

We used Heymann's microsphere technique to measure blood flow (9), as we have detailed elsewhere (10). Two differently labeled spheres (scandium-46 and ruthenium-103, New England Nuclear, Boston, MA) with an average size of $16.7 \pm 0.1$ $\mu$m were rechecked for size, shape, specific activity, radionuclide label purity, and leaching. In order to keep the distribution variability within 5%, the number of microspheres per injection was about $10^6$ (11). Before injection, the microspheres were mixed ultrasonically, warmed, strongly shaken, and flushed back and forth with a three-way stopcock between two syringes. They were injected into the left atrium within 30 seconds to guarantee homogeneous mixing in the blood. We withdrew the reference blood with a Braun perfusion pump at a speed of 10 ml/min for $\frac{1}{2}$ minute before injection, during injection, and for 1 minute after.

At the end of the experiment, the brain was removed, weighed, and stored in 4% formalin. Ten days later, we again weighed the brain, cut it into five horizontal slices, and further cut $5 \times 5 \times 5$-mm samples. Every specimen was weighed again and its activity counted with a gamma counter (Gammazint, Fa, Berthold, BF 5300) within 1 day. We corrected the activity of both isotopes for background activity. The ruthenium was also corrected for crosstalk radiation from scandium. The weight was corrected for change before and after storage in formalin.

We calculated CBF according to the following formula:

$$\text{CBF (ml/100 g/min)} = \frac{\text{ta} \times \text{rf}}{\text{ra}},$$

where ta is tissue activity, rf is reference flow, and ra is reference activity.

## Experimental Protocol

Six hours after clipping the MCA, we performed two CBF studies, with a time interval of 15 minutes between the measurements, one before and one during 5-minute inhalation of 30% xenon in oxygen. In the second study, withdrawal of the reference blood began after 4 minutes of xenon inhalation. One-half minute later, the microspheres were injected and the withdrawal of reference blood continued for another minute. We checked blood gases 1 minute before and 1 minute after inhalation, upon completing withdrawal of the reference blood.

## RESULTS

Mean (standard deviation) local CBF in the unaffected hemisphere was 66.2 (15.5) ml/100 g/min. In the ipsilateral cerebellar hemisphere, mean flow values were about 9% higher than mean values in the unaffected cerebral hemisphere

**TABLE 1.** *Territorial cerebral blood flow 6 hours after clipping of the middle cerebral artery in five baboons*

| | Mean values (±SD) (ml/100 g/min) | |
| --- | --- | --- |
| | Unaffected hemisphere | Affected hemisphere |
| Anterior cerebral artery | | |
| Study 1 | 65.7 (16.0) | 46.9 (10.1) |
| Study 2 | 57.5 (13.1) | 44.1 (11.4) |
| Middle cerebral artery | | |
| Study 1 | 67.6 (17.1) | 49.1 (9.2) |
| Study 2 | 58.5 (13.1) | 48.6 (12.4) |
| Posterior cerebral artery | | |
| Study 1 | 63.9 (14.3) | 57.3 (13.7) |
| Study 2 | 58.4 (12.7) | 51.3 (12.5) |
| Cerebellum | | |
| Study 1 | 65.3 (14.1) | 72.2 (19.8) |
| Study 2 | 59.3 (12.9) | 62.7 (17.0) |

Mean $PaCO_2$ was 37.96 mm Hg and 36.06 mm Hg in studies 1 and 2, respectively.

(Table 1). Mean values for the contralateral cerebellar hemispheres were significantly lower, consistent with the concept of cerebellar diaschisis (12).

The affected hemisphere had mean flow values of 52.8 (10.3) ml/100 g/min. In five of the six animals, we observed significant focal ischemia in the territory of the MCA. Mean CBF in the territory of the clipped MCA was 49.1 (9.2) ml/100 g/min, in comparison to 67.6 (17.1) ml/100 g/min on the unaffected side. We found a similar interhemispheric difference in the mean territorial flow of the anterior cerebral artery (ACA). We also observed a mild interhemispheric difference for the posterior cerebral artery (PCA).

During xenon inhalation, $PaCO_2$ decreased slightly, from 37.9 (3.8) mm Hg before inhalation to 36.1 (3.8) mm Hg after inhalation. However, blood gases were sampled from the same arterial line used to withdraw the reference blood. Therefore, we could not document $PaCO_2$ levels until 1 to 1.5 minutes after xenon inhalation ended, and it might be assumed that the amount of hyperventilation during the second CBF study was even greater than these values reveal.

During the second study, CBF decreased in the unaffected hemisphere, in both cerebellar hemispheres, in the PCA territory, and, to a lesser extent, in the ACA

**TABLE 2.** *Reduction in territorial blood flow from first study (before xenon inhalation) to second (during hyperventilation and xenon inhalation)*

| | Mean (%) reduction (SD) | |
| --- | --- | --- |
| | Unaffected hemisphere | Affected hemisphere |
| Anterior cerebral artery | 10.4 (19.2) | 5.2 (17.2) |
| Middle cerebral artery | 8.2 (19.1) | 1.0 (14.8) |
| Posterior cerebral artery | 6.8 (19.3) | 9.1 (15.8) |
| Cerebellum | 8.8 (17.7) | 8.8 (21.95) |

Mean $PaCO_2$ was 37.96 mm Hg and 36.06 mm Hg in studies 1 and 2, respectively.

(Tables 1 and 2). There was no change in blood flow in the MCA territory, suggesting some vasoparalysis in the infarcted tissue.

## DISCUSSION

The results of our first study were consistent with other reports of mean values in the unaffected hemisphere (9), contralateral cerebellar diaschisis (12), and a cerebellar-to-cerebral ratio of 1.09 (13). The interhemispheric difference for the ACA was similar to that for the MCA, which may have been partially a result of the operative procedure: enucleating the eye, opening the dura, and clipping the MCA may damage the integrity of blood flow in the ACA (14).

The purpose of the study was to investigate the influence of stable xenon on CBF after clipping the MCA. Nevertheless, the experimental design probably produced some hypocapnia during the second study, counteracting the expected increase in CBF during xenon inhalation. In all but the affected territories, there was a mild decrease in CBF. So, we assume that two opposite effects predominated in the experiment: an increase in blood flow due to xenon and a decrease in blood flow due to hyperventilation. Because we could not exactly quantify the degree of hyperventilation, we could not gauge these opposing effects individually. We assume that the net effect of a decrease was the result of hyperventilation. Although any conclusion concerning the effect of xenon must be drawn cautiously, we suggest that during xenon inhalation, vasoreactivity to hyperventilation is preserved qualitatively in the unaffected territories.

## ACKNOWLEDGMENT

This project was partially supported by the Deutsche Forschungsgemeinschaft DFG DE-425/89.

## REFERENCES

1. Hartmann A, Wassmann H, Czernicki Z, Dettmers C, Schumacher H, Tsuda Y. Effect of stable xenon in room air on regional cerebral blood flow and electroencephalogram in normal baboons. *Stroke* 1987;18:643–648.
2. Junck L, Dhawan V, Thaler T, Rottenberg DA. Effects of xenon and krypton on regional cerebral blood flow in the rat. *J Cereb Blood Flow Metab* 1985;5:126–132.
3. Gur D, Yonas H. Measurement of cerebral blood flow during xenon inhalation as measured by the microsphere method. *Stroke* 1985;16:871–874.
4. Yonas H, Gur D, Good WF, Maitz GS, Wolfson SK, Latchaw RE. Effects of xenon inhalation on cerebral blood flow: relevance to humans of reported effects in the rat. *J Cereb Blood Flow Metab* 1985;5:613–615.
5. Dettmers C, Hartmann A, Schuier FJ, Wassmann HD, Schumacher HW. Effect of stable xenon on CBF in normal baboons and normal volunteers. *J Cereb Blood Flow Metab* 1987;7(Suppl 1):556.
6. Hartmann A, Dettmers C, Schuier FJ, Wassmann HD, Schumacher HW. Effect of stable xenon

on regional cerebral blood flow and the electroencephalogram in normal volunteers. *Stroke* 1991;22:182–189.

7. Obrist WD, Jaggi J, Harel D, Smith DS. Effect of stable xenon inhalation on human CBF. *J Cereb Blood Flow* 1985;5(Suppl 1):557.

8. O'Brien M, Waltz AG. Transorbital approach for occluding the middle cerebral artery in baboons. *Stroke* 1973;4:201-206.

9. Heymann MA, Payne BD, Hoffman JIE, Rudolph AM. Blood flow measurements with radionuclide-labeled particles. *Prog Cardiovasc Dis* 1977;20:55–79.

10. Dettmers C, Hagendorff A, Nierhaus A, et al. Cerebral blood flow, tissue $PO_2$ and somatosensory evoked potentials after intravascular occlusion of the middle cerebral artery in baboons. In: Meyer JS, et al., eds. *Cerebral vascular disease 7.* New York: Elsevier, 1989:229–237.

11. Buckberg GD, Luck JC, Payne BD, Hoffman JIE, Archie JP, Fixler DE. Some sources of error in measuring regional blood flow with radioactive microspheres. *J Appl Physiol* 1971;31:598–604.

12. Baron JC, Bousser MG, Comar D, Castaigne P. "Crossed cerebellar diaschisis" in human supratentorial brain infarction. *Ann Neurol* 1980;8:128.

13. Pawlik G, Herholz K, Beil C, Wagner R, Wienhard K, Heiss WD. Remote effects of focal lesions on cerebral blood flow and metabolism. In: Heiss WD, ed. *Functional mapping of the brain in vascular disorders.* Berlin: Springer-Verlag; 1985:59–84.

14. Brassel F, Dettmers C, Nierhaus A, Hartmann A, Solymosi L. An intravascular approach to occlude the middle cerebral artery in baboons. *Neuroradiology* 1989;31:418–424.

*Cerebral Blood Flow Measurement with Stable
Xenon-Enhanced Computed Tomography,*
edited by Howard Yonas. Raven Press, Ltd.,
New York © 1992.

# Computer Simulation of the Effect of Xenon-Induced Flow Activation on Quantitative Results of Xenon-Enhanced Computed Tomography

Walter W. Lindstrom

*Picker International, Inc., 595 Miner Road, Highland Heights, Ohio 44143*

Recent ultrasonic measurements of blood flow velocities in the middle cerebral artery during 20% to 33% xenon inhalation indicate that delayed (1.5–2 minutes or more) increases in velocity occur in most patients (1). Others have found similar flow-activation effects caused by prolonged inhalation of xenon in similar concentrations, increases in velocity up to 40% have been reported. A key conclusion of these investigations has been the variation in magnitude and, particularly, the time of onset of these effects. Nevertheless, the relatively long delay (minutes) before these effects occur and the general tendency toward increased flow have been consistent findings, although in a minority of cases, minimal increases and even some small decreases have been noted.

In principle, it is possible to measure and correct for these effects during an examination with xenon-enhanced computed tomography (Xe/CT). In practice, however, this poses too many problems. The purpose of our investigation was to determine the degree of error that results from calculating flow using the standard algorithms (based on the Kety-Schmidt equation, which assumes time-invariant local flow during xenon uptake), even when flow activation is present.

## METHODS

For the purpose of this investigation, we assumed that global cerebral blood flow velocities can increase as much as 40%. We then computed the time course of xenon enhancement as expected from the Kety–Schmidt equation and used these data to obtain the flow and partition coefficient simultaneously. Figure 1 shows our assumed-flow graph; it was chosen to represent the maximum reported degree of xenon-induced flow activation. As illustrated, blood flow starts to elevate about 1.5 minutes after the beginning of xenon inhalation, increases

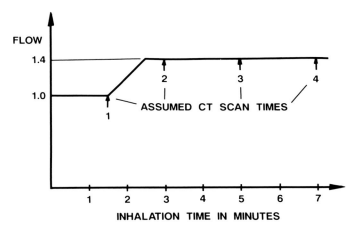

**FIG. 1.** Assumed flow increase. As shown, each initial flow is assumed to increase 40% from its desired pre-activation value.

40% to a constant level in the next minute, and subsequently remains at this enhanced level.

First, we computed the time course of xenon enhancement expected when blood flow increases. We could not use the usual Kety-Schmidt equation because of its inherent assumption of time-invariant local blood flow. Therefore, we returned to the basic assumption that the amount of xenon entering the tissue is equal to the amount delivered minus the amount that exits:

$$dC_{\text{Tissue}} = d\text{IN} - d\text{OUT} = \text{flow}\,(C_{\text{Artery}} - C_{\text{Vein}})d\text{TIME}$$

where $C_{\text{Tissue}}$ is the concentration of xenon in (brain tissue), $C_{\text{Artery}}$ is the concentration of xenon in (brain) arteries, $C_{\text{Vein}}$ is the concentration of xenon in (brain) veins, and flow is the rate of blood flow.

If we further assume that this process is slow enough that local tracer equilibrium is maintained between tissue and venous blood so that the ratio ($\lambda$) of tissue to venous concentration is a tissue-specific time invariant, we derive the following equation.

$$dC = \text{flow}\left(C_{\text{Artery}} - \frac{C_{\text{Tissue}}}{\lambda}\right)d\text{TIME}$$

This equation was used to calculate the expected xenon enhancements in the brain, that is, the simulated data. If we also assume that each local blood flow value would be time-invariant, then we can use the usual Kety–Schmidt integral.

$$C_{\text{Tissue}}(T) = Fe^{-(fT/\lambda)}\,0^T C_{\text{Artery}}(t)e^{-(ft/\lambda)}dt$$

This equation was used (indirectly) to analyze the simulated data for flow ($f$) and $\lambda$ as if flow were not time-dependent.

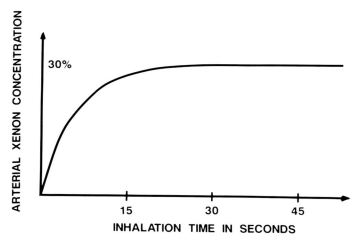

**FIG. 2.** Assumed arterial-blood xenon-uptake curve.

Figure 2 details the assumed arterial-blood xenon-uptake curve chosen for these simulations. This arbitrarily chosen curve for a healthy nonsmoker is a steady exponential.

Figure 3 illustrates what happens (with and without a 40% flow increase) to the expected gray-matter Xe/CT enhancement (in Hounsfield units [HU]) during 10 minutes of continuous xenon inhalation. Although there is little difference for the first 1.5 minutes, this situation was ensured by our assumption that flow

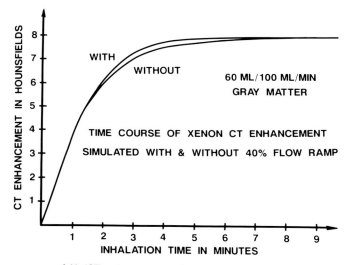

**FIG. 3.** Time course of Xe/CT enhancement, simulated for 60 ml/100 g/min "gray matter" ($\lambda = 0.8$) with and without the 40% flow increase.

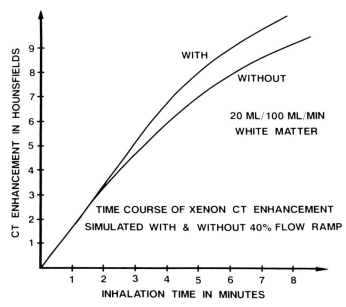

**FIG. 4.** Time course of Xe/CT enhancement, simulated for 20 ml/100 g/min "white matter" ($\lambda = 1.35$), with and without the 40% flow increase.

does not increase during this initial time. Note that for this typical gray-matter flow of 60 ml/100 g/min, the curves "with" and "without" the flow increase differ only slightly. Table 1 presents the calculated times to reach 10%, 90%, 95%, and 98% xenon saturation in gray matter ($\lambda = 0.8$). For flows above 40 ml/100 g/min, saturation is nearly reached in about 3 minutes; lower flows take longer.

Figure 4 and Table 1 show the situation for white matter. In this case, there is a large separation between the curves with and without a 40% flow increase (Fig. 4). This is explained by the long saturation times (Table 1). White matter requires much more time to reach 90% xenon saturation. For an area with a typical white-matter flow value of 20 ml/100 g/min, 90% saturation required 15.6 minutes, which is much longer than our clinical inhalation times of 5 to 7 minutes.

## RESULTS

Table 2 shows the final results of our simulation procedure. Here we calculated xenon tissue enhancement under the assumption of 40% flow activation and then used these simulated data to solve the usual Kety–Schmidt integral equation simultaneously for flow values and partition coefficients. The four columns reflect results obtained using the solution incorporated within the Picker Xe/CT system.

**TABLE 1.** *Time to near saturation of xenon*

| Blood flow | Time (minutes) to saturation of: | | | |
|---|---|---|---|---|
| (ml/100 g/min) | 80% | 90% | 95% | 98% |
| (λ = 0.8 for gray matter) | | | | |
| 120 | 1.2 | 1.6 | 2.1 | 2.7 |
| 90 | 1.5 | 2.1 | 2.8 | 3.6 |
| 60 | 2.2 | 3.2 | 4.1 | 5.3 |
| 40 | 3.3 | 4.7 | 6.1 | 7.9 |
| 30 | 4.4 | 6.2 | 8.1 | 10.5 |
| 20 | 6.5 | 9.3 | 12.1 | 15.7 |
| (λ = 1.35 for white matter) | | | | |
| 60 | 3.7 | 5.3 | 6.8 | 9.0 |
| 40 | 5.2 | 7.8 | 10.3 | 13.5 |
| 30 | 7.3 | 10.5 | 13.4 | 17.7 |
| 20 | 10.4 | 15.6 | 20.5 | 27.7 |
| 10 | 20.8 | 31.2 | 41.0 | 54.0 |

We obtained CT scans after 1.5, 3, 5, and (optionally) 7 minutes of xenon inhalation to get three or four data points for simultaneous flow and λ determinations. We called these scan times 1, 2, 3, and 4, respectively. For example, in the column headed "1, 2, 3," the first 5 minutes of xenon enhancement data were used; in the third column (1,3), only the 1.5- and 5-minute scans were used. A CT noise of 0.7-HU standard deviation (RMS) was used in these simulations.

## DISCUSSION

Our simulation found very small "errors" in the "initial" flow values. For gray-matter flow of 90 ml/100 g/min, for example, use of scan data for 1.5, 3, and 5 minutes led to an "error" of −2.8 in the "correct" early flow value. Although

**TABLE 2.** *Computed flow change with simulated 40% flow activation[a]*

| Xenon-induced blood flow | Scan times utilized[b] | | | |
|---|---|---|---|---|
| (ml/100 g/min) | (1, 2, 3) | (1, 2) | (1, 3) | (1, 2, 3, 4) |
| 90 (Gray matter) | −2.8 | −4.6 (−5%) | −3.8 | −2.2 |
| 60 (Gray matter) | +1.5 | +1.0 | +0.9 | +2.5 |
| 30 (Gray matter) | +0.5 | −0.1 | −0.9 | +1.1 |
| 30 (White matter) | +1.8 | −0.7 | +1.5 | +2.4 |
| 20 (White matter) | +2.0 | +2.2 | +2.3 | +2.4 (+12%) |

[a] Standard deviation = 0.7 Hounsfield units.
[b] Scan times indicate Xe/CT scans included in the computation; scan times 1, 2, 3, and 4 represent scans performed 1.5, 3, 5, and 7 minutes, respectively, after xenon inhalation; 7 minutes was included as an optional scan time, since not all methods prolong inhalation to that extent.

it may seem implausible that a negative error was derived with an assumed increase in flow, this occurred because both flow and λ values were determined simultaneously; the small mistakes made for λ were just enough to correct the flow. The reason for these mistakes follows directly from the assumption of time-invariant flows built into the Kety–Schmidt integral equation. This was most flagrant in the case of white matter at 20 ml/100 g/min, which showed a 10% increase. Yet, a flow error of 2 in 20 is relatively small. Even if the data for all 7 minutes are used (1, 2, 3, 4) so that the xenon-enhanced flow has been activated for even longer, the error in the "correct" early flow is only 12%.

Note that there was no advantage to using only the first two scans to avoid including the later times, when flow activation is greater. In fact, the disadvantage that results from not clearly separating white-matter from gray-matter data is potentially a much greater cause of inaccurate flow measurements. It should be remembered that one of the major advantages of the Xe/CT technique is its ability to determine flow and λ values simultaneously, which is valuable for both accurate flow measurement and clinical assessment of tissue function.

This unexpected ability of the "incorrect" Kety–Schmidt formulation to derive correctly early flow values is clinically important. It means that although xenon-induced flow activation may differ among individual patients as much as some have reported (1), and although the degree of activation may be unknown, as is usually the case in clinical practice, the Xe/CT method can be used safely to measure early (pre-activation) flows in patients.

## REFERENCE

1. Giller CA, Purdy P, Lindstrom WW. Effects of inhaled stable xenon on cerebral blood flow velocity. *AJNR* 1990;11:177–182.

*Cerebral Blood Flow Measurement with Stable Xenon-Enhanced Computed Tomography,* edited by Howard Yonas. Raven Press, Ltd., New York © 1992.

# Discussion

Participants:

Dr. Teiichi Takasago (Yamaguchi, Japan)
Dr. Joseph Horton (Pittsburgh, Pennsylvania, USA)
Dr. Mohammad-Nabi Nemati (Hannover, Germany)
Dr. Alexander Hartmann (Bonn, Germany)
Dr. Howard Yonas (Pittsburgh, Pennsylvania, USA)
Ms. Elizabeth Marks (Pittsburgh, Pennsylvania, USA)
Dr. Ralph Grenberg (Pearl River, New York, USA)
Dr. Walter Obrist (Pittsburgh, Pennsylvania, USA)
Dr. Walter Lindstrom (Cleveland, Ohio, USA)
Dr. David Gur (Pittsburgh, Pennsylvania, USA)

In responding to the procedural problems discussed by Dr. Takasago, Dr. Horton stressed the importance of a good rapport between the patient and the person directing a xenon-enhanced computed tomographic cerebral blood flow (Xe/CT CBF) study. He specified the need to make the patient aware in advance of what he or she may experience and noted that guiding patients through the study requires continuous verbal encouragement. Dr. Takasago agreed. He also noted that, in his experience, the incidence of problems significantly increases with the protraction of xenon inhalation beyond 5 minutes.

In response to Dr. Nemati's report that xenon caused only a slight electroencephalographic (EEG) alteration, Dr. Hartmann noted that he had seen epileptic activity in 3 of 11 normal subjects during xenon inhalation. Dr. Nemati replied that he had never seen evidence of increased seizure activity, even in patients with seizure disorders who were studied via depth electrodes during Xe/CT studies. Dr. Yonas added that Sclabassi (*Electroencephalogr Clin Neurophysiol* 1987;67:340–347) had found no significant EEG changes with 33% xenon inhalation.

Following the presentation by Ms. Marks on the time course and extent of transcranial Doppler-measured (TCD-measured) velocity changes that accompany xenon inhalation, Dr. Grenberg raised the concerns mentioned in Dr. Giller's article (Giller CA et al., *AJNR* 1990;11:177–182), questioning the reproducibility of Xe/CT-derived flow values due to the unpredictability of flow activation. Ms. Marks agreed that she had indeed found considerable variation between patients. Dr. Obrist added that velocity did not begin to change until 2 to 3 minutes after xenon inhalation, and significant change did not occur until after some 4.5 to 5 minutes. He said that in a recent study in which TCD and $^{133}$Xe CBF measurements were obtained during xenon inhalation ($CO_2$ was added to maintain the end-tidal $pCO_2$ levels, which normally fall 3–4 torr), a 25% to 30% flow augmentation was noted with both methods. Dr. Hartmann stated that he too had seen similar CBF changes using TCD and $^{133}$Xe and believed that such changes were due to the pharmacological activity of xenon.

In the final talk of the meeting, Dr. Lindstrom had presented computer simulation data demonstrating that a delayed xenon-induced flow augmentation (of 90 seconds) had a slight effect on fast flow and a moderate effect on slow flow. Dr. Obrist commented that this paper was an excellent example of how computer simulations can lend perspective to the independent observations made using $^{133}$Xe, TCD, and microspheres. Dr. Gur added, however, that Dr. Lindstrom's method was protocol-dependent and that scanning more frequently and earlier than three times at 1.5-minute intervals, as is done with the Picker system, can further lessen the impact of xenon activation on calculated flow values. Dr. Lindstrom responded that performing the initial scan 1.5 minutes after xenon inhalation begins causes a loss of only the ability to accurately record flow values above 120 ml/100 g/min. He cautioned that scanning too early would not be productive, because some time is needed for adequate amounts of xenon to diffuse into brain tissue and enhance images. Thus, scanning too soon after beginning xenon inhalation not only would be nonproductive, but would also expose the patient to unnecessary radiation.

# Subject Index